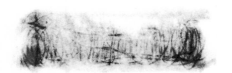

Automated Visual Field Testing

Techniques of Examination and Interpretation

David E. Silverstone, M.D.
Associate Clinical Professor of Ophthalmology and Visual Science
Yale University School of Medicine
New Haven, Connecticut

Joy Hirsch, Ph.D.
Associate Professor of Ophthalmology and Visual Science
Yale University School of Medicine
New Haven, Connecticut

APPLETON-CENTURY-CROFTS/Norwalk, Connecticut

0-8385-0500-7

Copyright © 1986 by Appleton-Century-Crofts
A Publishing Division of Prentice-Hall

86 87 88 89 / 10 9 8 7 6 5 4 3 2 1

Prentice-Hall of Australia, Pty. Ltd., Sydney
Prentice-Hall Canada, Inc.
Prentice-Hall Hispanoamericana, S.A., Mexico
Prentice-Hall of India Private Limited, New Delhi
Prentice-Hall International (UK) Limited, London
Prentice-Hall of Japan, Inc., Tokyo
Prentice-Hall of Southeast Asia (Pte.) Ltd., Singapore
Whitehall Books Ltd., Wellington, New Zealand
Editora Prentice-Hall do Brasil Ltda., Rio de Janeiro

Library of Congress Cataloging-in-Publication Data

Silverstone, David E.
   Automated visual field testing.

   Bibliography: p.
   Includes index.
   1. Perimetry—Handbooks, manuals, etc. 2. Perimetry—Data processing—Handbooks, manuals, etc. 3. Eye—Diseases and defects—Diagnosis—Handbooks, manuals, etc. I. Hirsch, Joy. II. Title. [DNLM: 1. Perimetry—methods. 2. Visual Fields. WW 145 S587a]
RE79.P4S55 1986   617.7'5'0287   86-7916
ISBN 0-8385-0500-7

Design: Jean Sabato-Morley
Cover: M. Chandler Martylewski

To our families and friends

Contents

Preface

Automated techniques of testing the visual field currently provide data that are accurate, reliable, and more flexible than ever before. At the same time, however, the interpretation and understanding of this data has presented new challenges to the physician. Results of tests performed using automated equipment do not resemble the results of tests obtained using traditional manual equipment, hence a new approach to reading automated visual fields is required. Although the automated data obtained are usually more exact and more complete than the manual data, computerized analyses are often necessary in order to extract the available information. The understanding of a new jargon, still unfamiliar to most practitioners, is a necessity.

The recent infusion of new information related to the visual field has not been accompanied by an equal effort to merge the benefits of new technology with the mainstream of clinical practice. The intent of this text is to serve as an interface between the technology and clinical practice for the growing numbers of people associated with automated visual field testing. To accommodate the wide range of backgrounds of our readers, we have tried to present the basics and at the same time achieve an overview useful for the more advanced audience. Both the scientific and clinical aspects of visual field testing have been covered. It is important for clinicians to have an understanding of the physics of light and principles of the human visual system in order to understand the rationale behind field testing hardware and software design. The different aspects of hardware design have been discussed so as to help readers understand the strengths and limitations of each of the available field testing machines. Much emphasis has been placed on software, as it is the software strategy which determines how the field will be tested and analyzed on a particular machine.

An important benefit of automated visual field data is the opportunity for computerized analysis of visual field test results. More sophisticated analysis strategies are capable of unlocking more field information. However, these new field "indices" complicate field interpretation, and this book is intended to facilitate the use of extended field information. Finally, the book focuses on the interpretation of field results including reliability and response bias measurements as well as different methods of data presentation.

We have cataloged for the reader the appearance of the major types of visual field defects as shown by various automated field reports. While doing this, we have striven to keep this new technology in perspective, as there are clinical situations in which manual methods of examining the field are appropriate. Automated methods are a valuable new technology, and to use them properly and to best advantage the examiner must be able to choose the method of testing from the entire spectrum of automated, semi-automated, and manual methods.

There are many different automated visual field testing systems on the market. Despite the number, they can be categorized according to certain characteristics that allow generalizations to be made that apply to many machines. Differences among machines are also important because they are the sources of each machine's strengths and weaknesses. In this text we have attempted to explore these similarities and differences in a manner that will allow generalizations to be made to other machines that have yet to be developed.

Clinicians need to be familiar with all of the major automated visual field testing devices. Hardware designs and the software strategies used by each machine must be understood in order to be able to read the visual field test results recorded by any one of the machines and to compare the results from one machine with those of another. This book provides that basis of understanding.

Ophthalmology is at the threshold of uncovering new facets of the visual field. Application of new technology and new ideas to the visual field testing process has already improved our ability to detect, analyze, and follow field defects. We look ahead to continued development of the many potential contributions that the automated visual field offers toward earlier detection and optimal disease therapy. Our goal is that readers of this book will be able to embrace the new technology and reap its clinical benefits.

Acknowledgments

Many people have helped in the production of this book, and we are grateful to all of them. Their support, their encouragement, and their assistance has helped make a monumental task a manageable one.

Our technicians Barbara White, Pamela Fox Torniero, Rebecca Green, and Jackie Gold do a masterful clinical job. For this book they also helped to select and prepare fields for publication. Their countless hours of meticulous attention to accuracy and detail are manifest throughout the book. Our typists Barbara Skolones and Debbie Tewksbury did a wonderful job. They could always be counted on to meet deadlines. Our research assistant C. Allen Waddle spent many hours researching the literature and trying to assure the accuracy of all the material presented. His hours of research in the Yale Medical Library are especially evident in the bibliography.

Our colleagues locally, nationally, and internationally have been very helpful in deciding what material to include and how to present that material effectively. Some contributed visual fields from their own collections and that has added to the depth of this text. Members of the Octopus Users' Society have been crucial to the development of that machine and have indirectly contributed to this book. The product managers of most of the visual field testing machines have been particularly helpful in confirming the data on each machine. Some have also contributed fields and have helped in defining our goals.

The Yale Octopus and visual field analysis service is partially supported by research grants. These include grants from Research to Prevent Blindness, the Connecticut Lions Eye Research Foundation and NEI EY00785.

Dr. Marvin L. Sears, Professor and Chairman of the Department of Ophthalmology and Visual Sciences at Yale deserves special mention. Not only is Dr. Sears one of the foremost figures in ophthalmic research today, he is also the founder of a unique ophthalmology department. At Yale, clinicians and research scientists on both the full-time faculty and the part-time faculty have been able, and indeed, have been encouraged to come together to solve clinical problems and enhance our knowledge of eye diseases. This book is a testament to the spirit of scientific inquiry and cooperation that he has fostered. It is particularly fitting that the publication of this book coincides with the opening and dedication of the Yale Eye Center for Clinical Research which he has worked so hard to construct.

We owe our greatest debt of thanks to our families and friends. They gave of their time and companionship, they put up with our extra hours of work and deadlines and truly sacrificed to help make this text a reality. It is to them that we dedicate our work.

David E. Silverstone
Joy Hirsch
New Haven, Connecticut
April, 1986

1

Principles of Light and Vision Applied to Visual Field Testing

Light is the basic material for vision. Appreciation of the extent to which light is capable of stimulating a visual response requires consideration of both the physical properties of light as well as the physiological properties of the eye. Because the fundamental task in visual field testing is the determination of sensitivity to small spots of light, this chapter is devoted to those specific principles of light and vision most relevant to the detection of light increments superimposed on a constant background level of illumination. It is divided into two main sections: (1) measurement of light and (2) properties of the visual system that influence the detection of light increments.

Measurement of Light[1-4]

Both the wave and particle natures of light are relevant to vision. The wave nature of light is the basis for selective absorption by photoreceptors, and the particle nature of light is the basis for intensity specifications.

THE VISIBLE SPECTRUM (WAVE NATURE OF LIGHT)

The range of the electromagnetic spectrum that is visible is specified according to the wave properties of light. Photoreceptors of the eye absorb and respond to wavelengths within a specific region (approximately 400 to 700 nanometers, nm) and are essentially insensitive to wavelengths in the ultraviolet (below 400 nm) and infrared (above 700 nm) regions.

The commonly used units for specifications of the wavelengths around and including the visible spectrum are angstroms, nanometers, and microns.

One angstrom is about the size of a hydrogen atom, and is the unit used to measure waves in the ultraviolet range, which is generally below the range that stimulates the sensation of light.

$$\text{angstrom (Å)} = 10^{-10} \text{ meters} \qquad (1-1)$$

One millimicron (nanometer) is about the size of a benzene molecule, and is used to measure that portion of the electromagnetic spectrum that stimulates the sensation of light.

$$\text{nanometer (nm)} = 10^{-9} \text{ meters} = \text{millimicron (m}\mu\text{)} \qquad (1-2)$$

One micron is about the size of a small bacterium, and is the unit used to measure lightwaves in the infrared region of the spectrum, which is generally above the range that stimulates the sensation of light.

$$\text{micron } (\mu) = 10^{-6} \text{ meters} \qquad (1-3)$$

For perspective it is interesting to note that the center-to-center spacing of photoreceptors in the central fovea of the human eye is approximately 3 μ.[5] Assuming that the aperture of each photoreceptor approximates the center-to-center spacing of photoreceptors in the central fovea, then the aperture is 3 × 10^{-6} meters (3 μ), which is about the size of 6 wavelengths of light at 500 × 10^{-9} meters (500 nm). Because the aperture must be large relative to the wavelengths to maintain separate optical channels, wavelength of light is one of the factors limiting the minimum photoreceptor spacing and consequently visual resolution.

QUANTIFICATION OF LIGHT INTENSITY (PARTICLE NATURE OF LIGHT)

To quantify *amounts* of light the particle nature of light is used in vision. Particles of light are called quanta and are emitted from hot sources such as the sun, a candle, or a wire filament. The amount of light energy emitted from a source, arriving at an extended surface, and reflected from the extended surface can be measured in both radiometric and photometric units.

Radiometric units are equally applicable to all wavelengths of the electromagnetic spectrum and are not discussed in detail here. The human visual system, however, is differentially sensitive to different wavelengths of light. That is, energy at some wavelengths appears brighter than equal energy at other wavelengths. Therefore, it is necessary to have a measurement system that specifies the visual effectiveness of a radiant source. These units are photometric units.

Photometric units have been developed to reflect the visual effectiveness of radiant energy. The human eye is maximally sensitive to light at wavelengths of 555 nm, and the visual effectiveness of the radiant energy falls off both above and below that point. This function (Fig. 1–1) is called the photometric luminosity curve and defines the visual effectiveness of any radiant source. In photometry, all physical measurements of light energy are weighted by the luminosity curve.

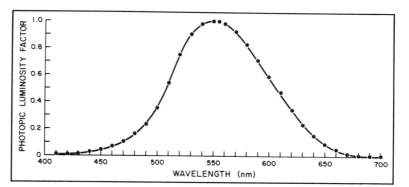

Figure 1–1. *Human photopic luminosity function. This function describes the relative visual effectiveness of wavelengths from 400 to 700 nm. The human cone system is most sensitive to wavelengths around 555 nm.*

Luminous Intensity: The Candle

Luminous intensity is the radiant energy emitted from a source corrected by the visual effectiveness of each wavelength. The basic unit of luminous intensity is the *candle*, which is defined as 1/60 of the intensity per square centimeter (cm^2) of a blackbody radiating at the temperature of melting platinum (2046°K). Light energy based on the candle can also be expressed as *luminance flux*, which is the amount (volume) of light energy transferred from a source to a surface over some unit of time.

Candle-based Measures of Luminance. Luminance refers to the luminous flux radiated from a spatially extended source. The luminance of a surface is measured in candles/meter^2 (cd/m^2), candles/centimeter^2 (cd/cm^2), millilamberts (mL), and footlamberts (ftL). Luminance can be measured directly either from a surface that is self-luminous, such as extended sources like cathode ray tubes (CRT) or light emitting diodes (LED), or from a surface that reflects light emitted from another source like the cupola of a projection perimeter.

If a point source with luminous intensity of 1 cd is spread over an area of 1 m^2, the luminance is 1 cd/m^2 (Fig. 1–2). Likewise, if a point source of 1 cd is spread over an area of 1 cm^2, then this area has a luminance of 1 cd/cm^2. The relationship between the two areas, cm^2 and m^2, is 10^4. That is, 1 cd/m^2 is equal to 10^4 cd/cm^2.

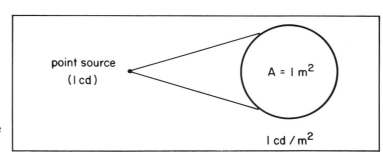

Figure 1–2. *A point source of luminous intensity equal to 1 cd spread over a surface area of 1 m^2 has a luminance L of 1 cd/m^2.*

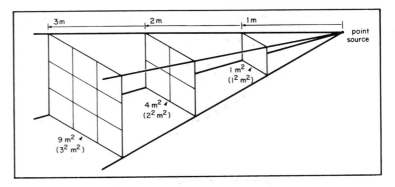

Figure 1–3. *Inverse square law of illuminance. Light that illuminates an area of 1 m² at a distance of 1 m from a point source will illuminate 4 m² at a distance of 2 m from the source and will illuminate an area of 9 m² at a distance of 3 m from the source.*

The luminance (*L*) of a surface area, which is illuminated by another source, depends upon two factors: the amount of light falling upon it (illuminance, *I*) and the reflectance (*R*) of the surface. The specific relationship is expressed as

$$L = IR \qquad\qquad (1\text{--}4)$$

where *R* is the ratio of light reflected to light incident on the surface. For example, 40 cd/m² radiating to an intercepting surface that reflects only 50 percent of the light has a luminance of 20 cd/m².

ILLUMINANCE

Illumination is the amount of light from a point source falling on an intercepting surface. As the distance between the source and the intercepting surface increases the illuminance at the surface decreases by the inverse square law (Fig. 1–3). For example, light that covers 1 m² at a distance of 1 m from a point source will cover 4 m² at a distance of 2 m from the point source and 9 m² at a distance of 3 m. More specifically, illuminance is equal to the candle power of the source specified in lumens over the square of the distance (d²) between the source and the surface. One lumen falling upon a surface area of 1 ft² is a footcandle (see below). The illuminance on a screen 2 ft from the

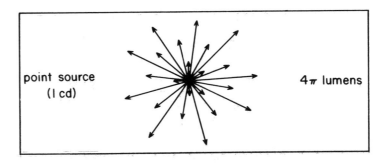

Figure 1–4. *A point source radiates energy in all directions forming a solid sphere. Because the solid angle of a sphere is 4π, the total flux emitted by a candle point source is 4π lumens or 12.57 lumens.*

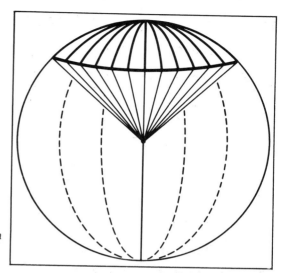

Figure 1–5. A unit solid angle (a steradian) can be isolated from a solid sphere of energy radiating from a point source. In radiometric units energy is often specified as watts/steradian.

point source of 40 lumens is equal to 40 lumens divided by 2^2 ft or 10 footcandles (ftcd).

$$\text{Illuminance (ftcd)} = \text{lumens/d}^2 \text{ (ft)} \qquad (1-5)$$

Lumen-based Measures of Luminance

Consider a point source with a luminous intensity of 1 cd. The point source radiates energy in all directions so that it becomes the center point of a solid sphere. If the point source emits a radiant flux uniformly in all directions (Fig. 1–4), then a solid angle is created. This unit solid angle is called a *steradian* (Fig. 1–5). Radiance, a radiometric unit, is the number of watts per steradian

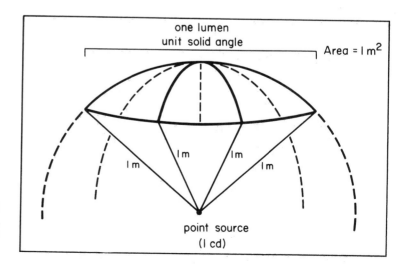

Figure 1–6. When the luminous intensity of the point source is 1 cd and the radius of the sphere is 1 m, a unit solid angle contains 1 lumen of flux.

emitted per square meter of some surface area. All radiant energy can be expressed as a unit of power (work per unit of time as in ergs per second). For example, the familiar watt is a unit of radiant flux equivalent to 10^7 ergs/sec. The luminance (the photometric equivalent of radiance) of a unit solid angle from a sphere radiating from a 1 cd point source with a radius of 1 m is 1 lumen (Fig. 1–6). Lumens can also be expressed as watts. For example, a common 52-watt incandescent bulb radiates an average of 800 lumens, and a 60-watt bulb radiates an average of 890 lumens. At a wavelength of 555 nm, one lumen is equal to 685 watts. The number of watts per lumen increases as the wavelength deviates from 555 nm due to the human luminosity function (Fig. 1–1).

RELATIONS AMONG COMMON PHOTOMETRIC UNITS

Historical precedent has left visual science with an array of photometric units. Table 1–1 summarizes the relationships among most of the common photometric units. The table is read by selecting any unit on the top row and reading down the column. The tabled numbers indicate the conversion from the selected top unit to the units listed in the left-hand column. For example, 1 cd/m^2 (second column) is equal to 10^{-4} cd/cm^2, 3.1416×10^{-4} lumens/cm^2, 3.1416 lumens/m^2 (apostilb, asb), and 3.1416×10^{-1} millilamberts. The first two columns cd/cm^2 and cd/m^2 are the units based on intensity per area of a circle.

TABLE 1–1. RELATIONS AMONG COMMON PHOTOMETRIC UNITS

	Candle/cm^2 (stilb)	Candle/m^2 (nit)	Lumen/cm^2 (lambert)	Apostilb (lumen/m^2) (lux)	Millilambert (mL)
Candle/cm^2 (stilb)	1	10^{-4} $1/10^4$	3.183×10^{-1} $1/\pi$	3.183×10^{-5} $1/\pi \times 10^4$	3.183×10^{-4} $1/\pi \times 10^{-3}$
Candle/m^2 (nit)	10^4	1	3.183×10^3 $10^4/\pi$	3.183×10^{-1} $1/\pi$	3.183 $10^4/\pi \times 10^{-3}$
Lumen/cm^2 (lambert)	3.1416 π	3.1416×10^{-4} $\pi/10^4$	1	10^{-4} $1/10^4$	10^{-3}
Apostilb (lumen/m^2) (lux)	3.1416×10^4 $(\pi \times 10^4)$	3.1416 π	10^4	1^*	10 $10^4 \times 10^{-3}$
Millilambert (mL)	3.1416×10^3 $\pi \times 10^3$	3.1416×10^{-1} $\pi/10^4 \times 10^{-3}$	10^3	10^{-1} $1/10^4 \times 10^3$	1^{**}

* 1 asb is equivalent to 0.0929 footcandles.
** 1 mL is equivalent to 0.922 footlamberts.
To convert from one unit to another locate the appropriate column and read the equivalent units along the column. For example, 1 asb (column 4) is equivalent to 3.183×10^{-1} cd/m^2 (row 2) and 10^{-1} mL. (*The general form of this table follows a similar table in Hurvich L, Jameson D: The Perception of Brightness and Darkness, Allyn and Bacon, 1966.*)

The last three columns, lumen/cm², lumen/m², and millilambert, are based on the number of lumens per area. In reading the table it will be helpful to recall that the area of a circle is equal to πr^2 where $\pi = 3.1416$ and r is the radius of the circle. Hence, 1 cd spread over a circular area of radius equal to 1 m has an area of πm². The geometrical rationale for each of the conversions is indicated below each conversion factor.

RETINAL ILLUMINATION: TROLANDS

Light from a stimulus must travel through the optical components of the eye to reach the photoreceptors. Therefore, the light that actually arrives at the retina may not necessarily be a constant portion of the stimulus intensity. Opacities along the optical path and/or a constricted pupil will reduce the expected retinal illumination. The effect of the optical opacities such as a cataract or clouded media on retinal illumination are not easily assessed. The effect of pupil size can be quantified, however, by correcting stimulus luminance by pupil size.

Assuming that the light passing through a pupil is proportional to its area, the product of stimulus luminance and pupillary area can be used to specify retinal illumination. Specificially, the troland is a unit of retinal illuminance that corrects stimulus luminance by pupil area. A troland is defined as the luminance of a stimulus (L) in cd/m² times the area of the pupil (A) in mm².

$$\text{Trolands} = L(A) = \text{cd/m}^2 \, (\text{mm}^2) \hspace{2cm} (1\text{-}6)$$

The relevance of the troland in visual field testing is shown by the following example. Suppose the reported value of a point determined on an Octopus is 20 decibels (dB), and the patient's pupil size is 1 mm in diameter (radius, r = 0.5 mm).

20 db corresponds to a threshold of 10 asb (Table 1–2)

10 asb is equivalent to 3.183 cd/m² (Table 1–1)

Therefore $L = 3.183$ cd/m²

Area of the 1 mm pupil is $\pi r^2 = 3.1415 \times 0.5$ mm²

Therefore $A = 0.785$ mm²

$$\text{Trolands} = 3.183 \text{ cd/m}^2 \times 0.785 \text{ mm}^2 = 2.5 \hspace{2cm} (1\text{-}6a)$$

However, if the pupil had a 2-mm diameter (r = 1 mm), the retinal illuminance would have been 10.00 trolands.

$$\text{Trolands} = 3.183 \text{ cd/m}^2 \times 3.1415 \times (1 \text{ mm})^2 = 10.00 \hspace{1cm} (1\text{-}6b)$$

Therefore, due to a constricted pupil, the retinal illumination was reduced by a factor of 4 (10/2.5) and it would be expected that measured sensitivity would also be reduced. This reduction in sensitivity, however, could be attributed to pupil size rather than eye disease. This example illustrates that the decision about whether the observed point is disturbed or not must include the fact that

TABLE 1–2. RANGE OF TEST SPOT INTENSITIES FOR THE OCTOPUS AUTOMATED PERIMETER

Asb	Log Asb	Sensitivity (dB)
	−2.1	51
	−2.0 to −1.6	50 to 46
0.008 to 0.25	−1.5 to −1.1	45 to 41
	−1.0 to −0.6	40 to 36
0.31 to 0.80	−0.5 to −0.1	35 to 31
1 to 2.5	0.0 to 0.4	30 to 26
3.1 to 8.0	0.5 to 0.9	25 to 21
10 to 25	1.0 to 1.4	20 to 16
31 to 80	1.5 to 1.9	15 to 11
100 to 250	2.0 to 2.4	10 to 6
315 to 800	2.5 to 2.9	5 to 1
1000	3.0	0

the stimulus was effectively dimmer than expected, and the expected normal value cannot apply.

Clinically, pupil size is a significant factor for the interpretation of fields. For example if a glaucoma patient who has been followed by consecutive visual field examinations is placed on a miotic and the pupil size is reduced, expected threshold values will rise (sensitivity, dB, will decrease). In this case, the pupil should be either dilated for the field examination to compare with previous examinations, or a new baseline examination should be started at the new pupil size.

SPECIFICATION OF LIGHT INTENSITY IN VISUAL FIELD TESTING

The Apostilb

The apostilb (asb) is the unit of light intensity most often used in automated visual field testing. The apostilb is one lumen of flux contained in one unit solid angle incident upon a surface area of 1 m² (Fig. 1–7). When the reflectance of the surface area is 100 percent, the apostilb is equivalent to 1 lumen/m² = 0.318 cd/m² (Table 1–1). If the reflectance of the viewing surface is less than 100 percent, however, illuminance (the amount of light falling on the intercepting surface) is not equal to luminance (the amount of light reflected from the intercepting surface). This constraint serves to emphasize the importance of the bowl surface in projection machines. If the reflectance properties of the surface deviate from the expected high reflectance matt-Lambertian surface, calibration of the test lights will be altered. This calibration problem does not apply to self-luminous light sources such as LEDs.

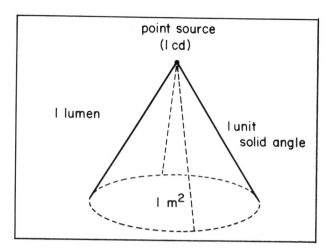

Figure 1–7. *The apostilb is a measure of illuminance (the incident flux per unit area). It is equivalent to 1 lux or lumen/m² of incident surface.*

The Apostilb to Decibels

The range of test light intensities used in automated field testing instruments is often measured in apostilbs and expressed in decibels (dB). This conversion is shown in Table 1–2 for the Octopus units, Table 1–3 for Humphrey units, and Table 1–4 for Dicon units. These three tables provide examples of each type of scale currently used for projection and LED automated perimeters, and are similar to other currently available automated perimeters.

In the case of the Octopus, a projection machine, the full range of test spot luminance is from 0.008 to 1000 asb (Table 1–2). In log units the equivalent range is from −2.1 to 3.0 encompassing a range of 5.1 log units. The decibel (dB) is a log unit subdivided by 10 so that the full range of test intensities for

TABLE 1–3. RANGE OF TEST SPOT INTENSITIES FOR THE HUMPHREY FIELD ANALYZER

Asb	Log Asb	Sensitivity (dB)
0.1 to 0.8	−1.0 to −0.10	50 to 41
1 to 2.5	0.0 to 0.4	40 to 36
3.2 to 8.0	0.5 to 0.9	35 to 31
10 to 25	1.0 to 1.4	30 to 26
32 to 79	1.5 to 1.9	25 to 21
100 to 251	2.0 to 2.4	20 to 16
316 to 794	2.5 to 2.9	15 to 11
1000 to 2512	3.0 to 3.4	10 to 6
3162 to 7943	3.5 to 3.9	5 to 1
10,000	4.0	0

TABLE 1–4. RANGE OF TEST SPOT INTENSITIES FOR THE DICON AUTOMATED PERIMETER

Asb	Log Asb	Sensitivity (dB)
0.13 to 0.25	−0.89 to −0.60	49 to 46
0.32 to 0.80	−0.49 to −1.10	45 to 41
1.00 to 2.50	0.00 to 0.40	40 to 36
3.20 to 8.00	0.50 to 0.90	35 to 31
10.00 to 25.00	1.00 to 1.40	30 to 26
32.00 to 80.00	1.50 to 1.90	25 to 21
100.00 to 250.00	2.00 to 2.40	20 to 16
320.00 to 800.00	2.50 to 2.90	15 to 11
1000.00 to 2500.00	3.00 to 3.40	10 to 6
3200.00 to 8000.00	3.50 to 3.90	5 to 1
10,000	4.0	0

the Octopus is 51 dB. Because sensitivity is the inverse of threshold, the dB scale (as shown in the last column of Table 1–2) is inverted so that the highest luminance (1000 asb) is associated with 0 dB and the lowest luminance (0.008 asb) is associated with 50 dB. Accordingly, a value of 20 dB corresponds to 10 asb and 15 dB corresponds to 31 asb.

In the case of the Humphrey Field Analyzer (Table 1–3), also a projection machine, the full range of test spot luminance is from 0.1 asb to 10,000 asb also encompassing a range of 5 log units of intensity and 50 dB. As shown on the last column, however, a value of 20 dB corresponds to 100 asb and 15 dB corresponds to 316 asb (a factor of 10 higher than the corresponding Octopus intensities). Although the Humphrey Field Analyzer and the Octopus logarithmic scales cover essentially the same range, the corresponding linear intensity scales (asb) are offset by a factor of 10.

The Dicon (Table 1–4), an LED machine, uses intensities similar to the Humphrey Field Analyzer. The full range of test spot luminance is from 0.13 to 10,000 asb encompassing 4.9 log units and 49 dB. Likewise other instruments employ similar scales.

Although sensitivity and threshold values are inversely related, this relationship is not directly obvious from the decibel scales shown on Tables 1–2, 1–3, and 1–4. For example, if a light increment threshold is 10 asb then we could theoretically represent sensitivity as 1/10. Due to the scaling conventions adopted in automated visual field testing, however, 10 asb corresponds to a sensitivity of 20 dB on the Octopus scale and 30 dB on most other automated perimeter scales. This is a result of the fact that the log scale is inversely related to the intensity scale so that the maximum intensity of either 1000 asb or 10,000 asb is associated with 0 dB.

Properties of the Visual System That Influence Sensitivity

The human eye is a highly versatile and sensitive light detection instrument. Perception of light is the result of a complex chain of events starting with the optical collection and focusing of light onto an array of photoreceptors distributed over the retina. These photoreceptors selectively absorb specific wavelengths of light (approximately 400 to 700 nm) and transduce light energy to neural signals, which are processed and transmitted to the brain. The detection and image reconstruction process of vision starts at the photoreceptor array on the retina. Figure 1–8 shows a photoreceptor array of a primate (*Macaca fascicularis*) that includes the central fovea.[5] The array of photoreceptors is cut perpendicular to the axis of the photoreceptor, and is shown at the level of the external limiting membrane near the photoreceptor entrance aperture. Figure 1–8 illustrates that vision is the result of light sampled by a two-dimensional array of discrete photosensitive cells.

Figure 1–9 is the fellow eye and the section is cut parallel to the photoreceptor axis.[6] Light enters the eye from the bottom, and passes through the inner neural (plexiform) layers consisting of the ganglion, bipolar, horizontal, and Mueller cells to reach the photoreceptor inner segment. The inner segment serves as a wave guide to pass the captured light energy onto the outer segment where the transduction of light energy to neural signals occurs. The signal is then transmitted back up along the cell body to the first synapse at the inner plexiform layer where the signal is contributed to the information

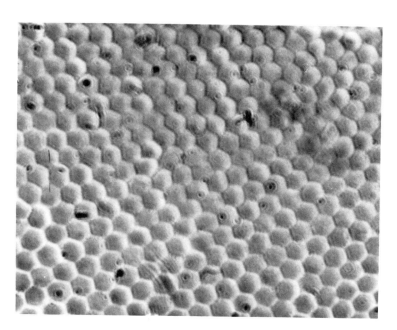

Figure 1–8. Foveal cone inner segments in the monkey retina (Macaca fascicularis) shown in a photograph of a 1-μm thick section at the external limiting membrane. (From Miller, WmH, 1979, with permission.[5])

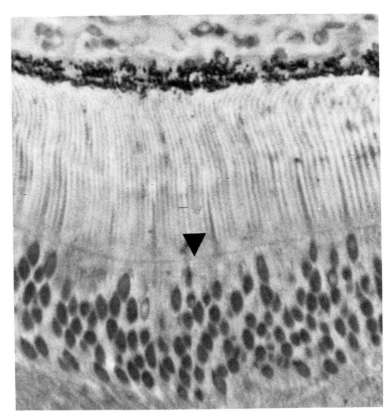

Figure 1–9. Foveal cones sectioned perpendicular to the external limiting membrane (Fig. 1–8) for the monkey (Macaca fascicularis). Light enters from the bottom and passes through the inner plexiform neural layer before entering the individual photoreceptors at the external limiting membrane indicated by the arrow. (From Miller, WH and Bernard, G, 1984, with permission.[6])

processes that ultimately results in the various image reconstruction tasks performed by the eye.[7]

Under optimal visual conditions only a few quanta of light are required to produce a visual effect. However, sensitivity of the eye varies depending upon a variety of visual conditions. These conditions include adaptive state of the eye, location of the stimulus on the retina, and optical factors such as pupil size and refractive error.

LEVEL OF LIGHT ADAPTATION: THE EFFECT OF BACKGROUND ILLUMINATION

The human eye is able to function over a very large range of luminances (Table 1–5). This is due in part to the fact that the retina consists of two types of photoreceptors, rods and cones. Rods are responsible for vision in dim illumination whereas cones are responsible for vision during daylight levels of illlumination. Ambient illuminance levels from 10^{-5} to 10^0 asb are not sufficient for cone activity, and are referred to as scotopic levels of illuminance. Illuminance values from approximately 10^2 to 10^8 asb stimulate only cones and are

TABLE 1–5. THE TOTAL RANGE OF LUMINANCE FOR THE HUMAN EYE IS APPROXIMATELY 13 LOG UNITS

Luminance (mL)		Illuminance (asb)
10^9	Damaging	10^{10}
10^8		10^9
10^7	- -	10^8
10^6	Photopic	10^7
10^5	(cones only)	10^6
10^4		10^5
10^3		10^4
10^2		10^3
10^1	- -	10^2
10^0	Mesopic	10^1
10^{-1}	- - - - - - - (rods and cones) - - - - - -	10^0
10^{-2}		10^{-1}
10^{-3}		10^{-2}
10^{-4}	Scotopic	10^{-3}
10^{-5}	(rods only)	10^{-4}
10^{-6}		10^{-5}

This range is shown for both units of luminance (mL) and illuminance (asb).

referred to as photopic levels of illuminance. The narrow range of illuminances between 10^0 and 10^1 asb, stimulates both rods and cones and is referred to as the mesopic range of illuminance. The total range of illuminance over which the human eye is capable of visual function is approximately 13 log units.

The feature of the visual system that allows vision over such a large range of luminances is called adaptation. At any given time a person is rarely confronted with a luminance environment that exceeds a range of more than 2 log units and the eye adjusts its sensitivity to whatever the range happens to be. Whenever a person quickly changes from one luminance environment to another (as in leaving a darkened movie theater on a sunny afternoon), a momentary "blindness" results until the eye becomes *adapted* to a new range of luminance. Effectively, the eye adjusts or adapts to a new dynamic range. In the case of light adaptation (adjusting to a brighter environment) the process takes only a few minutes. In the case of dark adaptation (adjusting to a darker environment) the process may take as long as 40 minutes until the eye reaches its maximum level of sensitivity.

The physiologic mechanisms underlying visual adaptation are complex and beyond the scope of this chapter. However, the two main operative influences are photochemical and neural. The photochemical basis for light and dark adaptation is best established in the case of rods. Rhodopsin, the photosensitive substance in rod outer segments, is bleached by light. Therefore in light conditions the concentration of rhodopsin is less than in dark conditions. Visual adaptation depends in part upon the balance between bleaching and restorative reactions of the photopigment.

The second main influence on visual adaptation is neural. It has been shown that changes in visual thresholds can occur as a result of adaptation even when there is no significant change in the concentration of visual pigment. Rushton[8] formulated a hypothesis of neural "pools" to account for neural regulation of visual sensitivity depending on the level of light stimulation. The neural basis for adaptation has also been confirmed by Dowling.[9]

LEVEL OF VISUAL ADAPTATION AND VISUAL FIELD TESTING

The primary significance of visual adaptation to visual field testing is that background luminance of the perimeter controls visual sensitivity. In general, an intense background luminance decreases visual sensitivity and a low background luminance increases visual sensitivity. In the case of a background luminance of 4 asb (as in the Octopus system) or 1 cd/m² (as in the Perimat 206) cone sensitivity is set at the lower limits of the dynamic range possible for cones (Table 1–5). In the case of a higher background luminance such as 31.5 asb (as in most other systems) the dynamic range of the eye shifts upward and threshold values are higher confirming that the eye is less sensitive. For example, when the reported dB levels of the Octopus and Humphrey machines are the same, it can be concluded that visual sensitivity at the Octopus 4 asb background level is greater than sensitivity at the Humphrey 31.5 asb background level (Tables 1–2 and 1–3). This difference in sensitivity is attributed to the different background levels of illumination and the resultant adaptive state of the eye.

ECCENTRICITY: EFFECT OF STIMULUS LOCATION

Sensitivity to small spots of light tends to fall off with eccentricity from the fovea. Figure 1–10 shows a plot of average sensitivity (dB) as a function of

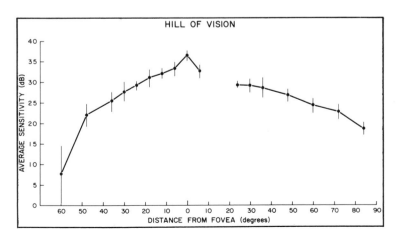

Figure 1–10. Average sensitivity (dB) as a function of retinal eccentricity in degrees of visual angle from the fovea. Values represent averages of eight eyes between 18 and 39 years old along the horizontal meridian. Error bars represent ± 1 SD and indicate the interindividual variation. (Values used to graph hill of vision were obtained from the Octopus Visual Field Atlas, 1978.)

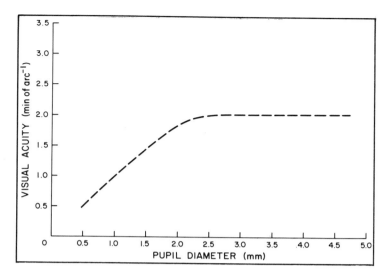

Figure 1–11. *The effect of pupil size on visual acuity.*

retinal eccentricity (deg) for normal observers (18 to 39 years) tested on an Octopus 201 instrument.[10] This general reduction in sensitivity is called the Hill of Vision. However, the slopes of the fall-off depend in part upon level of visual adaptation and spot size.

PUPIL SIZE

The pupil of the eye serves as the optical aperture that controls the amount of light that enters the visual system. That is, the retinal illuminance (light arriving at the photoreceptors) cannot necessarily be assumed equal to the light reflected or emitted from a stimulus. A constricted pupil will limit the effective (retinal) stimulus intensity (see section on retinal illuminance: trolands). Figure 1–11 shows visual acuity as a function of pupil diameter. Acuity falls off rapidly below approximately 2.0 mm and is approximately constant from 2.25 to 5 mm. As the pupil is reduced in size below approximately 2.0 mm, visual sensitivity is reduced due to the reduction in light that reaches the retina and due to the restricted field of view. Both factors are relevant to perimetry.

REFRACTIVE ERROR

Measurement of retinal sensitivity to light requires that the optical transmission of light to the retina be the highest quality possible. Otherwise, an observed field defect may be due to optical obstruction or poor image quality rather than a failure of the visual system. To assure that any refractive error is minimized, corrective lenses are added to the distance prescription for a patient prior to a central visual field examination. The amount of optimal correction

TABLE 1–6. RECOMMENDED OPTICAL ADDS

Age (yr)	Bowl Size		
	30 to 33 cm	*42 cm*	*50 cm*
30 to 35	1.00	0.75	0.50
36 to 40	1.25	1.00	0.75
41 to 45	1.50	1.25	1.00
46 to 50	2.00	1.50	1.25
51 to 55	2.50	2.00	1.50
56 to 60	3.00	2.25	1.75
61 +	3.25	2.50	2.00

depends upon the age of the patient and the size of the cupola on the perimeter. Table 1–6 shows recommended added corrections for both a 50-cm and a 30- to 33-cm bowl size for ages above 30 years.

The trial lens should be removed for a peripheral field examination beyond 30 degrees because the refractive correction is not effective for most patients in the peripheral field, and the ring of the lens may interfere with the test. A contact lens correction may be advisable for aphakic patients and patients with high myopia.

References

1. Hurvich L, Jameson D: The Perception of Brightness and Darkness. Boston, Allyn and Bacon, 1966.
2. Graham CH: Vision and Visual Perception. New York, Wiley, 1966.
3. Rainwater C: Light and Color. New York, Golden Press, 1971.
4. Riggs A: Vision, in Kling JW, Riggs LA (eds): Woodworth's and Schlosberg's Experimental Psychology. New York, Holt, Rinehart and Winston, 1971.
5. Miller WmH: Ocular Optical Filtering, in Handbook of Sensory Physiology, Vol. VII (6A). Berlin, Springer, 1979.
6. Miller WmH, Bernard G: Averaging over the foveal receptor aperture curtails aliasing. Vision Res 23:1365–1369, 1984.
7. Stein FH (ed): The Molecular Mechanism of Photoreception. Dahlem Konferenzen. Life Sciences Research Report. Berlin, Springer-Verlag, 1985.
8. Rushton WAH: Increment threshold and dark adaptation. J Opt Soc Am 3:104–109, 1963.
9. Dowling JE: The site of visual adaptation. Science 155:273–279, 1967.
10. Octopus Visual Field Atlas, ed 2. Schlieron, Switzerland, Interzeag, N2.9–N2.10, 1978.

2
The Evolution of the Visual Field Examination

The History of Visual Field Testing

The first mention of visual field defects was made by Hippocrates (460–380 BCE) who recorded the existence of a hemianopsia in a patient. According to Damianus, Ptolemy made the first attempt to measure the visual field in 150 BCE. Galen (131–179 CE) discussed scotomata.[1] Mariotte discovered the existence of the blind spot in 1668.[2] This caused considerable excitement and Mariotte was called before Charles II of England to demonstrate the blind spot. Mariotte incorrectly interpreted the presence of the blind spot to mean that vision was performed in the choroid rather than in the retina. Over 100 years would pass before Thomas Young would give the first exact measurement of the blind spot and nearly 200 years before Von Graefe would note the enlargement of the blind spot in disease.

The Dutch physician Boerhaave in 1708 mentioned the existence of scotomata.[3] In 1801 Thomas Young, an English physicist, was the first to make an exact measurement of the normal visual field and the blind spot.[4] This work was also done by Purkinje in 1825.[5]

Albrecht Von Graefe was the first to introduce visual field testing into clinical ophthalmology exploiting the qualitative or diagnostic information that can be obtained. Writing in 1856 he remarked that the visual field is as important a measurement of a patient's visual function as is central visual acuity. His "campimeter" was a 3- by 4-foot blackboard divided into 3-inch squares with a fixation point at the center. The patient was placed at a distance of $1\frac{1}{2}$ feet from the board. The test object was a piece of chalk and the patient would be instructed to maintain fixation at a central fixation spot.[6] In 1867 De Wecker designed a similar screen but with radial markings instead of Cartesian squares.[7]

Von Graefe recognized the contraction of the visual field that occurs with glaucoma and documented that this occurs prior to the loss of central acuity. He was probably the first to plot the paracentral field defects that occur in glaucoma and to use them for the evaluation of surgical results. He recorded the loss of the peripheral field in retinitis pigmentosa and the loss of selective areas of the visual field in central nervous system diseases. He recognized and described homonymous hemianopsias and bitemporal hemianopsias and used these defects to try to localize lesions. He remarked on the incomplete loss of an area of the visual field in retinal detachments.[8]

The first practical instrument for perimetry was developed by Richard Forster in 1869. He developed a 180-degree circular arc pivoted on a stand. Test objects of different sizes were moved in from the side. Mainly large sized test objects were used, however.[9] With the introduction of Forster's perimeter, there was a widespread abandonment of von Graefe's methods and the perimeter became the instrument of choice for studying the visual field.

Jannik Peterson Bjerrum introduced the Bjerrum screen in 1889. This led to the large scale analysis of the visual field and the concept of quantitative visual field testing. A 2-meter screen and a 2-meter test distance were used.[10] Test objects of various sizes and as small as 1 mm were used. Because the testing distance was increased from about 300 mm to 2 meters and because test object size was decreased to as small as 1 mm, test objects subtended very small visual angles increasing the sensitivity and accuracy of visual field testing.

Bjerrum was able to distinguish between relative and absolute scotomas and was able to characterize the scotomas of glaucoma that circle fixation and include the blind spot. He was also one of the first to recognize the importance of correcting refractive errors when testing the visual field, but interestingly he discounted the effect that a change in pupil size can make on the visual field.[11] Using the Bjerrum screen, and using modifications of it such as umbrella-shaped screens, significant contributions were made to the science of visual field testing by Roenne in Denmark (1909–1927),[12] Sinclair (1905–1906),[13] and Traquair (1914–1949)[14] in Scotland, and Walker (1913–1921)[15] and Peter (1916–1931)[16] in the United States.

In 1893 Groenouw[17] developed the concept of isopters of sensitivity. Using small test objects he would connect the points at which the objects first became visible.

Traquair introduced the concept of the visual field as an island of sight within a sea of darkness. This important analogy has remained with us to this day and is often called upon to explain the value of a three-dimensional conception of the visual field.[18]

Harvey Cushing was the first to appreciate the value of quantitative perimetry and to insist on it being an integral part of the neurologic investigation of intracranial disease. He quantified defects caused by chiasmal and cerebral lesions. Indeed the stimulus for visual field study was both neurologic and ophthalmologic.

Goldmann attempted to produce an instrument that would provide ideal conditions for visual field testing and introduced his projection perimeter in

1945. The spherical shape allowed easier testing of the complete field. The bowl rather than arc design provided for more even illumination. There was complete freedom of test object movement. Size, brightness, and color could be accurately controlled. The perimeter provided a pantograph for recording data adding to the accuracy of the written record of the test.[19]

The first practical instrument for static perimetry was designed by Professors H. Harms and E. Aulhorn of the University of Tubingen in Germany and introduced in 1962. Their perimeter allowed for an increase in light intensity in steps. Patients were tested along the horizontal, vertical, and two diagonal meridians at 1-degree intervals from fixation to 15 degrees and then at 5-degree intervals to the periphery. Kinetic perimetry could also be performed with the instrument to study areas where a defect was found by static testing techniques. Static perimetry was employed by them to study glaucomatous visual field defects.[20]

Several visual field screening devices have been introduced. Harrington and Flocks[21] introduced an instrument for presenting multiple spot patterns. Originally this was done with cards that would be shown with short pulses of blue light. Recently a television version of this test has been presented.[22] In the early 1970s Friedmann[23] introduced a visual field analyzer that also presented multiple test spots. These devices have only a screening function and are not designed for quantitative or qualitative analysis of the field.

Since the early 1970s, Fankhauser has worked on the automation of visual field testing and this has resulted in the Octopus perimeter. Various other devices including the Peritest, the Dicon, and the Fieldmaster have been developed in the past 10 years and these have been studied by many investigators. These automated machines are explored in depth in later chapters.

Representation of the Visual Field

The normal visual field of an eye is a slightly irregular oval. From its center it extends approximately 60 degrees superiorly, 75 degrees inferiorly, 105 degrees temporally, and 60 degrees nasally. The nasal field partially overlaps the contralateral temporal field.

Where the optic nerve enters the globe, no retina is present, resulting in an absolute visual field defect known as the blind spot. There is some slight variation from patient to patient but generally the blind spot is located in the temporal field with its center at about 15.5 degrees from fixation, just below the horizontal meridian. It is vertically oval and measures approximately 6 degrees by 8 degrees.

The sensitivity of the visual field is greatest in the center and decreases as the periphery is approached. Traquair has described this as an island hill of vision in a sea of darkness. The area of the island represents the extent of the field and the height of its sensitivity. The blind spot is seen as a cylindrical defect in Traquair's hill of vision.[24] Using data for normal Octopus threshold sensitivity across the horizontal meridian, this hill was demonstrated in Chapter 1 (Fig. 1–10).

The visual field can be measured using test objects of increasing relative intensity. The intensity of the test object determines the sensitivity that will be necessary for the eye to see it. Therefore, using Traquair's hill of vision conceptualization, a particular test object can be thought of as corresponding to a particular altitude, the smaller the test object the greater the altitude. The intersection of a plane through that altitude and the sides of the hill of vision will define a ring of equal sensitivity or an isopter.

The visual field can be tested by moving the test spot from an area of nonvision to an area of vision (kinetic technique) or increasing the test spot intensity until it can be seen at a fixed location (static technique). The results of the examination can be represented in different forms depending on whether kinetic or static techniques are used.

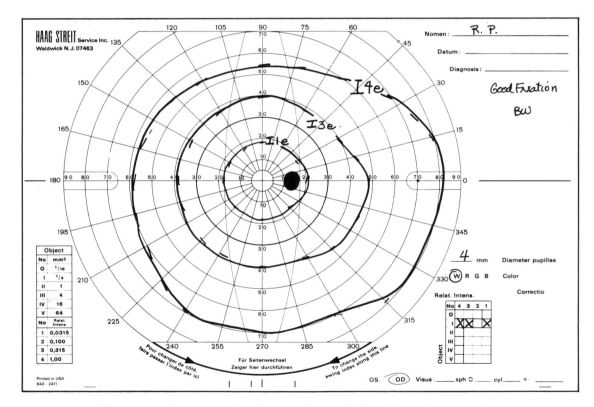

Figure 2–1. *The isopter plot of a normal visual field of the right eye as obtained on a Gold-mann-type bowl perimeter. The outermost isopter was obtained with an I4e test object, the innermost with an I1e test object. This type of visual field representation is analogous to a contour map.*

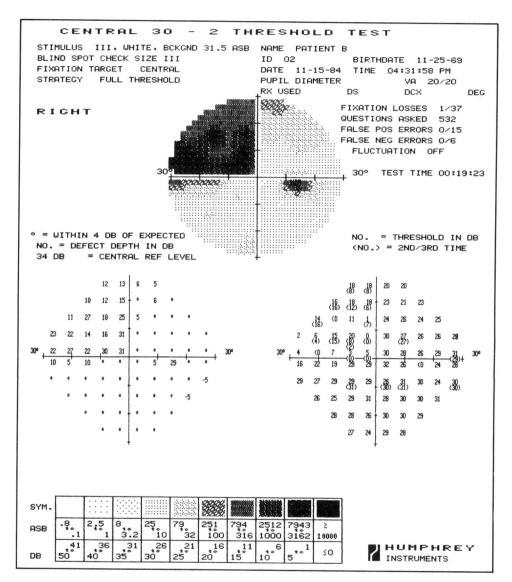

Figure 2–2. *The standard printout of a threshold visual field examination performed on a Humphrey Visual Field Analyzer contains the numeric threshold measurements at each spot tested, an interpolated grey scale derived from those measurements, and a symbolic matrix in which the threshold results are represented by symbols, each indicating the range the particular spot fell within.*

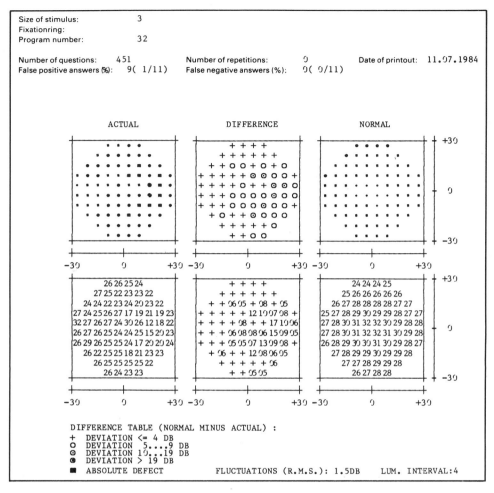

Figure 2–3. *Comparison printout from an Octopus 201 examination of the right eye of a patient with a right inferior quadrantanopia. The left-hand column represents the actual examination, the right-hand column the expected normal, and the center column the difference. Actual threshold measurements are indicated by the numbers in the bottom row. These numbers are converted to symbols in the top row. The meaning of the symbols in the central difference column is shown by the difference table at the bottom.*

A kinetic examination will produce a series of spots indicating where a particular test object intensity was first seen. Connecting these spots will produce an isopter plot for that test object intensity. If this process is repeated for several different test object intensities, a series of isopter plots will be produced. The collection of isopter plots will produce a contour map of the hill of vision. This is demonstrated by the visual field drawing as obtained on a Goldmann-type perimeter (Fig. 2–1).

A static examination reports the threshold intensity of a particular spot in the visual field. At the completion of the entire examination, a numerical threshold value is obtained for each spot tested. This can be reported in various ways. First, the values can be listed at their respective locations. Second, the values can be converted to a shade of grey ranging from solid black where the test spot could not be seen to white where the recorded threshold was very low. The spaces in between the recorded values are then given interpolated shades of grey and a "grey scale picture" of the visual field is produced. Third, different ranges of threshold sensitivity can be represented by different symbols. The printout shows these symbols at their respective locations along with an interpretation key. All three of these modes of printout are commonly available and are displayed on one sheet by the Humphrey Visual Field Tester (Fig. 2–2). Fourth, the values can be compared with expected "normals" and areas of deviation can be indicated. This is done in an Octopus comparison printout (Fig. 2–3). Fifth, if the spots tested are arranged along a meridian, a two-dimensional graph of intensity versus location can be drawn (meridional threshold). This can be obtained for an Octopus threshold examination (Fig. 2–4). Sixth, if the spots tested are arranged in a circle at a particular distance from fixation a similar type of intensity versus location graph can be drawn (circular threshold). Dicon makes such a testing pattern available (Fig. 2–5).

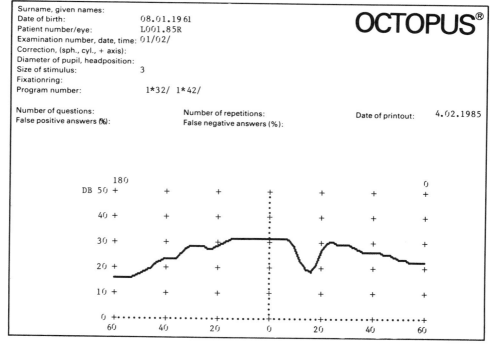

Figure 2–4. *Meridional threshold printout. After program 32 is performed on an Octopus 201 perimeter, the printout of a static cut through the thresholds can be obtained.*

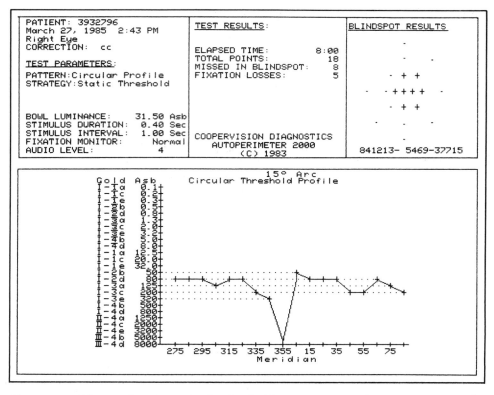

Figure 2–5. *When performing a circular threshold examination on the Dicon AP 2000, the examiner inputs the distance from fixation, the starting point on that circle, and the ending point. The graph generated plots the intensity on the Y axis and the position on the X axis. A normal result would be a nearly straight graph. The graph would dip down in the area of a scotoma. The dip in this graph represents the patient's physiologic blind spot.*

Seventh, if the spots tested are confined to a particular section of the field, such as along both sides of the vertical meridian, a symbolic plot of the area can be produced. This type of testing pattern highlights the area of interest to the examiner and is produced by the Octopus Series 70 software (Fig. 2–6).

Variations on threshold examinations produce other types of visual field representation. A suprathreshold examination combines the fixed location strategy of a threshold examination with the fixed test object intensity strategy of a kinetic examination. The patient's response at each test spot is a yes or no answer—the spot is either seen or not seen. Therefore the printout consists of an array of yes and no response indicators. The Fieldmaster 200, for example, performs threshold examinations and marks a preprinted test report form as to which spots were seen (Fig. 2–7).

A threshold-related examination is similar to a suprathreshold examination in that only one test spot intensity is used at each location. The intensity, however, is varied from one location to another increasing as the periphery is

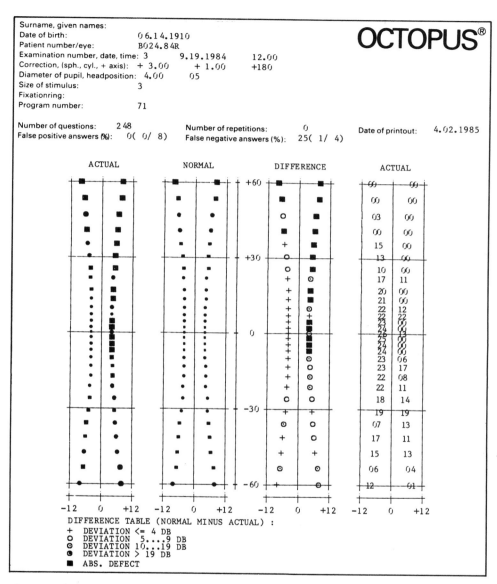

Figure 2–6. *The Octopus Program 70 studies the vertical meridian to try to demonstrate a neurologic field defect (specifically looking for a Chamlin step). Points are checked from fixation to the periphery at 12 degrees on either side of the vertical meridian. The threshold values are presented in the fourth column. They are converted to symbols in the first column; compared to "normal" values which are displayed as symbols in the second column, and the difference between normal and actual is displayed as symbols in the third "difference" column.*

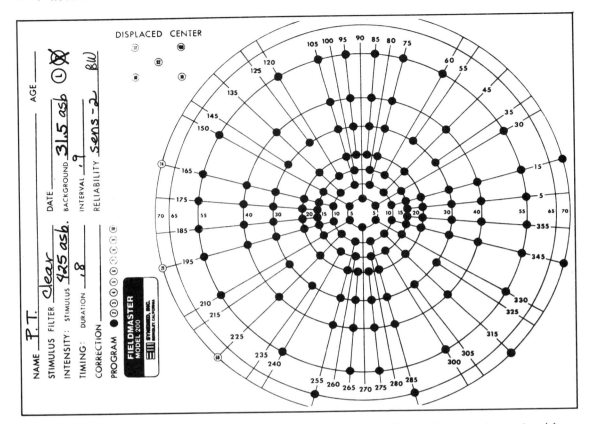

Figure 2–7. *The Fieldmaster 200 performs suprathreshold examinations. A preprinted form is placed in the machine. Spots seen are marked on the form. The software program (or distribution of spots) is also marked. Other variables including testing intensity, background intensity, stimulus duration, and test spot color are written on the form by the technician.*

approached. The patient's response, however, as in a suprathreshold examination, is limited to yes or no. Therefore the printout is a similar array of yes and no response indicators, however, the question asked at each spot is different as opposed to the questions asked at every spot in a suprathreshold examination being identical. The peritest screening mode for example uses this type of strategy. A key indicating the testing intensities used at each location is required for interpretation.

A suprathreshold examination and a threshold-related examination give no information as to the depth of a defect and minimal information as to the breadth of the defect because only one intensity is tested at any location. Stepped suprathreshold and stepped threshold-related examinations retest missed spots at successively greater intensities and therefore provide that missing information. Each spot tested is marked on the printout with a symbol representing the lowest intensity that the patient was able to see. Therefore the printout is a cross between the limited information printout of a suprathreshold examination and the numerical printout of a threshold examination. Several different symbols, the number dependent on the number of different intensities tested, are used for the printout. Dicon makes both of these testing strategies available. The printouts look similar except that the stepped threshold-related examination also contains a testing curve key (Figs. 2–8 and 2–9). The Peritest

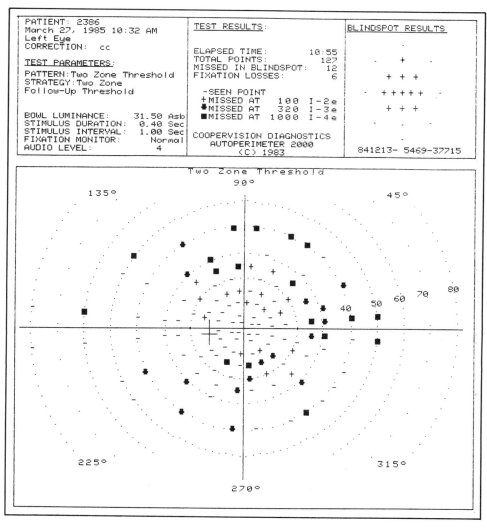

Figure 2–8. *The Dicon Two Zone Program uses a stepped suprathreshold testing logic. If a spot is seen at the starting intensity, a dash is displayed. If it is missed, but seen at the second intensity, a cross is displayed. If it is missed, but finally seen at the third intensity, a heavy cross is displayed. If missed at all intensities tested, a box is displayed.*

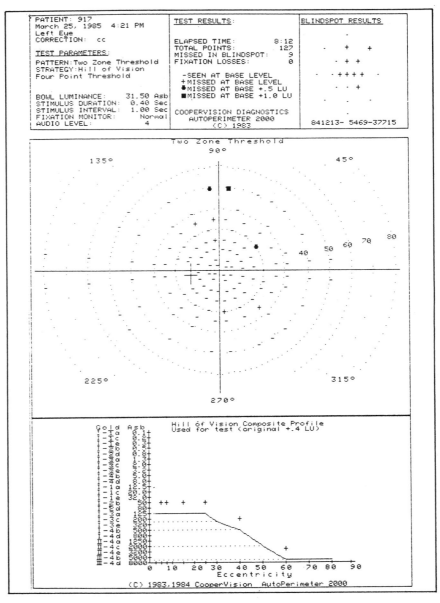

Figure 2–9. The Dicon Hill of Vision Program uses a stepped threshold-related testing logic. A hill of vision curve is first produced by a selected spot thresholding program. A testing curve is then calculated by both machine and operator input. The testing curve tells the examiner what starting intensity is used at each location. If spots are missed, they are reexamined at one-half and one log units above the starting intensity. The resulting printout is similar to the two-zone printout in Figure 2–8. Instead of the simple key indicating the exact intensity every spot was tested at, however, a more elaborate key, a testing intensity curve, is included. Symbols relate to the curve. A dash indicates that the test spot was seen at the intensity shown by the curve. The other symbols indicate a difference from the starting intensity.

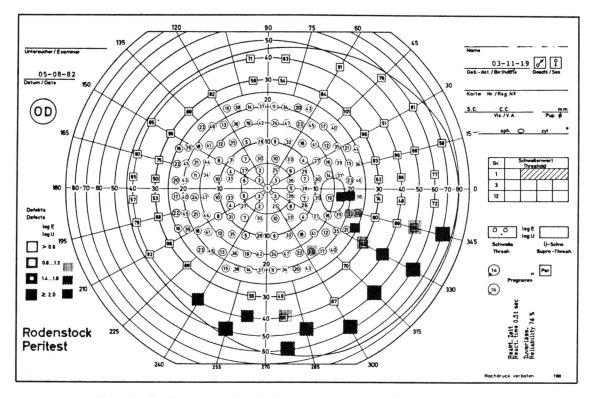

Figure 2–10. *The stepped threshold-related strategies used in the Perimat and Peritest employ a preprogrammed hill of vision curve. The user selects the number of steps he or she wants to evaluate. The results are printed onto a preprinted form using grey scale boxes indicating the depth of the defect obtained at each spot tested.*

and the Perimat stepped threshold-related strategy does not customize the hill of vision testing curve to the individual patient but does explore defects with more steps than the Dicon programs. Symbols of increasing grey scale intensity are used to indicate the depth of defects (Fig. 2–10).

Manual Methods of Examining the Visual Field

When reviewing a visual field report, either from a manual or automated testing device, the elegance of the representation often gives the impression that the results of the examination are as objective and as exacting as in an electrocardiogram or an electroencephalogram. The results, however, represent subjective responses and are influenced by many factors including the patient's mental status at the time of the examination and the limitations of the device used. Therefore, it is important to choose a method of testing the visual field that is appropriate to the clinical situation at hand. Often the method of choice is a manual one rather than an automated one.

Before actually starting a visual field examination it is important to get a patient history. It is necessary to know whether the patient has noticed a defect in his or her visual field or has been stumbling over objects. Perhaps the patient has had transient visual field loss or the scintillating scotomas of migraine. During the examination the patient might have "ignored" a portion of the visual acuity chart or a portion of color testing plates and this would be highly suggestive of a visual field defect in the area that the patient was "ignoring." It is also important to know whether anything in the clinical examination suggested a glaucomatous, a neurologic, or a retinal problem that could have a resulting visual field defect.

CONFRONTATION METHODS

Confrontation visual field tests are useful for quick screening and for bedside visual field testing. With confrontation methods, the examiner compares his or her visual field to that of the patient. The examiner presents objects to the patient and the patient has to respond as to whether he or she sees the objects or not. There are many methods for performing a confrontation visual field examination. The common element of all these methods is the fact that the examiner monitors fixation by direct observation with his or her opposite eye and compares the field of the patient to his or her own.

Finger counting fields are performed by presenting fingers in each of one or two of the four visual field quadrants. The patient is then asked to tell the examiner how many fingers were presented. It is a particularly effective way of eliciting the Riddoch visual field extinction phenomenon.

With a moving finger confrontation approach the examiner asks the patient to tell when the examiner's finger is first seen as it is moved from an area of nonvision to an area of vision. A similar field can be performed on a patient with very poor vision by using a large white object such as a box instead of the finger. Obviously the method will identify only large, absolute defects.

Light projection is a confrontation technique that is useful in patients with profoundly decreased vision. A focused light is presented from each of the four visual quadrants. The patient must identify where the light is coming from. Only large field defects can be identified by such methods.

Double simultaneous presentation of two similar objects in corresponding areas of the field can be useful for demonstrating relative (nonabsolute) visual field defects. Perhaps the most effective method is to present two identical red dropper bottle caps on either side of the midline. If they look identical, no field defect is demonstrated; if one looks dull or grey, it is probably in an area of depressed visual field function or a "relative" defect; if only one is seen then there is an absolute field defect.

Small central visual field defects can often be mapped with small red- or white-tipped matches. With these the examiner can plot the patient's blind spot and small central scotomas. The patient is asked to inform the examiner of the disappearance of the small match tip.

In confrontation visual field examinations, the "hardware" can be thought of as the examiner's fingers or the test objects that he or she is presenting. The "software" can be thought of as the examiner's decisions as to how to present his or her fingers or the objects to the patient. Fixation monitoring is done by eye-to-eye contact with the contralateral eye.

THE TANGENT SCREEN

In a tangent screen visual field examination the patient maintains fixation at a central point on a large black screen. Test objects are brought in from areas of nonvision to areas of vision. The patient reports to the examiner when he or she sees the test object.

Tangent screens are relatively easy to construct and therefore many variations have been designed over the years. The most common, however, is a screen that is approximately 1 m². The test is then performed at a distance of either ½ m, 1 m (most commonly), or 2 m from the tangent screen. Test objects can be small flat round discs on the end of a stick, small balls on the end of a stick, or illuminated discs at the end of a stick. The size of the test object can range from a fraction of a millimeter to 20 or more millimeters in diameter. The most commonly used sizes, however, are 1, 2, or 3 mm in diameter. Usually the test objects are white, but any color can be used.

At 1 m or 2 m the tangent screen only measures the patient's central visual field. At 1 m slightly more than 30 degrees can be measured and at 2 m about 20 degrees can be measured. If the screen is moved to only ½ m from the patient, however, the visual field can be measured out to 50 degrees. Even at 1 m, if the patient shifts his or her fixation to the right, to the left, up and down, 60 degrees can be added to the extent of the visual field. This allows for the entire visual field to be mapped, but obviously requires a great deal of work.

The "hardware" in the tangent screen is the screen and the test spots. The "software" is the examiner's decisions as to how to present the test spots. Fixation monitoring is done indirectly. Background illumination is kept constant by a controlled overhead light source.

BOWL AND ARC PERIMETERS

With a perimeter, the test spot is projected on a curved surface. The surface can be a bowl, such as the Goldmann-type perimeters, or an arc, such as the Aimark perimeter. The patient's head is placed in the center of the bowl or arc and test spots are presented on the surface of the bowl or arc. The entire visual field is covered by the bowl. The arc is rotated so that it can also cover the entire visual field.

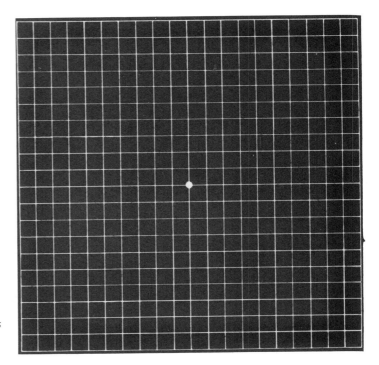

Figure 2–11. The Amsler grid. When held at a distance of 28 to 30 cm from the eye, the entire grid subtends 20 degrees on the retina. Each small box subtends 1 degree.

The advantage of the perimeter over the tangent screen is that the entire visual field can be tested without having to resort to fixation shifting tricks. Fixation is monitored with a periscope in the Goldmannn bowl-type perimeters and by observation in the Aimark arc-type perimeter. The visual field is recorded by a pantograph, which is calibrated with the movements of the test spot. The background is usually white instead of the black used in a tangent screen and the test object is a projected spot of light. Both the size and the color of the spot of light is varied. The surface of the perimeter is located closer to the patient's eye than the surface of the tangent screen. Most have a radius of approximately 33 cm. Some have a radius of up to 50 cm.

Because a projected light source is used, it is practical to do both static and kinetic examinations with a bowl-type perimeter. The projected test spot is moved from an area of no vision until it is seen in an area of vision in a kinetic examination. The test spot is kept at a constant position and the intensity is increased until it is seen in a static examination.

The "hardware" in a perimeter is the machine itself. The "software" is the examiner's decisions as to which test spots to present and what size and color the test spots will be. Fixation monitoring depends on the particular machine but is either by direct or indirect visualization of the patient's eye.

THE AMSLER GRID

The Amsler grid tests the patient's central vision. The grid consists of a 10-mm square white on black pattern of horizontal and vertical lines forming a large box subdivided into a 20 by 20 box grid (Fig. 2–11).

The chart is held at a distance of 28 to 30 cm from the patient. The pattern covers 20 degrees of field with each box representing 1 degree. The patient is instructed to look at the center of the grid. He or she needs to wear a refraction including a near correction for the 28- to 30-cm distance. Even lighting on the chart is necessary. The patient normally would use his or her fovea for fixation and the foveal area represents an oval that is approximately 8 mm in length and 6 mm in width. The area of the retina covered by the Amsler grid is shown in Fig. 2–12.

The patient is asked a series of questions. First, if he or she sees the white spot in the center of the square chart. Second, while keeping the gaze fixed on

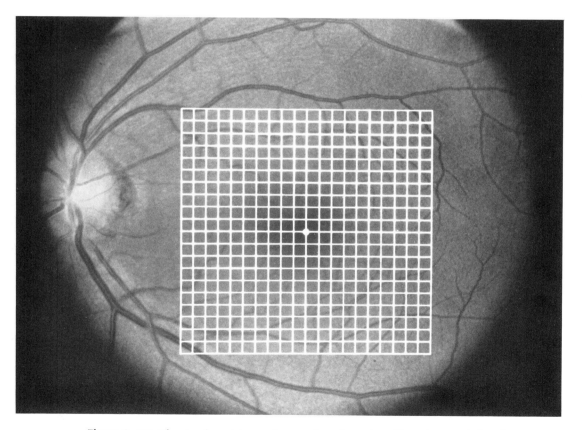

Figure 2–12. *The Amsler grid superimposed on the retina. Distortions and disturbances seen in the grid pattern by the patient are sensitive indicators of macular field loss.*

the white spot at the center, he or she is asked if the four corners of the chart and the four sides of the square are seen. Third, while keeping the gaze fixed on the central fixation point, he or she is asked if there are any places where the pattern is disrupted or blurred. Fourth, while looking at the central fixation point, he or she is asked if there is an area where the pattern is irregular or where the lines appear to curve. Using a replica of the chart, the patient is then requested to draw the areas of the visual disturbance.

The Amsler grid is an exceedingly powerful way of studying the patient's central foveal visual field. It is an excellent way of monitoring lesions in the retina or choroid near fixation that can be enlarging such as retinal edema or a melanoma. Lesions, which displace but do not destroy the retina, will cause the lines to curve. Lesions, which destroy the retina, will cause defects within the pattern. Small pocket-sized Amsler grids have been designed to enable a patient to monitor the progression of his or her macular disease on a daily basis.

Several variations on the chart have been designed to enhance the ability of the Amsler grid to bring out visual field patterns. A large X placed over the chart is useful when the patient has difficulty maintaining fixation on the central dot. Dots on the chart, rather than a grid pattern, can be useful for determining areas of absolute visual loss. Using a chart with only the horizontal or the vertical grid can be useful when measuring distortion of the vision. Using charts that are red on black rather than white on black can be useful when looking for an early central scotoma from optic neuritis.

The "hardware" for the Amsler grid is the chart. The "software" in the Amsler grid test is the questions that the examiner asks the patient. Fixation is monitored by indirect observation.

VISUAL FIELD SCREENERS

The Harrington Flock visual field screener and the Friedmann visual field analyzer both employ a similar principle of showing the patient several spots at once and asking the patient to inform the examiner how many spots he or she is seeing and where they are located. Screening tests are designed to determine if a patient has a field defect, not to quantify it. If a defect is found, a qualitative examination is then necessary. They are meant to be rapid and simple to perform.

The Harrington Flock screener flashes multiple patterns of visual field test spots. The spots are white in fluorescent sulfide ink on white cards. A $\frac{1}{4}$-second flash of ultraviolet light makes the spots shine against a dark background. The patient describes the pattern seen. Errors in the description indicate areas of field defects. The test has proven to be very effective for quick screening. A television version has been produced and has been used for large scale screenings.

The Friedmann visual field analyzer was first introduced in 1966 and is now available as the Mark II. It is a semi-automated screening perimeter that presents a series of multistimulus patterns in the central 25 degrees of the visual field.

The patterns are determined by two rotating templates. When holes in the two plates are aligned, two, three, or four stimuli are displayed simultaneously on the bowl in 20-millisecond flashes. Stimulus intensity is controlled by neutral density filters. Color filters are also provided. Stimuli increase in size toward the periphery. There is no provision for checking fixation.

The examiner selects a luminance level at which all of a test's stimuli are presented and manually selects each pattern to be presented. A test chart, placed on the console, is lit from behind by light emitting diodes (LEDs) that display each stimulus in its position as it is presented to the subject. The examiner marks the spots the patient reports seeing.

These devices have been useful as screening devices to determine whether there is a visual field defect or not. Formal visual field analysis is necessary, however, when a defect is demonstrated and to characterize the defect.

Automated Methods of Examining the Visual Field

All of the currently available automated visual field testing devices are based on either the tangent screen or the bowl-type manual devices. Test spots are produced by either a projected light, fixed LEDs, or fiberoptic light bundles. A computer controls the presentation of test spots. Each machine is a combination of hardware (the machine itself) and software (the instructions that govern the way in which the machine studies the field). Hardware design is discussed in Chapter 3. The principles on which software design is based are discussed in Chapter 4.

References

1. Duke-Elder Sir S: System of Ophthalmology, vol VII: The Foundations of Ophthalmology. London, Kimpton, 1962, p 394.
2. Mariotte PE: A new discovery touching vision. Translation by Justel, Royal Society of London. Philos Trans 3:668–671, 1668.
3. Duke-Elder Sir S: System of Ophthalmology, vol VII: The Foundations of Ophthalmology. London, Kimpton, 1962, p 394.
4. Young T: The Bakerian Lecture: On the Mechanism of the Eye. Philos Trans 92:23, 1801.
5. Purkinje: Beobachtungen u. Versiache z. Physiologie d. Sinne Berlin 2:6, 1825.
6. Von Graefe A: Examination of the visual field in amblyopic disease. Archives Fur Ophthalmologie 2:258–298, 1856.
7. De Wecker III Int Cong Ophthal Paris, 64, 1867.

8. Von Graefe A: Examination of the visual field in amblyopic disease. Archives Fur Ophthalmologie 2:258–298, 1856.
9. Kronfeld PC: Perimetry, in Duane TD (ed): Clinical Ophthalmology, Vol 3, Chap 41. Philadelphia, Harper & Row, 1981, p 6.
10. Bjerrum JP: An addition to the general examination of the field of vision. Skand O Mag 2:141, 1889.
11. Bjerrum JP: An addition to the general examination of the field of vision. Skand O Mag 2:141, 1889.
12. Roenne Uber das Gesichtfeld beim Glaukom. Klin Monatsbl f Augenheilk 47:12, 1909.
13. Sinclair AHH: Bjerrum's method of testing the field of vision, the advantages of the method in clinical work, and its special value in the diagnosis of glaucoma. Trans Ophthalmol Soc UK 25:384–412, 1905.
14. Traquair HM: The quantitative method in perimetry, with notes on perimetric apparatus. Ophthalmol Rev 33:65–83, 1914.
15. Walker CB: Color interlacing and perimetry. Trans Am Ophthalmol Soc 1916:14684–14718.
16. Peter KC: A simplified conception of visual field changes in chronic glaucoma Arch Ophthalmol 56:377, 1927.
17. Groenouw: Uber die Sehscharfe der Netzhautperipherie und eine neue Untersuchungsmethode der selben. Arch f Augenheilk 26:85, 1893.
18. Traquair HM: An Introduction to Clinical Perimetry, ed 6. St. Louis, CV Mosby, 1949.
19. Goldmann H: Demonstration unseres neven Projektionskugelperimeters samt theoretischen und klinischen Bemerkungen uber Perimetric. Ophthalmologica 111:187, 1946.
20. Aulhorn E, Harms H: Early visual field defects in glaucoma, in Glaucoma Tutzing Symposium, proceedings of the Twentieth International Congress of Ophthalmology. Basel, S. Karger, 1967, pp 151–186.
21. Harrington DO, Flocks M: Visual field examination by a new tachystoscopic multiple pattern method: A preliminary report. Am J Ophthalmol 37:719–723, 1954.
22. Flocks M: Visual Screening Via Television. Surv Ophthalmol 28:184–187, 1983.
23. Friedmann AI: Serial analysis of changes in visual field defects employing a new instrument to determine the activity of diseases involving the visual pathways. Ophthalmologica (Basel) 152:1, 1966.
24. Traquair HM: An Introduction to Clinical Perimetry, ed 6. St. Louis, CV Mosby, 1949.

3
Concepts in Automated Visual Field Testing Hardware Design

Although there are dozens of automated visual field testing devices, these devices can be compared on the basis of hardware, the machine itself, and software, the program that tells the machine what to do.

Hardware can be compared on the basis of:

1. Type of screen,
2. Type of light presentation system,
3. Background illumination control,
4. Method of monitoring fixation,
5. Method by which the operator communicates with the machine,
6. Method by which the machine communicates with the operator,
7. Type of printed output,
8. Provisions for storage of data, and
9. Provisions for changing software.

Type of Screen

Screens used in the automated field testers tend to parallel those used in manual devices. Automated machines using a flat screen are similar in concept to the tangent screen visual field system. The size of the screen and the distance from the patient's eye to the screen is kept constant in each automated device, although it varies from device to device.

The Digilab 350, for example, is a small screen field tester and the ATS-1 is a large tangent screen device. The patient is kept at 50 cm from the screen in the Digilab 350 and at 1 m from the screen in the ATS-1.

In bowl-based perimeters, the size of the bowl similarly can vary. For example, the Octopus 201 has a 51-cm radius bowl and the Ocumap a 10-cm radius bowl.

Those devices, which present test spots on a flat screen, can only test the central visual field unless the patient's gaze is shifted to the right, the left, the top, and the bottom. When the gaze is shifted, the entire visual field can be tested, but five examinations are required to cover the entire visual field.

When a bowl-type device is used, both the central and peripheral visual fields can be tested. Larger size bowls have a greater distance from the eye to the surface of the bowl. If smaller-sized test objects are then used, more detail can be obtained. In addition, the greater the distance of the surface from the eye, the less the effect of accommodation on the test results.

Type of Light Presentation System

Test spots either can be projected onto the screen or they can be fixed in position on the screen. With a projected light system, there is virtually an infinite number of spot locations that can be used for testing and the size of the test spots can be varied by controlling the aperture of the projection system. In addition, by placing a colored filter in front of the projected light, different colored test spots can be utilized. The Humphrey visual field tester, the Squid, and the Octopus are examples of three projected light systems.

Stationary light presentation systems are provided either by fiberoptic bundles drawing the rays of light to the screen from behind or by light emitting diodes (LED) fixed in position in the screen. The Fieldmaster 200 and the Tubinger automatic perimeter are examples of fiberoptic systems and the Dicon, Peritest, Keta Quantum 412, and Digilab 350 are examples of LED systems. With LED and fiberoptic presentation systems, the size of the test spot cannot be varied. In addition, the number of test spots is limited by the number of fiberoptic bundles or the number of LEDs placed in the screen. The color of the test spot can be varied in a fiberoptic system but it cannot be varied in an LED system. LEDs can be chosen that are of specific colors, however. The most common is approximately 570 nm which is close to where vision peaks in the human eye and is pale green in color. The Topcon field tester, however, uses red LEDs.

The limitation in the number of test spots in a fixed spot presentation system can be overcome by having a large number of spots present in the screen. Generally a bowl-type device having 300 or more spots will be adequate for any testing strategy. It should also be noted that with a projected light system, the number of test spot locations utilized is limited by the software. The spots are presented in fixed locations even though the hardware has the potential of having an infinite number of locations. Although the projected light systems would allow for the possibility of a kinetic presentation of the test spot, few of the devices currently available make use of this type of strategy.

It should be noted, however, that software usually allows for only one test spot size in any particular test in a projection system. The unchanging test spot size is compensated for by changing the intensity of the test spot.

Background Illumination Control

It is important for constant background illumination to be present. The entire screen should be evenly illuminated and at the desired intensity level. Room lights can be especially bothersome in the testing process and will have an effect on the screen background intensity. Most machines will recalibrate the background intensity when the ambient room lighting is changed. It is much easier to keep the background illumination even in a bowl-type device, however, than in a flat screen device. Although the background illumination level can be varied in some devices, it is always kept constant for the entire examination.

Method of Monitoring Fixation

Monitoring of fixation is exceedingly important. If fixation is not maintained, then the field is invalid. Only if fixation is maintained do the test spots study the locations in the field that are intended to be studied. No perfect method of monitoring fixation has been developed, but numerous methods are currently employed.

Some field testers use direct visualization of the pupil through a periscope. The examiner needs to monitor fixation and stop the test if fixation is lost. Video monitors are used by other field testers including the Octopus models. The examiner monitors fixation and stops the test if it is lost. The patient is then repositioned if necessary and the test is continued.

The Octopus also uses a corneal reflection system to monitor fixation. This system automatically excludes trials during periods of lost fixation and notifies the operator of the fixation loss.

Many of the Fieldmaster machines use a "mosaic monitor," a four-quadrant photodetector that is focused on the image of the patient's iris. It responds to the changes in light that are produced by eye movement. If the pupil moves, a change is detected, the examiner is notified, and the field test is stopped. The level of sensitivity of the device can be controlled.

Fixation can also be monitored by a software technique, the Heijl-Krakau method. First, the blind spot is mapped. Then, whenever it is decided to check fixation, a test spot is presented within the blind spot, which the patient should not be able to see. If the patient sees the test spot, fixation has been lost.

It is important to do more than just report the number of fixation losses. When fixation is improper, the field is invalid because test spots cannot then be correlated with retinal position. Therefore, it is important to reestablish fixation and retest all spots tested during the period of uncertain fixation. Some machines, which use the Heijl-Krakau method in their software to monitor fixation, do not retest spots during periods of lost fixation. Instead, they report the number of times fixation was found to be incorrect. Unless the number is exceedingly low (under 2), the examiner must assume that fixation was poor during enough of the examination to make the results invalid.

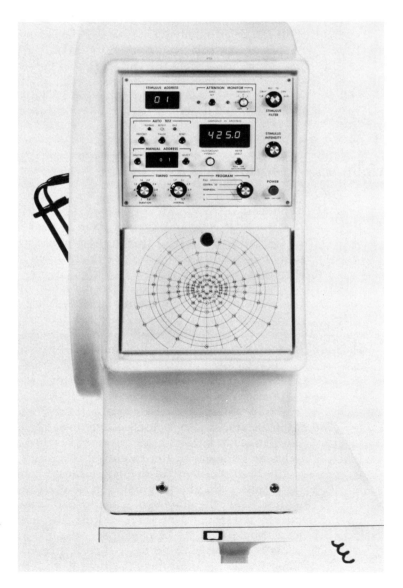

Figure 3–1. Instructions are communicated to the Fieldmaster 200 via a panel of control switches.

Method by Which the Operator Communicates with the Machine

A technician is required with all of the automated devices. The technician must communicate with the machine to tell the machine what software program to use and what options to employ. This can be done either by a panel of switches (Fig. 3–1), a typewriter-type keyboard, or a light pencil selecting options on a video screen. Of these, the panel of switches is the least flexible. As new software is developed and put into a machine, there must be a way of selecting it and its options. Keyboard and light pencil systems allow this flexibility.

Method by Which the Machine Communicates with the Operator

Many of the machines will tell the operator what is taking place as the machine is testing the patient. This can be done either by lights being illuminated on a

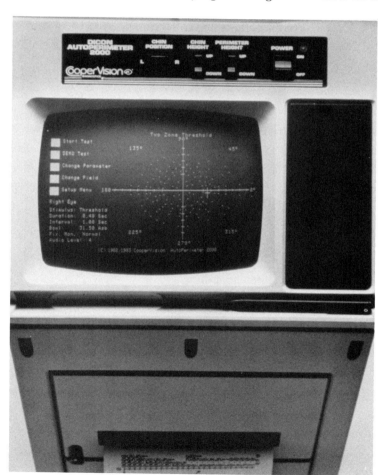

Figure 3–2. *The video screen in the Dicon AP 2000 is used to indicate what program the technician wants to use and to select appropriate parameters for the patient. An on-going report on the progress of the examination is displayed during the examination.*

panel indicating which test spots are being tested at a particular point in time (such as in the Peritest) or by a video screen that can indicate which test spots have been tested already, which have been missed, and whether the patient has had lapses of fixation (such as in the Dicon AP 2000, Fig. 3–2). In addition, buzzers are used to indicate fixation losses and the end of the test. Of these methods, the video screen is the most flexible. It allows the greatest amount of information to be presented and, as new software is developed, it allows for the display of additional information.

Type of Printed Output

At the completion of a test, a report is produced detailing the results obtained. The report needs to indicate what strategy and what test settings were used in addition to the results of the examination itself. Some machines print the report by making marks on preprinted forms. Most machines of more recent vintage print the data on blank letter-sized paper with a dot matrix printer. This enables the greatest amount of flexibility with respect to future software development and enables the generation of grey scales and special graphs.

Provisions for Storage of Data

The ability to store data enables the use of delta programs comparing the field examination to normal controls and previous studies of the same eye. Storage is either on a floppy disk or a hard disk. If the machine has an RS-232 port and is capable of transmitting the test data to an auxiliary computer, the field data could also be stored at the site of the auxiliary computer. Not all field testing machines have storage capabilities. If sophisticated analysis of the field is desired, however, it is necessary to perform all studies on a machine with storage capabilities.

Provisions for Changing Software

The software, or the instructions given to the hardware by the machine, controls the entire testing process. If new tests are added, new software must be added. Likewise, if new analysis methods are introduced, the software must be changed. If older testing strategies are improved or "bugs" are to be eliminated, the software also must be changed.

Changing the software is accomplished in different ways in different machines. Some machines maintain their software on floppy disks. When that

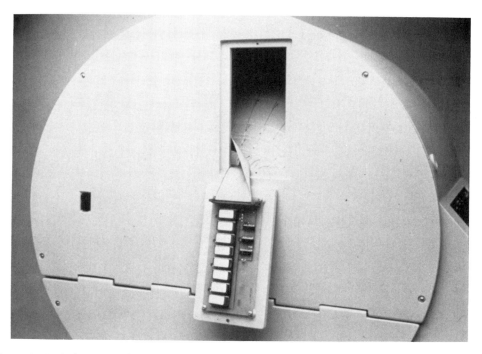

Figure 3–3. *Software in the Dicon AP 2000 is updated by replacing memory chips in the back of the machine.*

is the case, replacing the floppy disks with new ones will effect the change. Other machines maintain their software in the more permanent form of plug in memory chips. When that is the case, replacing the memory chips will change the software (Fig. 3–3). This is slightly more complicated than using a new floppy disk, but is easily accomplished. All other machines require factory modifications to be made each time the software is changed. Although these modifications can sometimes be performed by a repair technician, this is the most inconvenient and least flexible method of software modification.

4

Measurement of Visual Sensitivity to Light

Visual sensitivity to light is determined by the minimum amount of light energy necessary to elicit a detection response. The lower the minimum light intensity required for detection, the higher the sensitivity of the visual system. The intensity at which light is just barely detected is called a threshold. There is an inverse relationship between threshold light intensity and sensitivity. This relationship is expressed as

$$S = 1/t \qquad\qquad (4-1)$$

where S and t are sensitivity and threshold, respectively. Simply, the more light necessary to detect a spot, the less sensitive is the eye.

Threshold Determination

The concept of threshold is based upon the fact that the human visual system (like all biological detectors) gradually (not discretely) increases the probability of detecting a spot of light as the intensity of the light is increased. The expected shape of this psychometric function is illustrated in Figure 4–1.

As shown in Figure 4–1 a light increment threshold is defined as the luminance at which a target light can be identified above the background luminance on 50 percent of the trials. The determination of a 50 percent threshold requires many trials and random presentations of test lights at various luminances. Once the function is determined, the luminance corresponding to a 0.50 probability of a detection response is identified (Fig. 4–1). This luminance is called the threshold. Due to the characteristic gradual slope of the psycho-

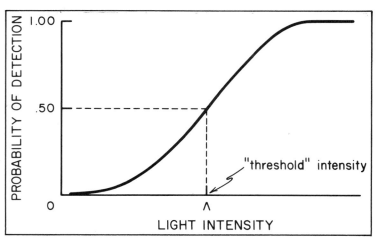

Figure 4–1. *A typical psychometric function can be obtained by plotting the probability that an increment of a test light is detected as a function of test light intensity. The higher the test light intensity the greater the probability that it will be detected. The psychometric function typically is characterized by a gradual rise from not seeing to seeing with some determined probability. Threshold is arbitrarily defined as the intensity that corresponds to a given probability of detection, usually 50 percent.*

metric function a visual threshold is not easy or simple to capture, and is associated with a number of assumptions and measurement error.

Obviously, the psychophysical function method of determining threshold is too time consuming to be useful in a clinical situation where thresholds are determined at about 100 locations in a 15-minute session. For a more practical (but less accurate) determination of threshold, various alternative strategies can be used.

Several different classes of strategies have been developed to determine thresholds appropriate for clinical practice. These strategies all involve a "tracking" logic where the luminance of the test light is adjusted according to the patient's previous response. Following is a very brief description of three commonly used general strategies for threshold determination. Specific details of these strategies depend on the particular machine, and some machines use combinations of all three strategies.

It must be kept in mind that in general the more trials that are used to determine a threshold the more reliable the value. There is a trade-off between accuracy and effort in threshold determination. Brief strategies such as those employed in fast bracketing and screening procedures yield only rough estimates of threshold values and should not be relied on for quantitative information regarding a visual field.

QUANTITATIVE THRESHOLD STRATEGIES

Quantitative strategies yield the most reliable threshold values. Threshold is approached by presenting a test spot in decreasing intensity steps (commonly 4 dB) until the spot is not seen. The light intensity is then increased on each trial until the spot is seen again. This process is repeated several times using smaller intensity steps (commonly 2 dB). The actual value listed on the patient report is determined from the final luminance at which the perception changes from seeing to not seeing. Clever strategies can be employed to quickly approach the threshold value by using information from a corresponding point on a previous examination, or by incorporating threshold information from nearby points on the same examination, or both.

A quantitative strategy is best applied in cases where early loss is suspected because it is the most sensitive method. Many practitioners prefer this type of strategy for all examinations due to the quality of information. A fundamental advantage to the quantitative strategies is that test–retest procedures during an examination can yield an estimate of the measurement error. (This estimate is commonly reported as a root mean square, RMS, and is discussed in detail later.)

Interpretation of a Quantitative Visual Threshold

It must be kept in mind that any measured threshold is associated with some measurement error (sometimes called short-term error), and therefore provides only an *estimate* of the "true" threshold at a particular retinal location. This statistical nature of a threshold can be represented by the following

$$P_{ijk} \text{ is estimated by } X_{ijk} \pm E_{ijk} \qquad (4-2)$$

where X represents the measured threshold value, P represents the real (actual) physiologic threshold, and E is the error due to the measurement procedure. The subscripts refer to the specific field location (i), the specific examination (j), and the specific patient (k). The real physiologic threshold, P_{ijk}, is what we want to know. However, P_{ijk} must be estimated from the observed threshold X_{ijk} and the error E_{ijk}. Given a normal distribution of thresholds it can be assumed that the true (actual) physiologic threshold P_{ijk} is contained in the interval between the observed threshold ± the measurement error. Specifically,

$$P_{ijk} \text{ is expected to fall between } X_{ijk} \pm 2E_{ijk}$$
$$\text{with a probability equal to 0.95.} \qquad (4-3)$$

For example, given an observed threshold of 20 dB with a standard deviation (RMS) of 3 dB (according to properties of a normal distribution), it can be assumed that the actual threshold P_{ijk} will fall between 20 dB ± 2(3) dB with a probability of 0.95. That is, the actual threshold P_{ijk} will be somewhere between 14 and 26 dB 95 percent of the time. Unfortunately the range between 14 and 26 dB is very large, i.e., greater than 1 log unit. This example demonstrates that an estimate of the error provides a critical tool for interpretation of thresholds. Further, single threshold values are generally not reliable sources of clinical information due to the measurement error. It will be demonstrated later that combining thresholds over some field area generally provides a more reliable report of the true physiologic condition over a more extended area.

FAST BRACKETING THRESHOLD STRATEGIES

Bracketing strategies fall somewhere in between the rigorous quantitative strategies for threshold determination described above and the rapid qualitative categorization of visual defects described below. Generally, the up–down procedure of test light presentations employs coarser steps than the more rigorous quantitative thresholds, and bracketed thresholds are estimated from fewer trials. Some instruments employ mixed strategies where "normal" values are bracketed and the more rigorous methods are employed only for "disturbed" points. The advantage to the fast bracketing strategies is a slightly shorter testing time, however, it is at the expense of somewhat less reliable threshold values. Unfortunately, due to the rapid bracketing procedure and coarse intensity steps, the measurement error is increased.

QUALITATIVE THRESHOLD STRATEGIES

Qualitative strategies, sometimes referred to as "screening strategies," employ time saving modifications that categorize visual sensitivity as "normal," "relative," or "absolute." Determinations are often estimated only when the first set of descending trials indicates that the threshold is out of the "normal range." All other thresholds are assumed to be equal to the expected value. If a threshold is determined to be "disturbed," then an up–down procedure is employed to categorize the defect as either absolute or relative. Although this method is definitely faster than the previous quantitative strategies, there is a greater risk of missing early field changes due to the rapid measurement strategy and the qualitative report. No measurement error is determined, and the results are provided in three symbols corresponding to normal range, relative defect range, and absolute scotoma.

Suprathreshold Strategies

Suprathreshold strategies present all test spots at one predetermined intensity. Strictly speaking, no threshold is determined. The information provided to the clinician is simply whether a given test light was or was not seen at the level of test light intensity. Only one light intensity is tested on one examination, however, the intensity of all the test lights can be changed on successive examinations. A pure suprathreshold examination is the static equivalent of a kinetic examination on a Goldmann-type perimeter in which only one isopter is plotted. Variations on suprathreshold strategies are available.

STEPPED SUPRATHRESHOLD STRATEGIES

Interpretation of suprathreshold field reports often requires that the field be measured at more than one level of intensity. As the intensity of the lights is decreased, regions of loss in sensitivity tend to become more obvious. If a defect is shallower than the intensity chosen, it will be missed. Likewise, if too weak an intensity is chosen, the field will look constricted. A suprathreshold examination can identify the presence of a defect, but provides little information as to the extent of the defect and no information as to its depth. This is partially corrected for in stepped suprathreshold strategies, which are the equivalent of doing multiple suprathreshold examination at successively higher test spot intensities.

To perform a semiautomated stepped suprathreshold examination, the operator needs to first determine a starting intensity and perform the field examination at that intensity. For the second examination the test spot intensity is increased (usually by $\frac{1}{2}$ log unit). For the third examination the test spot intensity is increased again (usually by an additional $\frac{1}{2}$ log unit). All missed spots are rechecked prior to moving on to the next intensity level. This stepped threshold strategy can be done on any machine that employs a suprathreshold strategy. Unfortunately, a separate test report is provided for each intensity and interpretation by comparison of the reports can be inconvenient. The Dicon two-zone program performs the stepped threshold examinations in a totally automated fashion. First, the initial intensity level is set by a four-dot identification procedure at approximately 15 degrees of eccentricity for the central field (0 to 25 degrees). A second initial intensity value is similarly determined for the periphery. The stepped threshold strategy is then applied separately for central and peripheral fields.

THRESHOLD-RELATED SUPRATHRESHOLD STRATEGIES

A threshold-related examination is performed in the same way as a suprathreshold examination is performed except that instead of each location being tested with the same intensity, the intensity used is varied depending on the distance of the location from fixation according to an estimate of the sensitivity fall-off with eccentricity (Fig. 1–10). There is an attempt to use the expected sensitivity fall-off with retinal eccentricity so that test lights increase in intensity with eccentricity to compensate for the expected fall-off in peripheral sensitivity. The Perimat 206, the Rodenstock Peritest, and the Tubingen automatic perimeter offer this type of threshold-related suprathreshold strategy.

Stepped Threshold-Related Suprathreshold Strategies
The most sophisticated version of this type strategy is the Dicon Hill of Vision program. A starting point is determined for each distance from fixation based on a determined threshold. A threshold-related examination is then performed to determine the initial testing level at each location. All missed spots are retested. The testing intensity of each spot is then increased by $\frac{1}{2}$ log unit and missed spots are tested again, spots still missed are retested. The testing intensity of each spot is increased by an additional $\frac{1}{2}$ log unit, missed spots are tested and if necessary, retested. The final printout shows the various intensities used and the responses at each test spot location.

Interpretation of Suprathreshold Fields

Suprathreshold strategies present one intensity at a given location. If the patient responds that he or she could see a spot that was actually not seen, it will not be rechecked and will be recorded as seen. If the patient responds that he or she did not see a test spot, most machines have an automatic or manual provision for rechecking the spot. Therefore false-positive responses are not rechecked whereas false-negative responses may be corrected during the retesting phase.

Keltner, Johnson, and Balistrery[1] have proposed standards for interpreting Fieldmaster suprathreshold fields. Similar criteria can be applied for stepped threshold and stepped threshold-related strategies employed by other manufacturers. Isolated missed test spots or test spots missed at one luminance level only are considered to be nondefects. Two or more adjacent missed spots, spots missed at different luminance levels, and marked contraction of a major portion of the visual field are considered to represent defects.

We have developed the following criteria for the analysis of defects obtained by the CooperVision Dicon two-zone strategy.

1. A single spot missed at the lowest intensity probably does not represent a scotoma.
2. Two adjacent spots missed at the lowest intensity represent a possible defect.
3. Three adjacent spots missed at two intensities represent a probable defect.
4. A single spot missed at two intensities represents a probable defect.
5. Two adjacent spots each missed at two intensities represent a highly probable defect.
6. A single spot missed at three intensities represents a highly probable defect.
7. Multiple spots missed in the periphery constitute a definite depression in that area.

Location of Test Spot

The particular distribution of test spots provides a probe for the determination of specific visual field loss. Properly chosen test locations can demonstrate field loss that could otherwise be confusing or missed. Optimal locations are dependent upon both the retinal region and the suspected eye disease. To examine the central 5 degrees, several spots should be tested in each central quadrant. In most machines it is mechanically impossible to test the very center unless the patient's fixation is altered, but the center can usually be approached within 2 degrees. (The Tubingen automatic perimeter routinely tests the very center of the field.)

A usual "central field examination" includes both the central 5 degrees and the arcuate areas. Because the arcuate area (the area between 5 and 25 degrees) is of particular interest in glaucoma, there should be an even and relatively dense distribution of test spots in this area. Likewise, the area near the blind spot should be carefully studied as should either side of the nasal horizontal meridian looking for a nasal step.

Test spot locations in the periphery do not need to be as closely spaced as test spots in the arcuate area. However, there should be a relatively dense distribution on either side of the vertical meridian (to look for a Chamlin step) and on either side of the horizontal meridian (to look for vascular and nerve fiber layer defects).

Some manufacturers have developed software with test spot locations designed to optimize the ability of the field machine to probe certain types of defects. For example neurologic field defects can be demonstrated by careful analysis of either side of the horizontal and vertical meridians. Octopus 70 series programs and the Dicon neurologic program selectively study these areas. The central macula area can be selectively studied by the Dicon macula threshold or macula tests, the Fieldmaster macula test, or Octopus program 61 which is a 15- by 15-degree field test that can be located at any desired field location. Glaucoma field tests generally concentrate on the central, arcuate, and nasal peripheral areas. Test spot location distributions are also available to study the blind spot area, the right side of the field, the left side of the field, the entire field with a minimal number of spots, or various concentric rings in the periphery.

Some instruments (such as Octopus and Humphrey) distribute spots according to a Cartesian coordinate system. Most other machines distribute test spots in a radial coordinate system. Whether there is a significant advantage to either system has yet to be determined.

It is important for the physician to know exactly where each test spot is located as test reports may display spots in a misleading pattern so as to condense the information onto one sheet of paper. It is also important to know whether there was a disadvantageous distribution of test locations. For example, if the physician suspects that a pituitary tumor might be causing a subtle superior bitemporal field defect, the defect might be missed if spots are presented directly on the 90-degree meridian rather than on either side of that meridian.

References

1. Keltner JL, Johnson CA, Balistrery FG: Suprathreshold static perimetry. Initial clinical trials with the Fieldmaster Automated Perimeter. Arch Opthalmol 97:260–272, 1979.

5
Automated Visual Field Testing Devices

There are dozens of available automated visual field testing devices. This chapter describes the key features of most of the devices available in the spring of 1986.

As with any state-of-the-art equipment, new machines are being developed monthly, older machines are upgraded, and some are discontinued. Therefore, it is impossible for a chapter such as this to be totally up-to-date. We have included it for the following reasons:

1. Many of the available machines have reached a point in their development that will establish them as standards. Thousands have been produced and are in daily use. New improvements will be introduced that will enhance their effectiveness but they will not be replaced.
2. Even when a device is discontinued, practitioners who have purchased the device will continue to use it. When fields obtained by that device are read, it is necessary to understand something about the machine to understand its visual field reports.
3. New machines will be developed and most will be based on the equipment described in this chapter. The advantages of these yet-to-be-developed machines will only be appreciated in the context of their predecessors.

The Automated Tangent Screens

Models: ATS-1 (Fig. 5–1A)
ATS-1A
ATS-2000 (Fig. 5–1B)
Manufacturer: The Computation Company
7748 Opportunity Road
San Diego, CA 92111
Screen Type and Size: 36- by 36-inch Tangent Screen (ATS-1 and 1A) 45- by 45-inch slightly concave Tangent Screen (ATS-2000)
Test Spots:
Type: LEDs
Size: 2 mm diameter (ATS-1 and ATS-1A); 1 mm diameter (ATS-2000)
Number Available: 114 (ATS-1 and ATS-1A); 172 (ATS-2000)
Locations: ATS-1 and ATS-1A: All spots are in an area 25 degrees from fixation horizontally and 15 degrees from fixation vertically. The ATS-1A allows fixation to be shifted so that the area tested can be expanded to 50 degrees by 30 degrees. ATS-2000: Spots are distributed in the central 30-degree field of the tangent screen; eccentric fixation is required for examination of peripheral field (approximately 60 degrees)
Color: Yellow
Intensity Range: ATS-1 and ATS-1A: 100 to 3000 asb in 252 steps; ATS-2000: 0 to 10,000 asb
Duration: Variable from 0.1 to 9.9 seconds (1.0 second is standard)
Interval: Programmable from 0.1 to 9.9 seconds. Standards are: ATS-1 = 0.5 seconds; ATS-1A = 0.3 seconds plus random amount (average is 0.5 seconds); ATS-2000 = 0.5 seconds
Fixation Monitor: By software (Heijl-Krakau method; spots tested during periods of presumed fixation loss are retested)
Background Illumination Level: Measured by photo cell but determined by room illumination with ATS-1 and ATS-1A; automatically provided (0 to 40 asb) with ATS-2000
Control of Background Illumination Level: Background illumination can be measured but not controlled with the ATS-1 and ATS-1A. A metering system is included so that the examiner can set the room illumination. There is automatic control with the ATS-2000
Testing Strategies Available: Suprathreshold (patient's "threshold" is manually determined); threshold related (Models ATS-1A and ATS-2000 only)
Test Spot Patterns Available: Central field (several densities are available); peripheral field (requires eccentric fixation and is not available on Model ATS-1); macula test, vision training test, blind spot only test, and neurologic test (not on Model ATS-1). Up to 20 custom tests can be user provided for the ATS-2000

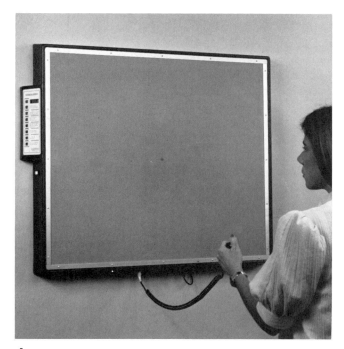

A

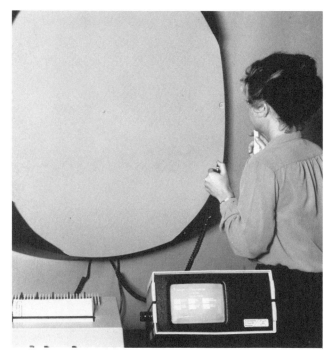

B

Figure 5–1A. ATS-1. *B.* ATS-2000.

Provisions for Delta Program Analysis: None

Technician Communication with Machine: ATS-1 and ATS-1A: Push button control panel; ATS-2000: Touch sensitive remote CRT display screen.

Machine Communication with Technician: ATS-1 and ATS-1A: During the test, there is a count down of the points remaining to be tested. At the end of the test, missed spots are displayed in the corner of the tangent screen. The ATS-2000 has a remote control console that monitors the progress of the test.

Type of Printed Output: ATS-1 and ATS-1A: Missed test spots are manually recorded by the technician on a preprinted form using a tracing method. The ATS-2000 prints out the results.

Provisions for Internal Data Storage and Retrieval: None

Provisions for Communication with External Computers: The ATS-2000 has an RS-232 port. Additional transmission software would be necessary.

Method of Changing Software: Models ATS-1 and ATS-1A provide for factory modifications only. Model ATS-2000 does allow for the entry of up to 20 user definable test patterns.

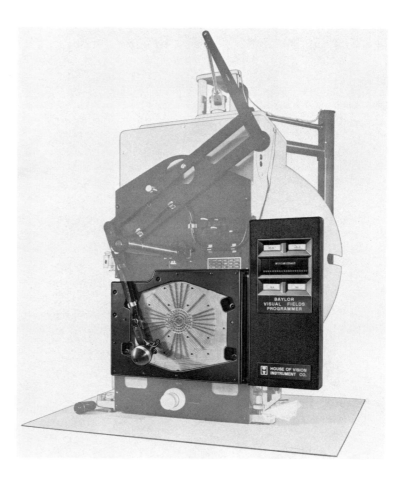

Figure 5–2. Baylor Visual Field Programmer.

Special Comments: A manual examination wand is included so that areas of the field can be examined manually. Results of the manual examination are not recorded by the machine

The Baylor Visual Field Programmer

Model: Baylor Visual Field Programmer (Fig. 5–2)
Manufacturer: WCO/HVO, Inc.
      925 26th Avenue East
      Bradenton, FL 33508
Screen Type and Size: Attachment for a Goldmann-type perimeter (33 cm bowl)
Test Spots:
  Type: Projected light
  Sizes: Standard Goldmann sizes
  Number Available: 69
  Locations: 69 in central 25 degrees; periphery is tested by manual kinetic techniques
  Colors: Standard Goldmann color filters
  Intensity Range: Limited only by the particular Goldmann-type perimeter used
  Duration: 1 second
  Interval: Manual control
Fixation Monitor: (optional) Light reflected off of cornea is measured and the operator is signaled if fixation is lost
Background Illumination Level: Determined by Goldmann-type perimeter used. Standard setting is 31.5 asb
  Control of Background Illumination Level: No provision
Testing Strategies Available: Suprathreshold
Test Spot Patterns Available: Basic screening, glaucoma, neurologic
Provisions for Delta Program Analysis: None
Technician Communication with Machine: Control panel and standard Goldmann-type perimeter controls
Machine Communication with Technician: The technician is led through the testing pattern chosen through an LED display. Spots are presented by the technician, however, and not the machine
Type of Printed Output: Visual display of results. Test report must be marked manually
Provisions for Internal Data Storage and Retrieval: None
Provisions for Communication with External Computers: An outlet port without software is provided
Method of Changing Software: None
Special Comments: This device attaches to a Goldmann-type perimeter and gives instructions to the operator. Therefore, test spot locations are controlled and standardized. The examination is performed by the operator, however, and not the machine.

The CooperVision/Dicon Autoperimeters

Models: Dicon AP 2000 (Fig. 5–3A)
Dicon AP 3000 (Fig. 5–3B)
Dicon AP 2500
Dicon AP 200 (Fig. 5–3C)

Manufacturer: CooperVision Diagnostic Imaging
7356 Trade Street
San Diego, CA 92121

Screen Type and Size: 33-cm bowl

Test Spots: Presented randomly

Type: LED (wavelength = 570 nm)

Size: 1.6 mm^2 (slightly larger than Goldmann size 2)

Number Available: 520 (AP 3000 and AP 2500), 372 (AP 2000), 196 (AP 200)

Locations: LEDs are distributed throughout the bowl, however, they are especially concentrated in the arcuate areas, on either side of the horizontal and vertical meridians, and adjacent to the blind spots.

Colors: Only 570 nm (pale green)

Intensity Range: 0 to 10,000 asb

Duration: 0 to 2 seconds (standard is 0.4 seconds)

Interval: 0 to 10 seconds (standard is 1 second)

Fixation Monitor: All models monitor fixation with the Heijl-Krakau software technique. All spots tested during periods of questionable fixation are retested. There is a periscope for patient alignment and operator fixation control. The AP 3000 has a video monitor for alignment and operator fixation control

Background Illumination Level: 0 to 45 asb (31.5 asb is standard)

Control of Background Illumination Level: Automatic

Testing Strategies Available: AP 2000, AP 2500, and AP 3000: Threshold, suprathreshold, threshold-related, stepped suprathreshold, stepped threshold-related; AP 200: Suprathreshold, stepped suprathreshold

Test Spot Patterns Available: Full field (with varying density), central, peripheral, neurologic, two-zone, custom diagnostic (any combination of areas selected by the examiner), right or left sided, macula, blind spot, glaucoma, meridional, circular, ZETA (programmable field pattern, AP 2500 and AP 3000 only), Esterman binocular disability pattern (AP 2000, AP 2500, and AP 3000)

Provisions for Delta Program Analysis: AP 2000, AP 2500, and AP 3000: Comparison with previous fields on that patient or comparison with user defined "normals."

Technician Communication with Machine: Light pen with CRT screen

Machine Communication with Technician: Menu options, progress of test, results of tests, and utility programs are displayed on CRT screen

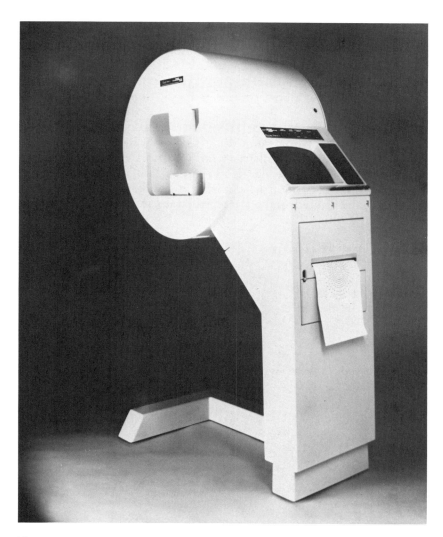

Figure 5–3A. *Dicon AP 2000.*

Type of Printed Output: AP 2000, AP 2500, and AP 3000: Dot matrix printer hard copy including graphics, grey scale, numeric and symbolic printouts; AP 200: Dot matrix thermal

Provisions for Internal Data Storage and Retrieval: Floppy disk drive in AP 2000, AP 2500, and AP 3000

Provisions for Communication with External Computers: RS-232 port with communications software for communication with IBM PC (AP 2000, AP 2500, and AP 3000)

Method of Changing Software: Replacement of chip in memory modules. Some software change can be accomplished with floppy disks in AP 2000, AP 2500, and AP 3000

Special Comments: All models are "user friendly" and contain special operator assistance ("help") program. Model AP 3000 includes automatically set clock. Software programs are often introduced on the AP 3000, later modified for the AP 2000 and finally adapted to the AP 200, if possible. Most of the features available on the AP 3000 are available at less cost on the AP 2500. CooperVision should be consulted on software program availability for a specific model at the present time

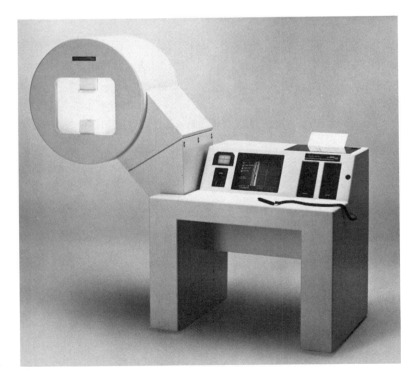

Figure 5–3B. *Dicon AP 3000.*

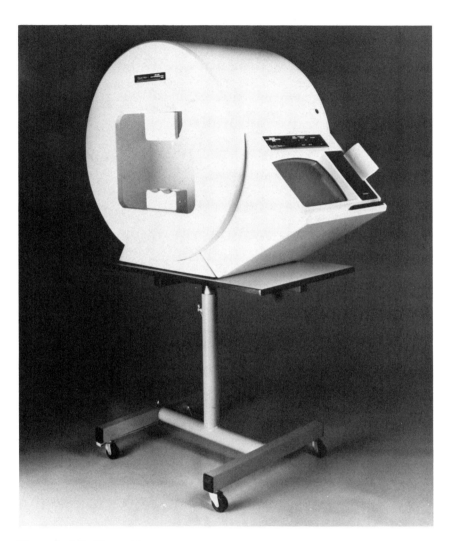

Figure 5–3C. Dicon AP 200.

The Digilab "Krakau" Perimeter

Model: Digilab Model 350 "Krakau Perimeter" (Fig. 5–4)
Manufacturer: Digilab Ophthalmics
Division of Biorad Laboratories, Inc.
237 Putnam Avenue
Cambridge, MA 02139
Screen Type and Size: Flat 35-degree tangent screen testing surface
Test Spots: Presented pseudorandomly
   Type: LED (rear projection)
   Size: 2 mm
   Number Available: 162
   Locations: 152 are in central 30 degrees. 10 are between 30 and 35 degrees. Field can be extended to 70 degrees by shifting fixation
   Color: Green
   Intensity Range: 0.3 to 1000 asb
   Duration: 0.25 to 1.0 seconds
   Interval: Not specified
Fixation Monitor: Heijl-Krakau software technique with number of fixation losses noted at the end of the test
Background Illumination Level: 0.315, 3.15, or 31.5 asb (standard is 3.15 asb)
   Control of Background Illumination Level: Automatic
Testing Strategies Available: Threshold and threshold-related
Test Spot Patterns Available: Central (20 or 35 degrees), peripheral (requires shifting of fixation and several tests), macula, blind spot, quadrants (eight available)
Provisions for Delta Program Analysis: None
Technician Communication with Machine: Keyboard
Machine Communication with Technician: None
Type of Printed Output: Printed numeric display of results
Provisions for Internal Data Storage and Retrieval: No
Provisions for Communication with External Computers: RS-232 port available
Method of Changing Software: Chip replacement
Special Comments: Based on original Heijl-Krakau design

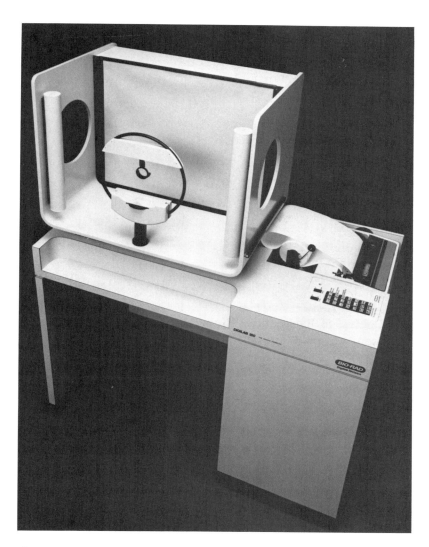

Figure 5–4. Digilab Model 350 ''Krakau Perimeter.''

The Digilab Bowl Type Machines

Models: Digilab Model 750 "Competer" (Fig. 5–5)
     Cambridge Perimeter
Manufacturer: Digilab Ophthalmics
     Division of Bio-Rad Laboratories, Inc.
     237 Putnam Avenue
     Cambridge, MA 02139
Screen Type and Size: 33 cm hemispherical bowl
Test Spots: Presented randomly
    Type: LED (rear projection)
    Size: 2.0 mm
    Number Available: 256
    Locations: Distributed throughout the bowl with 17 in each blind spot area
    Color: Green
    Intensity Range: 0.03 to 1000 asb
    Duration: 0.25 to 1 second
    Interval: Random
Fixation Monitor: Heijl-Krakau software technique with number of fixation losses noted during and at the end of test
Background Illumination Level: 3.15 or 31.5 asb (3.15 is standard)
    Control of Background Illumination Level: Automatic
Testing Strategies Available: Suprathreshold, threshold-related, threshold
Test Spot Patterns Available: Central 30 degrees, peripheral, full field, macula, blind spot, quadrant (eight available). Custom patterns are available on the Model 750
Provisions for Delta Program Analysis: Model 750 only
Technician Communication with Machine: Keyboard operation
Machine Communication with Technician: Cambridge perimeter: LCD display; Model 750: Via IBM PC display screen
Type of Printed Output: Dot matrix printer (grey scale and numeric)
Provisions for Internal Data Storage and Retrieval: Model 750: floppy disk is provided with IBM PC and hard disk storage is available; Cambridge perimeter: None
Provisions for Communication with External Computers: Model 750: Via IBM PC included; Cambridge perimeter: RS-232 port available
Method of Changing Software: Model 750: Floppy disk; Cambridge perimeter: Chip replacement
Special Comments: The Model 750 is controlled by an IBM PC, therefore the power of the microcomputer is potentially available for visual field analysis

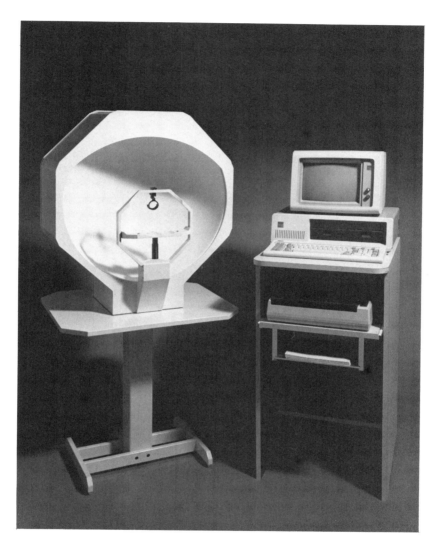

Figure 5–5. Digilab Model 750 ''Competer.''

The Fieldmaster Fiberoptic Perimeters

Model: Fieldmaster Model 101 PR (Fig. 5–6A)
　　　Fieldmaster Model 200 (Fig. 5–6B)
　　　Fieldmaster Model 225 (Fig. 5–6C) (no longer available)
Manufacturer: Bausch and Lomb Ophthalmic Instruments, Inc.
　　　1234 Ninth Street
　　　Berkeley, CA 94710
Screen Type and Size: 30 cm radius bowl
Test Spots: Pseudorandomized
　Type: Fiberoptic light bundles
　Size: 1 mm
　Number Available: 99 (Model 101 PR), 133 (Model 200), 149 (Model 225)
　Locations: Distributed in a radial coordinate system. Model 101 PR has spots directly on the horizontal and vertical meridian. Models 200 and 225 have an enhanced spot distribution with spots on either side of the horizontal and vertical meridians and a higher concentration of spots in the arcuate areas
　Colors: White, red, yellow, green, and blue
　Intensity Range: 40 to 10,000 asb; Model 225 extends to 100,000 asb
　Duration: 0.2 to 3.6 seconds; Model 225 extends to 9.9 seconds
　Interval: Variable from 0.3 to 3.7
Fixation Monitor: Synemed Mosaic Monitor
Background Illumination Level: 0 to 45 asb
　Control of Background Illumination Level: Automatically controlled in Model 225, measured in Models 101 PR and 200
Testing Strategies Available: Suprathreshold, threshold (Model 225 only)
Test Spot Patterns Available: All models: Full field, central, peripheral, blind spot, glaucoma screen; Models 200 and 225 only: Hemifields, macula, centrocecal, neurologic; Model 225 only: Meridian profile cuts, user definable
Provisions for Delta Program Analysis: None
Technician Communication with Machine: Panel of switches
Machine Communication with Technician: Test settings and spot being tested are displayed
Type of Printed Output: Models 101 PR and 200: Thermal printer marking preprinted form; Model 225: Thermal dot matrix printer
Provisions for Internal Data Storage and Retrieval: None
Provisions for Communication with External Computers: None
Method of Changing Software: Factory; Model 225 has computer memory space for 81 user definable programs

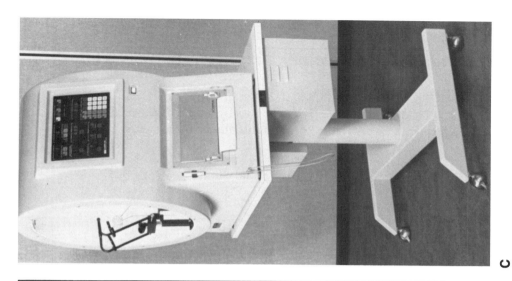

C

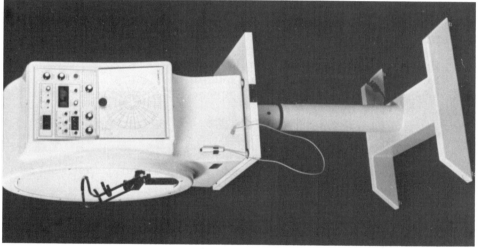

B

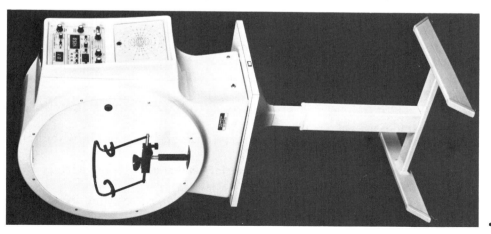

A

Figure 5–6A. Fieldmaster 101 PR. *B.* Fieldmaster 200. *C.* Fieldmaster 225.

The Bausch and Lomb/Fieldmaster Projection Perimeters

Models: Bausch and Lomb S/K 275 (Fig. 5–7A)

Fieldmaster Squid 300 (Fig. 5–7B) (no longer available)

Manufacturer: Bausch and Lomb Ophthalmic Instruments, Inc.

1234 Ninth Street

Berkeley, CA 94710

Screen Type and Size: 50 cm bowl (Squid 300)

30 cm bowl (S/K 275)

Test Spots: Pseudorandomized

Type: Projection

Sizes: 0.47 mm to 15.5 mm (Squid 300)

Goldmann sizes I to V (S/K 275)

Number Available: Limited only by software

Locations: Limited only by software

Colors: White, red, yellow, green, blue

Intensity Range: 1 to 10,000 asb (Squid 300)

0.1 to 2000 asb (S/K 275)

Duration: User controllable (no standard)

Interval: User controllable (no standard)

Fixation Monitor: TV monitor for alignment and positioning of patient, Video Mosaic Monitor (Model 275)

Background Illumination Level: Model 275: 4 to 50 asb; Model 300: 5 to 300 asb

Control of Background Illumination Level: Automatic

Testing Strategies Available: Threshold, suprathreshold, stepped suprathreshold. Has kinetic testing capability for periphery

Test Spot Patterns Available: Full field, central, peripheral, hemifield, macula, blind spot, glaucoma, centrocecal, neurologic

Provisions for Delta Program Analysis: Model 275: Comparison with normal previous field (up to 3) and previous fields performed on other instruments (projected capability). Model 300: Comparison to age-related thresholds and previous examinations

Technician Communication with Machine: Model 300: Keyboard and joy stick; Model 275: CRT screen with light pen

Machine Communication with Technician: CRT screen display of menu options, test progress, and test results

Type of Printed Output: Dot matrix printer with numeric table, grey scale, and special graphics

Provisions for Internal Data Storage and Retrieval: Model 275: $3\frac{1}{2}$ shutter protected diskette; Model 300: Hard disk

Provisions for Communication with External Computers: RS-232 port. Model 300 gives complete access to source code

Method of Changing Software: Model 275: $3\frac{1}{2}$ shutter protected diskette; Model 300: Floppy disk

Special Comments: Model 275 has internal clock/calender; Model 300 is no longer available

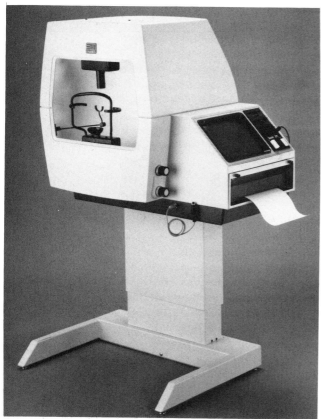

A

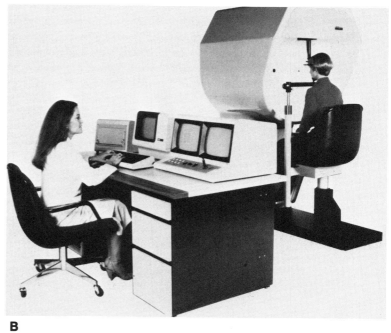

Figure 5–7A. *Fieldmaster Squid 275.* **B.** *Fieldmaster Squid 300.*

B

The Fieldmaster "LED" Perimeter

Model: Fieldmaster Model 50 R (Fig. 5–8)
Manufacturer: Bausch and Lomb Ophthalmic Instruments, Inc.
    1234 Ninth Street
    Berkeley, CA 94710
Screen Type and Size: 30 cm bowl
Test Spots: Presented pseudorandomized
  Type: LED
  Sizes: 1.5 mm
  Number Available: 360
  Locations: Meridional distribution
  Colors: 570 nm (pale green)
  Intensity Range: 1 to 10,000 asb
  Duration: 0.6 to 9.9 seconds
  Interval: User adjustable (0.8 seconds is standard)
Fixation Monitor: TV monitor for alignment and manual fixation control, Heigl-Krakau software method, and Video Mosaic Monitor
Background Illumination Level: 0.5 to 50 asb
  Control of Background Illumination Level: Automatic
Testing Strategies Available: Suprathreshold, threshold (optional)
Test Spot Patterns Available: Macula, vertical meridian, central, centrocecal, glaucoma, peripheral, central, full, meridian
Provisions for Delta Program Analysis: None
Technician Communication with Machine: CRT screen with light pen
Machine Communication with Technician: Menu options, progress of test, results of tests, and utility programs are displayed on CRT screen
Type of Printed Output: $8\frac{1}{2}$ by 11 inches thermal graphics impact printer
Provisions for Internal Data Storage and Retrieval: Custom tests stored in battery-powered RAM. Field test results cannot be stored
Provisions for Communications with External Computers: RS-232 port
Method of Changing Software: Factory modification only

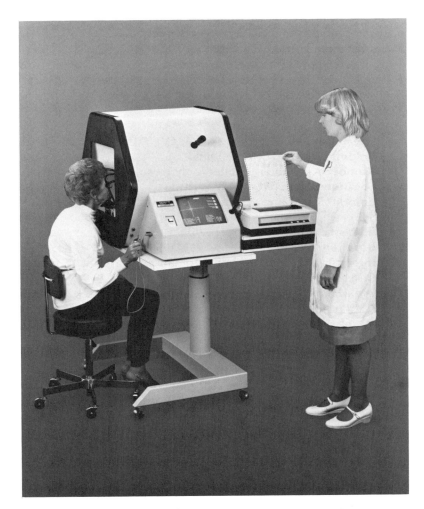

Figure 5–8. Fieldmaster Model 50 R.

The Humphrey Field Analyzers

Models: Humphrey Field Analyzer Model 605
Humphrey Field Analyzer Model 610
Humphrey Field Analyzer Model 620 (Fig. 5–9)
Humphrey Field Analyzer Model 630

Manufacturer: Humphrey Instruments
3081 Teagarden Street
San Leandro, CA 94577

Screen Type and Size: 33 cm bowl

Test Spots: Presented randomly

Type: Projection

Sizes: Goldmann sizes I, II, III, IV, V (Models 610, 620, and 630)
Goldmann size III (Model 605)

Number Available: Limited only by software

Locations: Limited only by software

Colors: Red, blue, green, white (Models 610, 620, and 630) White (Model 605)

Intensity Range: 0.08 to 10,000 asb

Duration: 0.2 seconds

Interval: Randomized but automatically varies with patient response time. Fast or slow speed can be set

Fixation Monitor: A telescope is mounted at the back of the bowl for manual observation in Models 605, 610, and 620. A video eye monitor is used instead of the telescope in Model 630. Heijl-Krakau software technique monitors fixation and lists number of fixation losses at end of test

Background Illumination Level: 31.5 asb

Control of Background Illumination Level: Automatic

Testing Strategies Available: All models: Suprathreshold, threshold-related, stepped threshold-related, combined threshold-related, and threshold. Models 610, 620, and 630 also will do a threshold examination. Models 620 and 630 also will do full threshold from prior examination data and fast thresholding

Test Spot Patterns Available: Central, peripheral, full field, glaucoma, temporal crescent, nasal step, meridian, arc, single point, neurologic, macula, and stored user definable tests

Provisions for Delta Program Analysis: Models 620 and 630 provide for comparison between fields. An optional statistical package (STATPAC) is scheduled to be available in late 1986

Technician Communication with Machine: Light pen with CRT screen

Machine Communication with Technician: CRT screen displaying progress of test, menu options, results of tests, etc.

Type of Printed Output: 80-column impact printer, plot of seen/missed targets, grey scale, numeric, profile graph, symbol notation, and difference between expected and actual results. A special 3 in 1 printout of reduced grey scale, numeric and defect depth formats on one sheet is available

Provisions for Internal Data Storage and Retrieval: Dual disc drive (Models 620 and 630)

Provisions for Communication with External Computers: RS-232 port

Method of Changing Software: Plug in modules

Special Comments: Machine is menu driven. Important steps cannot be missed inadvertently. Help screens are available for all aspects of the field testing process. Direct linkage with Humphrey office computer system is planned. Modular software design allows for upgrading all models.

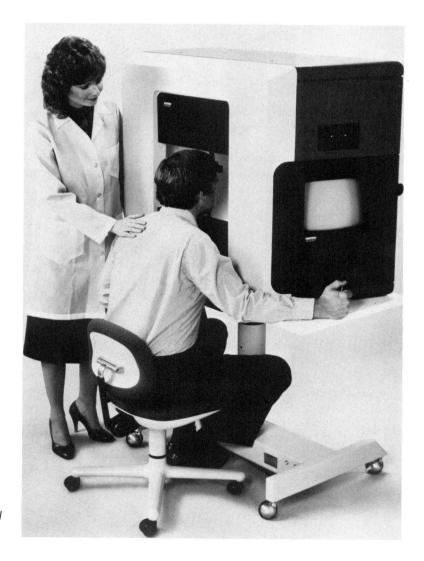

Figure 5–9. *Humphrey Visual Field Analyzer Model 620.*

The Keta Perimeter

Model: Keta Quantum 412 (Fig. 5–10)
Manufacturer: Keta Corporation
9 Canal Street
Danvers, MA 01923
Screen Type and Size: 33 cm bowl with polymer film over LEDs
Test Spots:
Type: LED (rear projection with uniform coating designed to eliminate the "black hole" phenomenon)
Size: 2.25 mm (Goldmann size III)
Number Available: 412
Locations: Radial distribution
Colors: 565 nm only (pale green)
Intensity Range: 0 to 1000 asb
Duration: 0.10 seconds (default), 0.25, 0.5 seconds
Interval: 1.0 seconds (default), 2.0, 3 seconds
Fixation Monitor: Heijl-Krakau every four to eight trials; if fixation is lost, some previous trials are retested
Background Illumination Level: 4 asb (31.5 asb available)
Control of Background Illumination Level: Buzzer indicates if intensity is greater than specified level
Testing Strategies Available: Suprathreshold, threshold, pseudokinetic
Test Spot Patterns Available: Full field, central, peripheral, meridional, macula, blind spot, and small discrete areas
Provisions for Delta Program Analysis: Planned for the future
Technician Communication with Machine: Computer keyboard
Machine Communication with Technician: CRT screen report of test progress
Type of Printed Output: Dot matrix silent ink jet graphics printer with numeric, symbolic, and grey scale modes
Provisions for Internal Data Storage and Retrieval: On floppy or hard disk
Provisions for Communication with External Computers: RS-232 port
Method of Changing Software: Disk
Special Comments: Practice program available

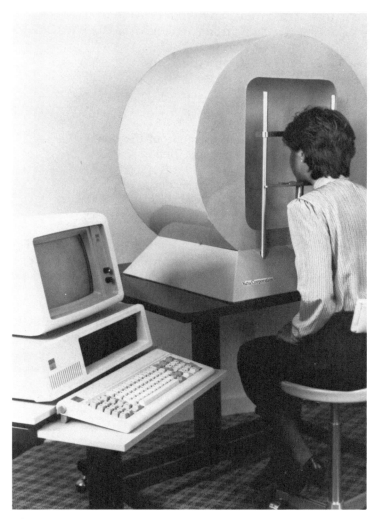

Figure 5–10. Keta Quantum 412.

The Kowa Perimeter

Model: Kowa AP-340 Automatic Perimeter SBP-1000 (Fig. 5–11)
Manufacturer: Kowa Company, Ltd.
            Electronics and Optics Division
            No. 3, 3-chrome, Nihonbashi-Honcho, Chuo-ku
            Tokyo 103, Japan
Screen Type and Size: 30 cm radius bowl
Test Spots:
     Type: LED
     Sizes: 1 mm
     Number Available: 340
     Locations: Distributed throughout the bowl
     Colors: Wavelength not specified
     Intensity Range: 13 to 3400 asb
     Duration: 0.6, 0.8, 1.0, 1.2 seconds
     Interval: 0.7, 0.9, 1.1, 1.3 seconds
Fixation Monitor: Kowa method (infrared sensor)
Background Illumination Level: 31.5 asb
     Control of Background Illumination Level: Automatic
Testing Strategies Available: Suprathreshold, meridional threshold
Test Spot Patterns Available: Full field, central 25 degrees, peripheral, macula, glaucoma, meridional, vertical meridian, diagnostic
Provisions for Delta Program Analysis: None
Technician Communication with Machine: Light pen with CRT screen
Machine Communication with Technician: Menu options, progress of test, results of test are displayed on CRT screen
Type of Printed Output: Dot matrix printer with $4\frac{3}{8}$-inch wide roll paper
Provisions for Internal Data Storage and Retrieval: None
Provisions for Communication with External Computers: None
Method of Changing Software: By factory

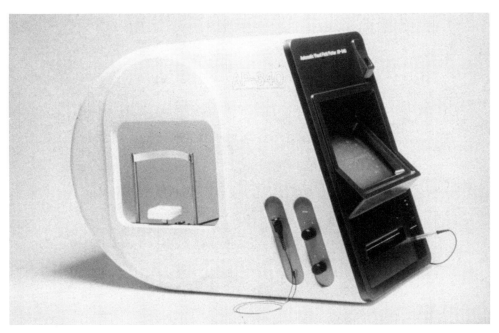

Figure 5–11. Kowa AP-340 Automatic Perimeter SBP-1000.

The Octopus Perimeters

Models: Octopus 201 (Fig. 5–12A)
Octopus 2000 R (Fig. 5–12B)
Octopus 500 E (Fig. 5–12C)
Manufacturer: Interzeag A.G.
Rietbachstrasse 5
CH-8952 Schlieren
Switzerland
Screen Type and Size: 51 cm bowl (201); 42 cm (2000 R/500 E)
Test Spots:
Type: Projected lights
Sizes: Goldmann I–V (201); Goldmann III & V (2000 R); Goldmann III (500 E)
Number Available: unlimited
Locations: unlimited
Color: White
Intensity Range: 0.008–1000 asb
Duration: 0.1 second (standard)—cannot be changed
Interval: 0 to 2 seconds (adaptive to patient response); 4 seconds (201)

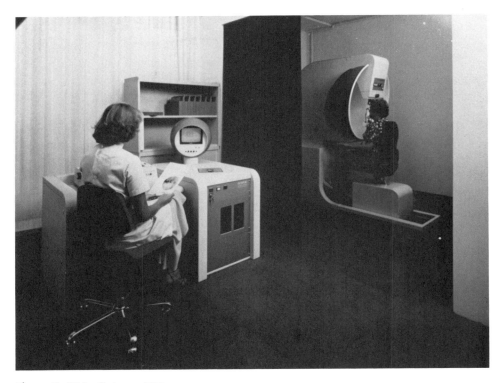

Figure 5–12A. Octopus 201.

Fixation Monitor: IR sensitive camera that disregards nonfixated point

Background Illumination Level: 4 asb

Control of Background Illumination Level: Automated

Testing Strategies Available: Two-level threshold-related test, fast threshold strategy, normal threshold strategy

Test Spot Patterns Available: Central, peripheral, full field, custom

Provisions for Delta Program Analysis: Delta/Trend over time; performed on machine (201 and 2000 R) and by transmission to an IBM PC (500 E)

Technician Communication with Machine: Keyboard (201, 2000 R); light pen (500 E)

Machine Communication with Technician: Printer (201), CRT (2000 R, 500 E)

Type of Printed Output: Dot matrix impact (201, 2000 R); thermal 500 E. Can obtain dot matrix from external PC

Provisions for Internal Data Storage and Retrieval: 201, 2000 R internal on floppy disk. External on 500 E

Provisions for Communication with External Computers: All machines transmit. External storage for 500 E on IBM PC

Method of Changing Software: Diskette (201, 2000 R). Plug in modules (500 E)

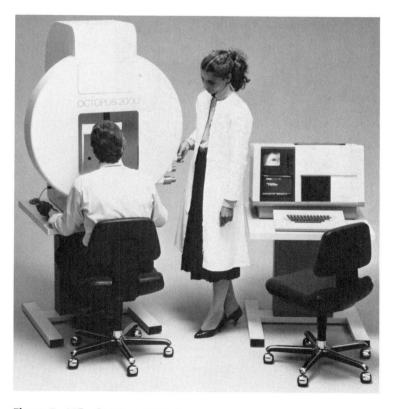

Figure 5–12B. Octopus 2000 R.

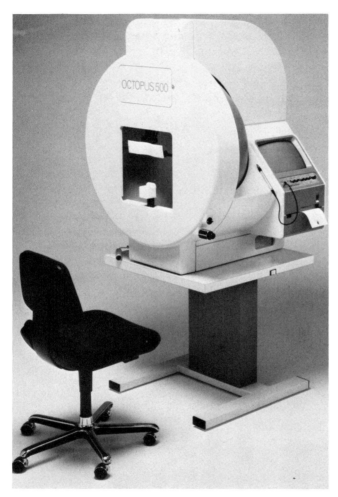

Figure 5–12C. *Octopus 500 E.*

The Ocumap Small Bowl Perimeter

Model: Ocumap
Manufacturer: SRD Ltd.
　　　　　　　D.N. Bikat Beit Kerem 20170
　　　　　　　Israel
Screen Type and Size: 100 m radius dome
Test Spots:
　　Type: Projection
　　Sizes: O–V diameters, corresponding to Goldmann stimuli
　　Number Available:
　　Locations: Test spot can be projected to any point within approximately $\frac{1}{2}$ degrees
　　Colors: White, red, green, blue
　　Intensity Range: 0 to 5000 asb, with computer-controlled increments corresponding to standard Goldmann stimuli
　　Duration: 0.1 to 1 second
　　Interval: Not specified
Fixation Monitor: Automatic fixation monitoring. Direct visual and automatic fixation monitoring with infrared light
Background Illumination Level: 0 to 30 asb controlled manually
　　Control of Background Illumination Level: Adjustable
Testing Strategies Available: Suprathreshold and threshold
Test Spot Patterns Available: Full kinetic examination; full static examination of region selected by operator; static and kinetic scotoma mapping; interactive operator-controlled static and kinetic tests
Provisions for Delta Program Analysis: None
Technician Communication with Machine: Keypad
Machine Communication with Technician: Printed output
Type of Printed Output: Isopter plot in Goldmann format, pseudogrey scale, missed/detected points, numerical
Provisions for Internal Data Storage and Retrieval: Internal memory
Provisions for Communication with External Computers: RS-232C with control software
Method of Changing Software: Plug-in modules

The Rodenstock Perimeters

>*Models:* Peritest (Fig. 5–13A)
>Perimat 206 (Fig. 5–13B)
>*Manufacturer:* G. Rodenstock Instrument Co.
>Drachenseestrasse 12
>Postfach 701560
>D-8000 Munchen 70
>West Germany
>*Screen Type and Size:* 30 cm bowl
>*Test Spots:*
>**Type:** LED
>**Sizes:** 30 ft diameter III Goldmann
>**Number Available:** 206
>**Locations:** 151 points. Within central 25 degrees points have 3 degrees intensity
>**Colors:** 560 nm (pale green)
>**Intensity Range:** 0.1 to 250 cd/m^2

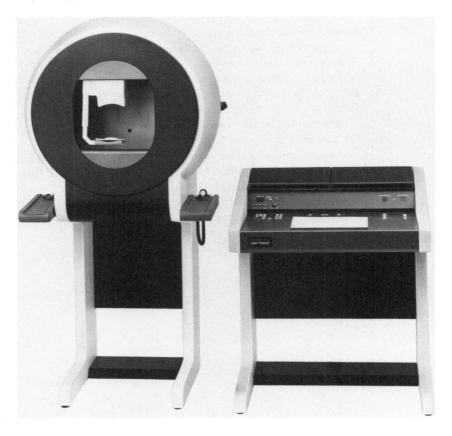

Figure 5–13A. Peritest.

Duration: 0.2 seconds
Interval: Not specified
Fixation Monitor: Direct visual observation
Background Illumination Level: 1 cd/m²
Control of Background Illumination Level: Not specified
Testing Strategies Available: Stepped threshold-related
Test Spot Patterns Available: Peripheral, central 30 degrees with single and double density, 10 degrees double density
Provisions for Delta Program Analysis: None
Technician Communication with Machine: Panel of switches
Machine Communication with Technician: LED monitor during test allows visual follow-up of examination results
Type of Printed Output: Peritest: Test data is printed on preprinted form. Perimat: Test data is generated by graphics printer
Provisions for Internal Data Storage and Retrieval: Storage capability on host computer memory
Provisions for Communication with External Computers: RS-232 port
Method of Changing Software: Factory modifications only

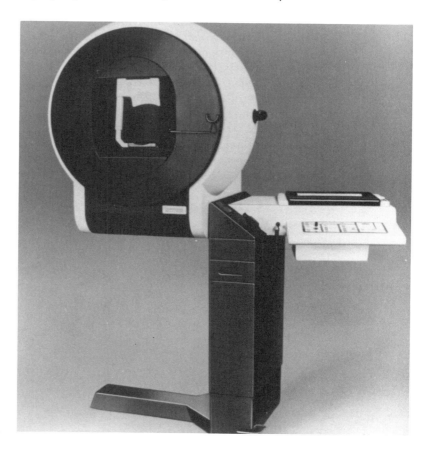

Figure 5–13B. Perimat 206.

The Topcon Perimeter

Model: Topcon Computerized Perimeter SBP-1000 (Fig. 5–14)
Manufacturer: Topcon
Screen Type and Size: 33 cm radius bowl
Test Spots:
    Type: LED
    Size: 2 mm
    Number Available: 257
    Locations: Distributed
    Colors: 585 nm (pale green)
    Intensity Range: 0 to 425 asb
    Duration: 0.2, 0.4, 0.8, 1.2, 3.2 seconds
    Interval: 0.2, 0.4, 0.8, 1.2, 3.2 seconds
Fixation Monitor: Heijl-Krakau method with built in television patient observation system
Background Illumination Level: 31.5 asb
    Control of Background Illumination Level: Automatic
Testing Strategies Available: Suprathreshold, threshold
Test Spot Patterns Available: Full field, central 30 degrees, peripheral, macula, glaucoma, nasal step, circular, meridional, hemianopic
Provisions for Delta Program Analysis: None
Technician Communication with Machine: Light pen with CRT screen
Machine Communication with Technician: Menu options, progress of test, results of test are displayed on CRT screen
Type of Printed Output: Thermal printer
Provisions for Internal Data Storage and Retrieval: None
Provisions for Communication with External Computers: None
Method of Changing Software: None

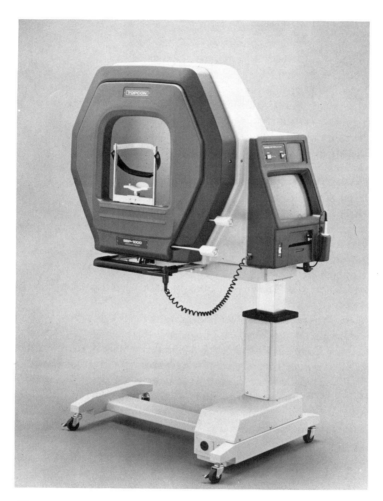

Figure 5–14. Topcon Computerized Perimeter SBP-1000.

The Tubinger Automatic Perimeter

Model: Tubinger Automatik Perimeter (Fig. 5–15)
Manufacturer: Oculus Optikgerate GmbH
　　　　　　　　Dutenhofen
　　　　　　　　D.6330 Wetzlar 17
　　　　　　　　West Germany
Screen Type and Size: 33 cm radius bowl
Test Spots:
　　Type: Fiberoptics rear projection with cover so that spots cannot be seen unless presented (designed to eliminate the "black hole" effect)
　　Sizes: 10 ft diameter
　　Number Available: 249
　　Locations: Distributed throughout the bowl
　　Colors: White (red, yellow, blue and green are available as an option)
　　Intensity Range: 0.32 to 5000 asb
　　Duration: 0.50/0.80
　　Interval: 0.6, 0.9, 1.2 seconds
Fixation Monitor: Automatic fixation control retests threshold value in the central area throughout the test
Background Illumination Level: 32 asb
　　Control of Background Illumination Level: Computer calibrated
Testing Strategies Available: Stepped threshold-related; threshold is available as an option
Test Spot Patterns Available: Total, central 30 degrees, custom diagnostic
Provisions for Delta Program Analysis: None
Technician Communication with Machine: Push button, control panel
Machine Communication with Technician: Via control panel
Type of Printed Output: Siemens printer onto preprinted DINA4 forms
Provisions for Internal Data Storage and Retrieval: None
Provisions for Communication with External Computers: Optional PC interface is available and integrated PC programs are available for testing and storage of data
Method of Changing Software: Factory modifications only unless PC interface is included
Special Comments: Operator may chose an area of special interest to test if desired

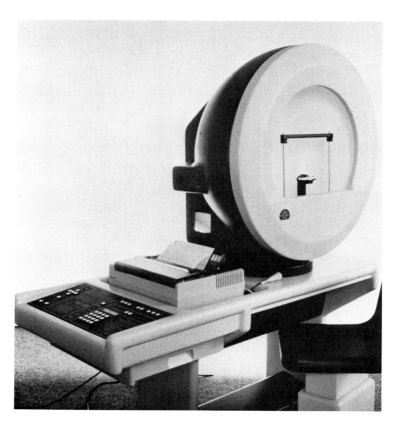

Figure 5–15. Tubinger Automatik Perimeter.

6
Analysis of the Visual Field

The report from an automated visual field examination can be confusing due to the variety of methods and symbols, statistical terms, and unfamiliar format. In this chapter our goal is to assist the reader to interpret various types of automated field reports and summaries from threshold visual fields. Visual field indices are statistics that summarize some aspect of threshold values and provide the physician with documentation to supplement clinical decisions. However, many physicians are not familiar with how a particular statistic should be applied or how to assess the limits of a particular report. The analysis of a visual field report requires a careful study of all of the data presented. The physician must ascertain how accurate the data are and decide whether or not the field is normal. If abnormal, the type or types of field defects need to be characterized. If previous fields are available, it is advantageous to compare the new field with previous fields over time. These clinical questions can be addressed by appropriate summaries of the field. In this chapter we provide an overview of many currently used field indices for threshold fields.

Determination of the Accuracy of Field Reports

ROOT MEAN SQUARE: ESTIMATE OF SHORT-TERM ERROR

One strategy to determine the accuracy of an examination is to determine the test–retest reliability of individual thresholds. Root mean square (RMS) provides an index of threshold variability in a given examination. The RMS is calculated from the thresholds determined more than once in each examination, and indicates overall how much the thresholds measured at the same location differed from each other.

A low RMS results when the multiple thresholds are similar and indicate that the examination is reliable (small error). A high RMS results when the error in the threshold determination is high, i.e., multiple determined points are not similar. A good rule of thumb is that an RMS equal to or less than 3.0 indicates a reliable examination, and RMS values above 3.0 indicate progressively less reliable examinations.[1] In cases with a moderate to advanced level of pathology, RMS values of 4 or 5 can be expected due to the higher variability of a diseased area. Occasionally, however, the RMS will be 0.0 on a field with very advanced loss. This means that the patient always responded the same way on the multiple determined points (there was no variation among the points because they were all in the areas of absolute loss).

Figure 6–1 shows a value table (Octopus 201, program 32) and indicates the 10 threshold locations determined twice. An example of the RMS determination for this examination is shown on Table 6–1.

Calculation of the Pooled Variance, RMS²

From Figure 6–1 and Table 6–1 it can be seen that 10 double determinations were made (m = 10) and the total variance ($S_{..k}^2$) is 44.00. Therefore, RMS² is

TABLE 6–1. DOUBLE DETERMINATIONS FOR THE VALUE TABLE SHOWN IN FIGURE 6–1 FOR OCTOPUS PROGRAM 32 THRESHOLD (dB) DETERMINATION

No. i	Location (x, y)	1st X_{i1k}	2nd X_{i2k}	Mean $\overline{X}_{i.k}$	Variance $s_{i.k}^2$
1.	(−3, 27)	17	13	15	8.00
2.	(3, 27)	9	11	10	2.00
3.	(15, 15)	17	19	18	2.00
4.	(−9, 9)	17	21	19	8.00
5.	(−27, −3)	22	16	19	18.00
6.	(27, 3)	26	26	26	0
7.	(−3, −9)	23	21	22	2.00
8.	(3, −9)	24	22	23	2.00
9.	(15, −15)	24	26	25	2.00
10.	(−15, −21)	24	24	24	0
				Total $S_{..k}^2$	44.00

The first column (i) indicates the number of the double determination. The location (x, y), second column, refers to the coordinates of each point. First and second threshold determinations at each location are listed in the next two columns. Column 5 shows the mean ($\overline{X}_{i.k}$) of the two determinations at each location (.) for patient k. The last column, variance ($s_{i.k}^2$) is the squared standard deviation of the two thresholds in the corresponding row. Total variance ($S_{..k}^2$) is the sum of the variance column. The subscripted dots indicate a variable that is summed. For example, $S_{..k}^2$ is summed over location (i) and examination (j) but not over patient (k).

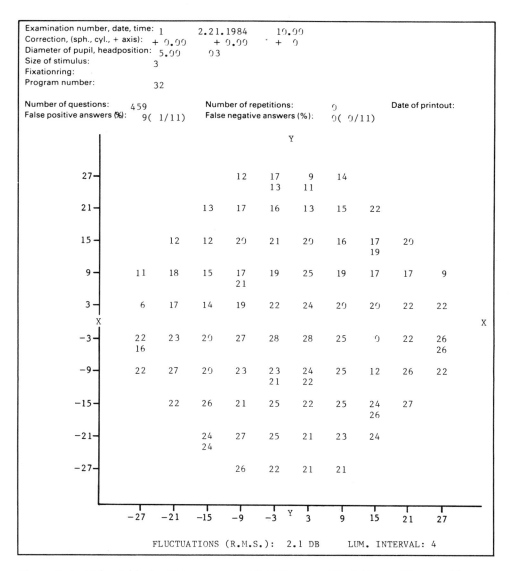

Examination number, date, time: 1   2.21.1984   10.00
Correction, (sph., cyl., + axis): + 0.00 + 0.00 + 0
Diameter of pupil, headposition: 5.00 03
Size of stimulus: 3
Fixationring:
Program number: 32

Number of questions: 459   Number of repetitions: 0   Date of printout:
False positive answers (%): 9(1/11)   False negative answers (%): 0(0/11)

FLUCTUATIONS (R.M.S.): 2.1 DB   LUM. INTERVAL: 4

Figure 6–1. Value table for Octopus central field Program 32, right eye, 71-year-old patient. Points that are determined twice are indicated by two threshold values. Coordinates have been superimposed on machine printout.

equal to

$$\text{RMS}^2 = \frac{\text{Total variance}}{\text{m}} = \frac{44}{10} = 4.4 \qquad (6\text{--}1)$$

and the RMS for the above example is equal to

$$\text{RMS} = \sqrt{4.4} = 2.1 \qquad (6\text{--}2)$$

RMS can be interpreted as the estimate of measurement error (in standard deviation units) associated with each threshold determination. That is, if we assume that the "pooled RMS" determined above provides an estimate of the error expected on each individual threshold in that same examination, then each threshold (shown on the value table of Fig. 6–1) ± 2 RMS has a 95 percent chance of including the true (actual) physiologic threshold P_{ijk}.*

$$\text{Pr} = 0.95 \left\{ X_{ijk} \pm 2 \text{ RMS includes } P_{ijk} \right\} \qquad (6\text{--}3)$$

For example consider the upper left threshold X_{ijk} on Figure 6–1. The value is 12 dB. The overall or pooled RMS value for the examination is 2.1 dB. It can be assumed therefore that the true (actual) physiologic threshold P_{ijk} is probably ($P = 0.95$) included in the interval:

$$12 \pm 2(2.1) \text{ dB}$$

$$12 \pm 4.2 \text{ dB} \qquad (6\text{--}4)$$

$$9.8 \text{ dB to } 14.2 \text{ dB}$$

This example demonstrates that RMS is an extremely important index for both determining the accuracy of a field and estimating the true physiologic significance of a single threshold.

Response Bias: False-Negative and False-Positive Answers

An important problem in field testing is to extract the influence of a patient's *response bias* from the patient's sensory (visual) limits. For example, it is possible for the patient to report that a light was seen on each trial regardless of what was actually seen, or it is possible for a patient to report that a light was never seen regardless of what was actually seen. The problem can be conceptualized as a 2 by 2 contingency table as shown in Table 6–2. The two types of correct responses are indicated on Table 6–2. However, it can also be seen that there are two types of errors: false-positive and false-negative errors.

False-Positive Responses and Catch Trials. As can be seen from the response/stimulus contingency table (Table 6–2), a false-positive response results when the patient reports seeing a stimulus that was not presented. In each Octopus examination, a small number of *catch trials* are presented to check for a positive response

---

* *Refer to Equations 4–2 and 4–3.*

TABLE 6–2. RESPONSE BIAS

| | | Stimulus | |
		Present	Not Present
Patient Response	**Seen**	correct	false-positive error
	Not Seen	false-negative error	correct

bias (or tendency to say "yes"). These catch trials consist of trials where the test luminance is set at 0 and a trial is indicated usually by a brief sound cue. If the patient reports "seeing" a substantial number of these positive catch trials then it can be assumed that the results of the examination are biased. That is, the examination results represent the true visual field as slightly better than it really is.

False-Negative Responses and Catch Trials. The remaining category shown on the contingency table is the type of error called false-negative responses. This type of error occurs when the patient reports not seeing a stimulus when it was present at some definitely seeable level (predetermined earlier in the examination). A response bias, or predisposition to report that a stimulus was not seen, "biases" the field results so that the examination report will show more field loss than is actually present. This type of response bias is measured by presentation of a few *negative catch trials* randomly throughout the examination.

Neither the negative nor the positive bias can be eliminated, but when they are identified and quantified, the field examination can be interpreted accordingly. In the example shown on Figure 6–1 one false-positive response occurred out of 11 catch trials and no false-negative responses occurred out of 11 catch trials. It can be concluded that results were not significantly influenced by either type of response bias.

It is possible for a reliable field examination (low RMS) to be strongly biased either toward positive or negative answers. Adequate evaluation of the accuracy of a field requires assessment of test–retest stability as well as response bias.

Is the Field Normal?

After the accuracy of the examination is assessed, it must be established whether or not the field is normal. The value table in Figure 6–1 supplies an exact and complete summary of the visual field examination and it is important to bear in mind that no further analysis can provide more information. However, detailed interpretation of the value table is difficult because it presents a two-dimensional matrix of raw (unprocessed) numbers. Therefore, it is convenient to have other, more readable, methods of looking at the data. Two strategies can be employed to answer the question, "Is the field normal?" The first is an evaluation of internal consistency and the second is a comparison with a normal population average. The Octopus automated perimeter provides both strategies and all other current machines use a form of the internal consistency method.

EVALUATION OF INTERNAL CONSISTENCY

The Grey Scale
The grey scale converts the value table into a pictorial summary of the observed sensitivities over the entire region tested. In general the dB scale is converted to a grey level scale and regions in between the actual data points are interpolated. Conventionally, regions of high sensitivity are indicated by the light grey levels and lower sensitivities are indicated by darker grey levels. The grey scale provides an immediate qualitative impression of sensitivity over the entire spatial extent of the field.

One way to evaluate if the internal consistency of the field is normal or not is to look for unexpected losses in sensitivity over some selected region of the field. For example in Figure 6–2 the grey scale corresponding to the value table in Figure 6–1 is shown. By using this grey format it is much easier to observe that the upper half of the field appears darker (less sensitive) than the lower half, and that the upper nasal quadrant appears more affected than the upper temporal quadrant. Therefore, this print mode provides a very useful and qualitative summary of the internal consistency of the visual field.

It is reasonable to conclude from the grey scale that the field is probably not normal. The evidence is primarily that the upper and lower hemispheres do not show equal sensitivities as would be expected from a normal field. For further evaluations, however, a variety of sensitivity statistics may be useful.

Sensitivity Statistics
Threshold statistics have the advantage of a purely empirical report of the field. These statistics condense or package information from the visual field into single numbers that provide useful summaries. They include mean sensitivity $\overline{X}_{.jk}$, sensitivity variance $S^2_{.jk}$, and sensitivity standard deviation $SD_{.jk}$.

Mean sensitivity, $\overline{X}_{.jk}$. The average visual sensitivity over a sample of I thresholds:

$$\overline{X}_{.jk} = \frac{\sum_{i=1}^{I} X_{ijk}}{I} \tag{6-5}$$

where I is the total number of thresholds included (each i is assumed to be at a unique location), X_{ijk} is a single threshold value at location i for session j and

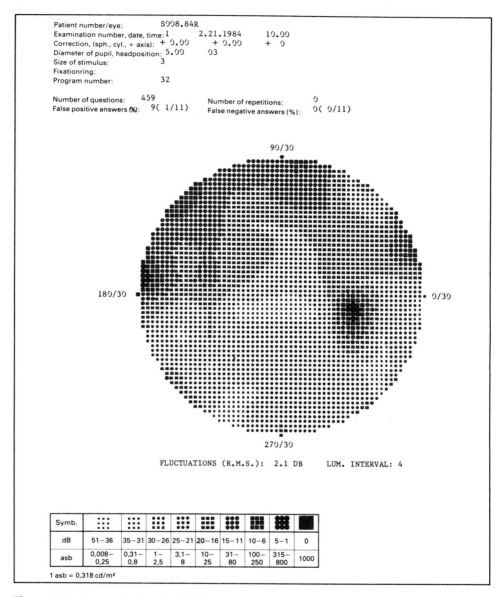

Figure 6–2. Grey scale for the field shown in Figure 6–1.

patient k. The mean threshold provides a reasonably stable estimate of overall sensitivity. This index can be provided for any region of the field. In the case of the Octopus DELTA program (Series mode) the average threshold (mean sensitivity) is provided over regions of the whole field, each of the four quadrants, and for three concentric rings of the examination area as shown in Figure 6–3. If not provided by a manufacturer these statistics can be easily determined from the value tables produced by the threshold examination.

For the example shown in Figures 6–1, 6–2, and 6–3, the average over the whole field is 20.1 dB. If one further divides the field into four quadrants, a mean can be determined in each one of the quadrants. These values are as shown in Table 6–3 as well as on the DELTA series mode printout in Figure 6–3.

This summary of mean sensitivity over four quadrant regions of the field confirms our general impression from the grey scale that sensitivity is reduced in the upper hemisphere. However, we have now provided a quantitative assessment of the actual sensory levels in four regions of the field.

Sensitivity Variance, $S_{.jk}^2$ and Sensitivity Standard Deviation, $SD_{.jk}$.

$$S_{.jk}^2 = \frac{(X_{ijk} - \overline{X}_{.jk})^2}{I - 1} \tag{6-6}$$

$$SD_{.jk} = \sqrt{S_{.jk}^2} \tag{6-7}$$

The sensitivity variance of a set of thresholds indicates how much the thresholds tend to differ from each other. It is reasonable that one sign of early pathology may be an increased variation in the thresholds over an affected region. The standard deviation is the square root of the variance and restores our original units, dB. Hence, standard deviation is the more convenient index of threshold variation. The standard deviation for the four quadrants of the above examination are listed in Table 6–4.

It can be seen from the sensitivity variation table (Table 6–4) that the original conclusion that the upper field showed greater loss of sensitivity compared to the lower field is also consistent with the analysis of variation. The thresholds in the upper field are *more variable* than the thresholds in the lower field. For example, in the upper temporal quadrant the thresholds tended to vary ±4.4 dB whereas in the corresponding lower field the thresholds varied ±2.2 dB. In suspect or borderline fields, the standard deviation between thresholds (over some regions of the field) may provide useful information.

Comparison With a Normal Standard

A normal visual field can be defined as a set of discrete test locations with known average sensitivity and variance determined from a sufficient sample of nonpathologic eyes to make inferences to a normal population. Clinically it is very useful to compare a measured patient field against a known standard. However, determination of the range of sensitivities found in the normal

```
                                              EX1

             DATE OF EXAM : DAY          02.21
                            YEAR          1984
             PROGRAM / EXAMINATION       32/01




             TOTAL LOSS (WHOLE FIELD)     249

             MEAN LOSS (PER TEST LOC)
                WHOLE FIELD                3.4
                QUADRANT UPPER NASAL       7.4
                         LOWER NASAL       0.6
                         UPPER TEMP.       4.7
                         LOWER TEMP.       0.7
                ECCENTRICITY   0 - 10      2.3
                              10 - 20      4.0
                              20 - 30      3.4


             MEAN SENSITIVITY
                WHOLE FIELD  (N: 24.1)    20.1
                QUAD.UPP.NAS.(N: 23.4)    15.7
                    LOW.NAS.(N: 24.4)     23.6
                    UPP.TMP.(N: 23.5)     17.9
                    LOW.TMP.(N: 25.1)     23.2
                ECC.  0 - 10 (N: 26.9)    23.5
                     10 - 20 (N: 24.9)    19.7
                     20 - 30 (N: 23.0)    19.4


             NO. OF DISTURBED POINTS       31
             R.M.S. FLUCTUATION           2.1
             TOTAL FLUCTUATION
```

Figure 6–3. Series mode of the Octopus DELTA program. Summary statistics are listed for the field shown in Figures 6–1 and 6–2.

TABLE 6–3. MEAN SENSITIVITY OVER FOUR QUADRANTS (FROM FIG. 6–1)

	Nasal Field	Temporal Field
Upper Field	$\overline{X}_{.jk} = 15.7$ dB	$\overline{X}_{.jk} = 17.9$ dB
Lower Field	$\overline{X}_{.jk} = 23.6$ dB	$\overline{X}_{.jk} = 23.2^*$ dB

* Two points in the blind spot region are omitted.

TABLE 6–4. SENSITIVITY VARIATION OVER FOUR QUADRANTS (FROM FIG. 6–1)

	Nasal Field	Temporal Field
Upper Field	$SD_{.jk} = 4.1$ dB	$SD_{.jk} = 4.4$ dB
Lower Field	$SD_{.jk} = 2.7$ dB	$SD_{.jk} = 2.2^*$ dB

* Two points in the blind spot region are omitted.

population is a major undertaking. The results of one effort from the Octopus test laboratory in Bern, Switzerland, are described.

Determination of Sensitivity Ranges in the Normal Population. A sample of 12 normal patients was studied in the Octopus test laboratory, Bern, Switzerland, using a standard Octopus 201 automated perimeter.[2] The patients (24 eyes) were divided into three groups: 18 to 39 years, 40 to 59 years, and 60 years or older. Four individuals (eight eyes) for each age group participated in the control studies which consisted of 10 examinations per eye. The average threshold values (expressed as sensitivity in dB) and standard deviation (the index of interindividual variability) are shown on Figures 6–4, 6–5, and 6–6 for each point tested in examination 31 (0 to 30 degrees), and Figures 6–7, 6–8, and 6–9 for each point tested in examination 41 (30 to 60 degrees).

Based on these average normal values for the three age groups, a set of standard thresholds have been determined for Octopus fields. The matrices of values chosen for the youngest and most sensitive age group (≤ 24 years) are shown on Figures 6–10 and 6–11 for programs 32 and 42, respectively.

Age Correction Constant. Results of the normal population study from the Bern laboratory suggested that light sensitivity tends to decrease with age. Therefore, to determine whether a particular point is disturbed, it must be compared to the expected normal value for the appropriate age group. The age correction constant employed by Octopus is approximately 0.1 dB decrease per year after 24 years. Specifically, no correction is used for patients who are 24 years old or younger. For each decade above 24 years, however, 1 dB is subtracted from each standard threshold value. These corrections are shown in Table 6–5. For example, if a patient is 35 years old, then the appropriate normal values (for program 32) are those shown on Figure 6–10 where each value is reduced by 2 dB as shown in Table 6–5.

Error Due to Estimation of a Normal Value from a Population Mean. A normal value based on a population mean is associated with an interindividual variance (Figs.

TABLE 6–5. AGE CORRECTION CONSTANTS

Decade (years)	Age Correction (dB)
≤ 24	0
25 to 34	−1
35 to 44	−2
45 to 54	−3
55 to 63	−4
64 to 74	−5
75 to 84	−6
85 to 94	−7
95+	−8

Figure 6–4.

Eccentricity in degrees											
30	24	18	12	6	0	6	12	18	24	30	
					25.8 / 2.6						30
		26.5 / 0.7	26.5 / 1.3	27.6 / 1.5	26.9 / 1.9	26.9 / 1.8	26.4 / 1.8	27.5 / 2.1			24
	28.5 / 0.7	28.2 / 1.5	27.1 / 2.0	28.7 / 1.8	28.3 / 1.8	29.1 / 1.6	28.8 / 1.8	28.6 / 2.0	29.0 / 1.4		18
	28.1 / 2.2	28.8 / 2.3	29.2 / 2.1	30.4 / 1.4	30.4 / 1.9	28.9 / 2.4	29.3 / 1.7	29.2 / 1.7	28.6 / 1.3		12
	28.4 / 1.4	29.2 / 2.2	30.8 / 1.6	31.5 / 1.8	31.8 / 1.3	31.6 / 1.4	28.7 / 2.5	29.2 / 2.1	29.1 / 2.1		6
27.8 / 2.0	29.2 / 0.8	31.2 / 1.6	32.2 / 1.2	33.2 / 1.6	36.5 / 1.3	32.8 / 1.6	20.2 / 1.1	9.5 / 10.4	29.6 / 0.9	29.3 / 1.4	0
	28.7 / 1.4	29.7 / 1.3	31.6 / 1.3	31.9 / 1.5	32.3 / 1.3	32.3 / 1.7	30.6 / 1.4	28.5 / 3.0	29.7 / 1.9		6
	27.3 / 1.6	29.8 / 1.4	30.0 / 1.3	29.9 / 1.4	31.3 / 1.8	31.0 / 1.0	28.7 / 1.8	30.1 / 1.9	28.3 / 1.5		12
	27.5 / 0.7	28.1 / 2.6	28.6 / 2.0	29.6 / 1.8	29.4 / 1.6	30.6 / 1.6	29.4 / 2.2	29.8 / 1.7	29.0 / 1.4		18
		28.0 / 2.8	27.2 / 2.2	28.9 / 1.1	28.5 / 1.9	28.9 / 2.2	28.8 / 2.5	29.5 / 0.7			24
					27.5 / 1.8						30

Mean Inter–Individual Variation (RMS) = 2.1 dB

Figure 6–4. Average central field sensitivities (top values) and interindividual variation (bottom values) of eight normal eyes between ages 18 and 39 years. (From The Octopus Visual Field Atlas, 1978.[2])

Figure 6–5.

Eccentricity in degrees											
30	24	18	12	6	0	6	12	18	24	30	
					22.1 / 2.7						30
		23.7 / 4.0	25.6 / 3.1	24.5 / 3.2	23.5 / 4.0	23.8 / 3.2					24
		24.5 / 4.5	26.2 / 3.4	25.6 / 3.0	27.5 / 2.5	25.6 / 4.2	26.5 / 2.9	25.8 / 1.9			18
	23.8 / 4.6	25.9 / 4.1	27.6 / 1.8	28.8 / 2.1	29.6 / 2.1	28.0 / 1.4	27.7 / 2.6	27.1 / 2.6	26.6 / 3.1		12
	25.7 / 3.4	28.1 / 1.8	29.6 / 1.4	29.5 / 2.1	29.6 / 1.7	29.4 / 1.7	27.9 / 1.7	28.9 / 1.7	27.2 / 2.2		6
24.9 / 2.7	26.3 / 3.1	29.9 / 1.7	31.4 / 1.7	31.9 / 1.1	35.1 / .20	31.4 / 1.3	23.7 / 9.6	10.4 / 10.4	28.5 / 1.1	27.8 / 1.9	0
	26.6 / 3.0	28.8 / 1.7	30.3 / 1.8	31.5 / 1.0	31.8 / 1.5	30.8 / 1.3	28.2 / 2.4	26.9 / 2.2	27.9 / 1.6		6
	26.1 / 2.4	27.0 / 1.5	28.8 / 1.5	27.9 / 1.5	29.7 / 1.7	29.9 / 1.1	28.5 / 1.3				12
		25.4 / 1.9	27.0 / 2.0	26.7 / 1.8	27.9 / 1.3	27.9 / 1.1					18
					25.0 / 2.5						24

Mean Inter–Individual Variation (RMS) = 2.9 dB

Figure 6–5. Average center field sensitivities (top values) and interindividual variation (bottom values) of eight normal eyes between ages 40 and 59 years. (From The Octopus Visual Field Atlas, 1978.[2])

Figure 6–6

Eccentricity in degrees

30	24	18	12	6	0	6	12	18	24	30	
					19.4						
					4.5						30
			20.8	22.6	23.3	22.3	22.6				
			3.3	3.0	3.0	3.0	3.1				24
		21.4	22.7	24.3	25.0	23.9	24.1	24.2			
		3.6	3.6	2.9	3.3	2.7	2.3	2.9			18
	22.4	23.4	24.9	25.9	27.0	26.7	26.2	24.4	24.8		
	3.4	3.1	1.4	2.0	3.2	2.1	2.3	3.0	3.9		12
	23.9	26.3	27.6	29.8	29.7	28.5	25.7	26.5	26.1		
	2.4	2.8	2.1	1.0	1.8	1.8	2.4	2.7	2.2		6
22.1	23.6	26.9	29.3	31.1	32.8	30.6	20.1	15.8	27.1	26.7	
2.9	2.8	3.1	2.2	1.3	1.3	1.6	9.9	9.8	1.8	1.8	0
	23.2	26.4	28.9	29.9	30.3	29.8	27.1	25.1	27.0		
	2.9	3.3	1.9	1.7	1.3	1.3	2.9	2.3	1.9		6
	22.4	26.3	27.3	27.8	28.6	28.1	2.5	27.4	26.8		
	2.1	2.2	1.9	2.4	1.9	1.9	1.5	2.4	2.2		12
		24.3	25.6	26.9	27.3	27.3	27.0	26.3			
		2.4	1.8	2.0	1.6	2.0	2.1	2.0			18
			24.4	25.1	25.9	26.8	25.3				
			2.0	2.3	2.0	1.8	2.0				24
					24.9						
					2.7						30

Mean Inter–Individual Variation (RMS) = 2.9 dB

Figure 6–6. Average central field sensitivities (top values) *and* interindividual variation (bottom values) *of eight normal eyes from patients 60 years and older. (From The Octopus Visual Field Atlas, 1978.*[2]*)*

Figure 6–7

Eccentricity in degrees

60	48	36	24	12	0	12	24	36	48	60	
				3.4	5.7	10.8					
				5.5	6.3	5.7					60
		7.6	15.0	16.7	17.6	19.1	19.2	19.1			
		4.1	6.6	4.9	7.1	4.5	5.4	3.3			48
	9.7	17.8	20.9	23.4	23.3	23.4	23.5	22.5	20.9		
	7.1	7.2	4.5	2.4	2.8	2.0	1.5	2.5	2.3		36
	18.2	23.0	26.6				25.8	24.5	23.6		
	7.2	2.5	2.2				2.1	2.2	1.3		24
10.8	22.5	25.6						27.3	24.8	22.9	
7.1	2.5	2.0						2.3	1.9	1.6	12
7.8	22.1	25.6						28.8	27.0	24.4	
8.4	2.1	1.9						2.0	1.4	1.8	0
2.6	19.5	25.7						28.3	26.3	24.3	
4.6	8.1	1.9						1.8	1.5	1.9	12
	5.5	19.3	25.0				27.4	26.6	25.8		
	9.0	9.8	2.4				1.6	1.5	1.6		24
	0.0	1.7	24.4	25.8	26.7	27.1	25.9	25.5	24.4		
	0.0	5.7	3.0	1.8	2.1	1.8	2.0	1.2	1.4		36
			0.0	16.8	22.6	23.8	24.7	24.3	24.1		
			0.0	6.7	1.7	1.9	1.7	2.1	1.1		48
					19.1						
					4.0						60

Mean Inter–Individual Variation (RMS) = 4.2 dB

Figure 6–7. Average peripheral field sensitivities (top values) *and* interindividual variation (bottom values) *of eight normal eyes from patients between 18 and 39 years. (From The Octopus Visual Field Atlas, 1978.*[2]*)*

Figure 6–8. Average peripheral field sensitivities (top values) and interindividual variation (bottom values) of eight normal eyes from patients between 40 and 59 years. (From The Octopus Visual Field Atlas, 1978.[2])

Eccentricity in degrees

60	48	36	24	12	0	12	24	36	48	60	
				1.9 / 3.4	3.8 / 5.3	4.3 / 5.6					60
		4.2 / 5.0	10.1 / 6.4	14.1 / 5.2	15.1 / 4.9	15.3 / 5.3	15.2 / 5.3	13.5 / 4.3			48
	9.0 / 6.6	17.5 / 4.6	19.4 / 4.0	22.1 / 2.8	21.7 / 3.4	19.7 / 3.8	22.0 / 3.2	20.6 / 2.7	17.0 / 3.9		36
	17.0 / 3.8	20.9 / 3.6	24.1 / 3.1				24.8 / 1.9	24.4 / 1.3	22.3 / 2.1		24
9.7 / 7.7	20.3 / 3.1	22.7 / 4.3						26.5 / 1.3	24.6 / 1.5	22.0 / 1.7	12
10.4 / 8.8	21.1 / 2.8	24.7 / 2.1						27.4 / 1.3	25.7 / 1.5	23.8 / 1.7	0
4.4 / 5.8	16.9 / 8.8	24.1 / 2.7						27.4 / 1.9	25.4 / 1.9	23.8 / 1.4	12
	7.9 / 9.8	18.9 / 8.7	23.8 / 3.4				26.4 / 1.5	26.3 / 1.4	24.7 / 1.7		24
1.4 / 4.1	8.0 / 10.3	18.6 / 8.0	24.3 / 2.1	24.8 / 2.3	26.1 / 1.7	25.5 / 1.7	24.9 / 2.3	23.2 / 1.7			36
		0.7 / 2.8	11.6 / 9.8	21.1 / 1.7	22.1 / 2.4	24.1 / 1.7	23.2 / 2.2	22.6 / 1.7			48
					18.6 / 2.8						60

Mean Inter–Individual Variation (RMS) = 4.5 dB

Figure 6–9. Average peripheral field sensitivities (top values) and interindividual variation (bottom values) of eight normal eyes from patients 60 years and older. (From The Octopus Visual Field Atlas, 1978.[2])

Eccentricity in degrees

60	48	36	24	12	0	12	24	36	48	60	
				2.3 / 4.0	4.0 / 4.5	4.8 / 5.5					60
		5.1 / 5.7	9.4 / 5.3	11.0 / 5.9	13.9 / 5.9	13.8 / 4.9	12.5 / 6.3	10.9 / 5.4			48
	5.9 / 4.9	11.5 / 5.4	16.9 / 4.2	19.4 / 4.7	20.4 / 4.0	17.9 / 4.7	19.3 / 3.4	15.2 / 6.6	16.3 / 2.4		36
	12.1 / 5.1	15.8 / 4.6	20.1 / 4.5				22.6 / 3.5	21.5 / 2.6	20.0 / 2.9		24
7.4 / 5.8	15.4 / 5.1	20.9 / 1.8						24.8 / 2.4	23.3 / 1.7	29.4 / 2.4	12
5.3 / 6.4	15.5 / 5.9	20.5 / 3.7						26.3 / 1.9	24.6 / 1.9	21.6 / 2.2	0
1.8 / 4.3	12.1 / 7.8	21.2 / 2.7						26.0 / 2.3	23.8 / 1.7	21.4 / 1.1	12
	3.1 / 5.8	12.1 / 8.6	21.5 / 2.7				25.6 / 1.7	25.1 / 1.8	22.6 / 1.4		24
	0.0 / 0.0	3.4 / 7.3	14.9 / 6.9	22.1 / 3.1	23.1 / 1.7	24.2 / 2.5	22.9 / 2.0	22.5 / 1.4	21.9 / 1.6		36
		0.0 / 0.0	10.1 / 8.3	20.8 / 1.5	19.3 / 2.6	21.1 / 1.7	21.5 / 2.6	20.5 / 1.7			48
					14.2 / 6.3						60

Mean Inter–Individual Variation (RMS) = 4.4 dB

Eccentricity in degrees											
27	21	15	9	3	0	3	9	15	21	27	
		25	25	25	26						27
	26	27	27	27	27	27					21
	27	28	29	29	29	29	28	28			15
26	28	29	30	31	30	30	29	28	28		9
28	29	31	32	33	33	31	30	29	29		3
											0
28	29	31	32	33	32	32	31	30	29		3
27	29	30	31	31	32	31	30	29	28		9
	28	29	30	30	31	30	30	29			15
		28	28	29	30	30	29				21
			27	28	29	29#					27

Figure 6–10. Central field (program 32, right eye) normal values employed by Octopus for ages less than or equal to 24 years.

6–4 to 6–9). Assuming that sensitivity is distributed normally in the normal population, it can be assumed that 95 percent of normal cases will fall within the range of the population mean $\pm$ two standard deviations. For example, if the expected interindividual variation (RMS) is 2.1 dB (Fig. 6–4), then the expected range for a population mean of 25 dB $\pm$ 2 (2.1 dB) is 20.8 to 29.2 dB (nearly a log unit). That is, it can be assumed that this interval represents the "normal population" interval ($P = 0.95$). In the case of the 30- to 60-degree field (Fig. 6–7), the overall interindividual variation (RMS) is 4.2 dB (ages $\leq$ 39 years). The expected range for a population mean between 30 and 60 degrees eccentricity of 25 dB would be 25 ± 2 (4.2) dB or 16.6 dB to 33.4 dB.

Eccentricity in degrees											
54	42	30	18	6	0	6	18	30	42	54	
			8	10	12	13					54
	9	14	18	20	20	21	20	18			42
7	17	21	23	24	25	24	24	22	21		30
13	22	24					26	25	23		18
16	23	26					28	27	25		6
											0
14	23	26					28	27	25		6
8	18	24					28	27	25		18
	8	18	25	27	28	27	27	26			30
	2	11	21	24	25	26	25	24			42
			4	14	21	23	24	23			54

Figure 6–11. Peripheral field (program 42, right eye) normal values employed by Octopus for ages less than or equal to 24 years.

This range is approximately $1\frac{1}{2}$ log units. That is, threshold variation is apparently somewhat higher in the peripheral field than in the central field.

The above example illustrates that the practice of estimating a single normal value for a particular patient from a group average yields a significant source of error. This problem is represented in symbols as:

$$\underset{\substack{\text{True normal}\\\text{value for patient } k}}{\mu_{ijk}} \quad \text{is estimated by} \quad \underset{\substack{\text{Average normal}\\\text{value for a population}}}{\overline{N}_{i..}} \quad \pm \quad \underset{\substack{\text{Interindividual}\\\text{variation}}}{\text{SD}_{i..}} \qquad (6-8)$$

where μ_{ijk} is the actual "true" normal value for a particular location i, session j, and patient k, $\overline{N}_{i..}$ is the estimated normal population value at location i based on averages from a sample of patients, and $\text{SD}_{i..}$ is the interindividual variation about the mean normal value. As can be seen from the example above, this source of error (interindividual variation) can be greater than 1 log unit of sensitivity.

Loss Statistics

One class of loss statistics compares each visual threshold with a normal value determined from a population average and summarizes the subset of points that have been recognized as disturbed. This class of statistic depends on both the specific definition of a disturbed point and the reliable estimates of the normal values. Examples of this type of loss statistic are reported on the Series mode of the Octopus DELTA program and include total loss and mean loss (Fig. 6-3). These loss statistics vary from examination to examination with respect to the sample sizes on which they are based. That is, if a given examination results in a large number of disturbed points then the loss statistics will be based on a larger sample size than those from an examination with only a few number of disturbed points. In general, due to their complexity and potential for error, applications of these statistics for interpretation of visual fields require caution.

Number of Disturbed Points. The number of disturbed points (d) is the count of thresholds that are lower than the expected normal value by a specific amount. This count depends entirely upon the specific definition of a disturbance. In the case of the Octopus system, a point (threshold) is considered to be disturbed when the measured threshold deviates from the tabled normal value ($\overline{N}_{i..}$) by more than 4 dB. (This value originates from the interindividual variation found for the normal central field population 2(2.1 dB) as described in the previous section (Fig. 6-4). The count of the points considered disturbed in a given examination provides a rough global index of the spatial *extent* of visual loss present in the field. For example, the Octopus program 32 determines 76 thresholds. If 38 thresholds were defined as disturbed, then it would be concluded that 50 percent of the sampled area showed a sensory loss due to a pathologic disturbance. However, this conclusion is fundamentally dependent upon two sources of error: measurement error and error from the estimate of the true normal values. Bebie and Fankhauser[3] have determined that the number of disturbed points is a highly variable index in test–retest situations especially for cases where sensitivity is only slightly below normal. It appears, therefore, that count or frequency descriptions of the visual field should be applied with caution.

Total Loss. Total loss (in terms of the Octopus DELTA system) is the sum of all threshold values that are considered disturbed in a specific region of the visual field. Because total loss only includes the subset of thresholds that are considered disturbed, the statistic is classified as restricted. In symbols, total loss (TL) is represented as

$$TL = \sum_{i=1}^{d} D_{ijk} \qquad (6-9)$$

where d is the number of disturbed thresholds D_{ijk}. The total loss index is a global indication of the overall level or depth of loss. However, it is associated with measurement error, error on the estimate of a normal value, and possibly a small sample size.

Mean Loss. The mean loss (ML) can be determined for any region over which a total loss (TL) has been calculated:

$$ML = \frac{TL}{d} \qquad (6-10)$$

where d is the number of disturbed points.

The mean loss field index provides the average loss over any specific area of the field, and is a more stable and sensitive estimate than total loss. However, mean loss is also dependent upon the accuracy of the normal values and may be based on a small sample size that tends to decrease the accuracy of the mean. This statistic is currently provided on the Series mode printout of the Octopus DELTA program for the whole field area, the four quadrants, and three concentric rings. (Fig. 6-3).

What is a Disturbed Point?

A disturbed point is a specific threshold measurement whose value is significantly depressed due to underlying eye pathology. The decision about whether a point is actually disturbed based on field measurements is statistical.

ESTIMATE OF A THRESHOLD DISTURBANCE USING A NORMAL VALUE TABLE

The extent of sensitivity reduction for a single threshold ($\alpha_{i..}$) can be evaluated from the normal value ($\overline{N}_{i..}$) (estimated from group norms) and the measurement error (E_{ijk}) (estimated for each threshold by the RMS). Assume that a measured threshold (X_{ijk}) $\pm$ measurement error (E_{ijk}) theoretically contains the true threshold (P_{ijk}).

$$P_{ijk} \text{ is within } X_{ijk} \pm E_{ijk} \qquad \textit{(from Eq. 4-2)}$$

Both P_{ijk} and E_{ijk} can be estimated. The true threshold component (P_{ijk}) can be subdivided into the "true" normal value $(\mu_{i..})$ minus the effect of eye diseases (α_{ijk}):

$$(\mu_{i..} - \alpha_{ijk}) \text{ is estimated by } X_{ijk} \pm E_{ijk} \qquad (6-11)$$

The true normal value $(\mu_{i..})$ is estimated by the population average $\overline{N}_{i..}$ and interindividual variation (ϵ_n) as shown below.

$$\mu_{i..} \text{ is estimated by } \overline{N}_{i..} \pm \epsilon_n \qquad (6-12)$$

Measurement error for a given point (E_{ijk}) is estimated from the pooled variance RMS^2.

$$E_{ijk} \text{ is estimated by } RMS_{.jk} \qquad (6-13)$$

Combination of the two sources of error (associated with Eq. 6–11) yields the following description of the pathologic contribution (α_{ijk}) for a particular location

$$\alpha_{ijk} = (\overline{N}_{i..} - X_{ijk}) \pm \sqrt{\epsilon_n^2 + RMS^2} \qquad (6-14)$$

where all symbols are as described above and the two sources of error are combined.

The above equation shows that the pathologic component of a single threshold (α_{ijk}) can be expressed as the observed threshold (X_{ijk}) compared to the expected normal value $(\overline{N}_{i..})$ $\pm$ the sum of all sources of error.

It can be seen from Eq. 6–14 that the estimate of a disturbed threshold is associated with at least *two* sources of error: (1) error on the estimate of the normal value (ϵ_n) (roughly estimated at $\pm$ (2 dB) for the Octopus system) and (2) threshold measurement error, (E_{ijk}) (roughly estimated by the RMS). (There is also error on the estimate of the threshold measurement error but this error is not known and is not included here.) Accordingly, the best estimate of a threshold disturbance will be associated with the error limits from all combined sources. It can be seen from these equations that inferences about the physiologic condition underlying a visual threshold are dependent upon the quality of the estimates of the normal value and measurement error.

INTERPRETATION OF A DISTURBED THRESHOLD

The first point on Figure 6–1 (value table) shows a measured threshold value (X_{ijk}) of 12 dB, the associated normal value $(N_{i..})$ is 20 dB (Fig. 6–10). The age correction constant for a 71-year-old patient is -5 dB (Table 6–5), the RMS is 2.1 dB, and the best estimate of the interindividual error, ϵ_m, is 2.9 dB (mean interindividual variation for normal population over 60 years [Fig. 6–6]).

Evaluation of Equation 6–14 shows

$$\alpha_{ijk} = 20 - 12 \pm \sqrt{2.9^2 \text{ dB} + 2.1^2 \text{ dB}} \qquad (6\text{–}14a)$$

$$\alpha_{ijk} = 8 \text{ dB} \pm \sqrt{8.4 \text{ dB} + 4.2 \text{ dB}} \qquad (6\text{–}14b)$$

$$\alpha_{ijk} = 8 \text{ dB} \pm 3.6 \text{ dB} \qquad (6\text{–}14c)$$

The visual loss attributed to a true physiologic condition for this threshold can be estimated to be 8 dB ± the combined errors. We can conclude that the confidence interval of 8 ± 2(3.6) or 8 ± 7.2 dB has a 95 percent chance of containing the true visual loss. This case establishes a *conservative* confidence interval because the error on the estimate of the measurement error is not included and reflects the situation usually found in clinical practice where that source of error is not available.

The example again demonstrates the fundamental problem of interpreting single threshold loss statistics. The absolute difference between the expected normal and the observed threshold was 8 dB. At first glance it may appear that 8 db would be a significant loss of sensitivity. However, the true loss was conservatively estimated (by assuming the RMS is a perfect estimator of the true measurement error) as anywhere between approximately 0.9 to 15.2 dB (95 percent of the time). Obviously, the physiologic/clinical significance of a 1-dB loss is much different than the physiologic significance of a 15-dB loss. Unfortunately, it is not possible to discriminate between these two extreme values on the basis of a single threshold approach.

Loss Over Specific Regions of the Field

Although the single threshold approach is necessary to establish the theoretical framework on which to base analyses of the total field, as demonstrated above, it does not prove to be a reliable clinical strategy. One approach to improve the clinical usefulness of visual field information is to extend the area over which estimates are made and summarize over a region of threshold values.

The above example is from the field (Fig. 6–1, value table, Fig. 6–2, grey scale, and Fig. 6–3, DELTA, series mode, and the specific comparison with normal values is shown on the comparison printout (Fig. 6–12). The value table of actual thresholds (X_{ijk}) is shown on the lower left matrix, the age corrected normal value table ($\overline{N}_{i..}$) is shown on the lower right matrix [the age of this patient was 71 years old, and therefore the age correction constant is -5 dB (Table 6–5) from the standard table (Fig. 6–10)]. The loss scores ($\overline{N}_{i..} - X_{ijk}$) are shown on the lower center matrix. From the above example, we know that each loss score in this field is expected to be associated with ± 7.1 dB of error ($P = .95$). However, the observation that the highest loss scores tend to *cluster* in the upper region of the field substantially increases the confidence that the field loss is disturbed in the upper region. The average loss score for the 38 upper points is 6.61 dB ± 0.57 dB (standard error of the mean, SEM).

$$\text{SEM} = \text{SD}/\sqrt{n} = 3.54/\sqrt{38} = 0.57. \qquad (6\text{–}15)$$

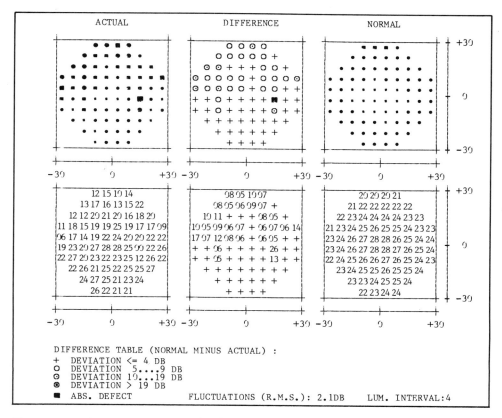

Figure 6–12. *Comparison printout for the field shown in Figures 6–1, 6–2 and 6–3, right eye, 71-year-old patient.*

That is, because the sample size is large (n = 38), the error on the average (6.61 dB) is relatively small (0.57 dB), and we can be very certain that even with the substantial single threshold error, that the regional conclusion of a field loss is highly probable.

The average loss score for the 36 lower points (two points in the blind spot region are excluded) is 0.94 dB ± 0.43 dB indicating that the lower half of the field overall probably is not substantially reduced in sensitivity. The increased certainty in these conclusions is at the price of extending the area (number of thresholds) over which the information is pooled.

Comparison of Visual Fields Over Time

One of the features that the introduction of the computer brought to automated visual field testing is the ability to recall a series of related examinations for analyses over time. This feature creates the opportunity to analyze a series of

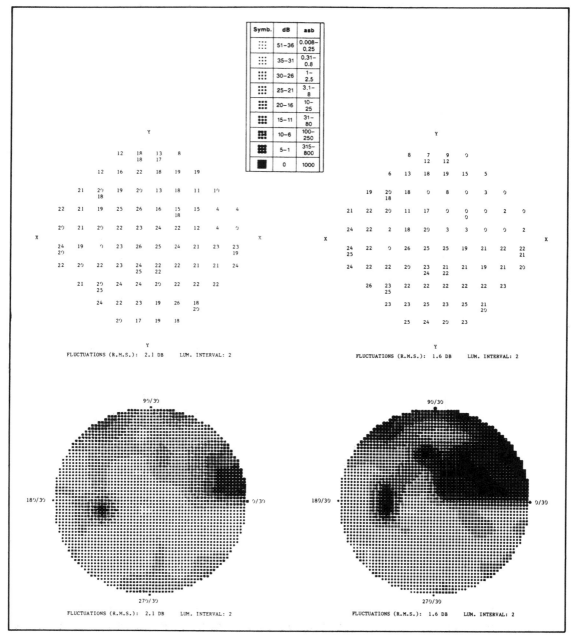

Figure 6–13. Octopus grey scale and value table for two left eye field examinations approximately 3½ years apart.

TABLE 6–6. NORMAL VALUE TABLE AND LOSS SCORES FOR TWO EXAMINATIONS SHOWN IN FIGURE 6–13

Normal Value Table,
$\overline{N}_{i..}$
(age, 71 years)

```
            21 20 20 20
         22 22 22 22 22 21
      23 23 24 24 24 24 23 22
   23 23 24 25 25 26 25 24 23 21
   24 24 25 26 28 28 27 26 24 23
   24 25 26 27 28 28 27 26 24 23
   23 24 25 26 27 26 26 25 24 22
      24 25 25 26 25 25 24 23
         24 25 25 24 23 23
            24 24 23 22
```

Loss Scores ($\overline{N}_{i..} - X_{ijk}$) (7/14/81)

```
            9  2  5 12
        10  6  0  4  3  2
      2  4  5  4 11  6 12 12
   1  2  5  0  0 10  9  9 19 17
   4  3     4  5  4  5 14 20 23
   2  6     1  3  3  3  5  1  2
   1  4  3  3  3  4  4  4  3  2
      3  3  1  2  5  3  2  1
         0  3  2  5  3  4
            4  7  4  4
```

Loss Scores ($\overline{N}_{i..} - X_{ijk}$) (2/21/84)

```
            13 11 10 20
         16  9  9  4  7 16
      4  4  6 24 16 24 20 22
   2  1  4 14  8 26 25 24 21 21
   2  2     8  8 25 24 26 24 21
   0  3     0  2  3  8  5  2  2
   1  2  3  6  4  5  5  6  3  2
      2  1  3  4  3  3  2  0
         1  2  0  0  0  3
            0  0  3  0
```

fields obtained over many examinations. In the previous section the important clinical issues addressed were, "Is the field normal?" and "What is a disturbed point?" The clinical question associated with comparison of multiple visual fields over time is, "Are there visual field changes over time that suggest changes in the underlying visual physiology?"

COMPARISON OF TWO VISUAL FIELDS: PAIRED T-TEST[4]

Statistical comparison of any two like fields (or any two groups of like fields) can be achieved by a paired t-test. The paired t-test involves a point-by-point comparison of two fields (or groups of like fields) where the values of one set of data are subtracted from the corresponding values of the other set of data. (Because the t-distribution is symmetrical, the order of subtraction is not relevant for this analysis.) In the case of Octopus fields corresponding loss scores ($\overline{N}_{i..} - X_{ijk}$) are subtracted. Figure 6–13 shows both the grey scales and value tables for two left eye visual fields approximately $3\frac{1}{2}$ years apart. Table 6–6 shows the normal value table and point-by-point differences (loss scores) between the value table and the two examination values. Figure 6–14 shows

```
                      - 4   - 9.  - 5    - 8

              - 6   - 3   - 4:   1:  - 4.  -14.

        - 2:   0:  - 1   -20.  - 5   -18   - 8   -10

  - 1:   1:   1.  -14.  - 9.  -16   -16   -15   - 2   - 4

   4:   1:       - 4.  - 3   -21.  -19   -12   - 4    2

   2:   3.        3:  - 1:   0:  - 5.    0  - 1:    0:

   2:   2:   0:  - 3.  - 1:  - 1.  - 1.  - 2.    0:  - 4:

   5:   2:  - 2:  - 2:   2.    0:    0:   1:

        - 1:   1:   2:   4.  - 1:   1:
```

DIFFERENCE TABLE : MEAN B MINUS MEAN A (NEGATIVE VALUES: DECREASED SENSITIVITY)
0-0 ALL RESULTS ZERO   <> LOW NORMAL VALUES
DOTS INDICATE THAT SOME (.) OR ALL (:) RESULTS ARE IN NORMAL RANGE (FULLY VALID)

CONFIDENCE INTERVAL FOR MEAN DIFFERENCE / T-TEST
(1) PATHOL. AREA (UNDOTTED)   - 7.5 ± 2.8 (T-TEST: ALTERATION IS INDICATED)
(2) WHOLE FIELD   - 3.1 ± 1.5 (T-TEST: ALTERATION IS INDICATED)

Figure 6–14. Octopus DELTA program (change mode) showing the difference between the two loss score matrices shown in Table 6–6. Corresponding points on the 2/21/84 field are subtracted from the 7/14/81 field.

the difference matrix for the two examinations where the corresponding loss scores (Table 6–6) are subtracted from each other. The resulting set of difference values is tested against the hypothesis that the average of the resulting sample of differences is equal to zero. If the t-test does not support the zero or null hypothesis, then the conclusion is made that there is a difference between the average threshold value of examination 1 and examination 2.

The specific test is defined below:

$$ t = \frac{\overline{d}_{..k}}{\frac{SD_{..k}}{\sqrt{n}}} \qquad df = n - 1 \qquad\qquad (6\text{--}16) $$

where $\overline{d}_{..k}$ and $SD_{..k}$ represent the mean and standard deviation of the set of difference values, respectively shown in Figure 6–14, and n is the number of pairs from which the difference values were obtained. The test statistic is based on n − 1 degrees of freedom (df).

In the case of the difference matrix (Fig. 6–14), the mean difference for all 74 values, $\overline{d}_{..k}$, is −3.08 ± 6.38 dB. The t score is

$$t = \frac{-3.08}{\frac{6.38}{\sqrt{74}}} = \frac{-3.08}{.742} = 4.15 \qquad (6-17)$$

which suggests that the thresholds for examinations 1 and 2 are not the same ($P = .05$, df = 73, critical value = 1.991).

DESCRIPTION OF THE CONFIDENCE INTERVAL

The confidence interval for the paired t-test is the range within which the true difference between the two examinations is expected to fall. The exact definition for the confidence level is

$$\overline{d}_{..k} \pm t_{\alpha/2} \times \frac{SD_{..k}}{\sqrt{n}} \qquad (6-18)$$

where all symbols are as described in Equation 6–16 and $t_{\alpha/2}$ indicates the t-score (1.99) corresponding to the desired confidence level ($\alpha = 0.05$) using a two-tailed test.

Consider the example from Figure 16–14 showing a difference table from the Octopus DELTA change mode. The mean of difference values ($\overline{d}_{..k}$) is −3.08 dB with a standard deviation ($SD_{..k}$) of 6.38 dB and the number of difference pairs (n) is 74. The confidence interval is

$$-3.08 \pm t_{\alpha/2} \times \frac{6.38}{\sqrt{74}} \qquad (6-19)$$

At the 95 percent level of confidence ($\alpha = 0.05$) the $t_{\alpha/2}$ value is 1.99. (This value is obtained from a table of t-scores and assumes a two-tailed test and n − 1, degrees of freedom.) The resulting confidence interval therefore is

$$-3.08 \pm 1.99 \times \frac{6.38}{\sqrt{74}}$$
$$-3.08 \pm 1.48 \qquad (6-20)$$

and is printed at the bottom of the printout in Figure 16–14. The actual confidence interval therefore ranges from −4.56 to −1.60.

INTERPRETATION OF THE CONFIDENCE INTERVAL

The confidence interval (−4.56 to −1.60) statistically speaking has a 95 percent chance of including the true mean threshold difference between examination 1 and examination 2. Because this interval does not contain 0, the "zero hypothesis" described above is rejected in favor of the conclusion that the data tend to indicate that threshold values between the two examinations are (on the average) not the same. That is, alteration is indicated. The direction of the alteration is negative suggesting progression of sensitivity loss from one examination to the other.

LIMITATIONS OF THE T-TEST

By definition, the paired t-test limits the comparison to only two examinations or groups of examinations. When using the paired t-test to compare fields the physician is often faced with the arbitrary decision of deciding which of several alternative examinations should be compared. Further, data from comparisons of only two examinations are not sufficient to make inferences regarding either a trend in the visual field or a change in the underlying physiologic mechanisms.

A statistically significant difference between two field examinations does not necessarily imply that the change in sensitivity was due to a corresponding change in the underlying physiologic mechanisms of eye disease. For example, it might be argued that the significant difference between the two examinations as indicated by the paired t-test may be due to changes in some type of *experimental error* or artifact instead of true physiologic changes. The t-test provides no way to discriminate between alternative possible causes for an apparent change in sensitivity or isolate various sources of error. *The complexities of threshold measurements limit the usefulness of the t-test as a statistical technique to probe the effects of true physiologic changes.* Applied properly, however, it does provide one source of information regarding field changes.

COMPARISON OF TWO OR MORE VISUAL FIELDS

Detailed statistical analyses to compare visual fields over time are currently in experimental and developmental stages, and most clinicians do not have access to these techniques. The Octopus DELTA and TREND programs offer the only commercially available descriptive summaries over multiple fields. The long-term analysis problem is demonstrated in Figures 6–15 through 6–20 which show Octopus field examinations for a glaucoma patient over a 3-year period. The fields are approximately 6 months apart. Grey scales, value tables, and comparison printmodes (Octopus) are shown for each examination in these figures. For this patient the grey scales are sufficient to conclude that the defect has increased in both area and depth during this period. However, in more subtle clinical cases the change over time may not be so clear and more quantitative documentation will be required. The series mode of the Octopus DELTA program packages both the grey scales and a few summary statistics for each field over time on a single page. The six fields shown on Figures 6–15 to 6–20 are summarized on Figure 6–21. Each column in Figure 6–21 contains a set of summary statistics that describe a separate examination. The last column combines all examinations into a composite summary. Each row contains a type of field index that describes some aspect of the field.

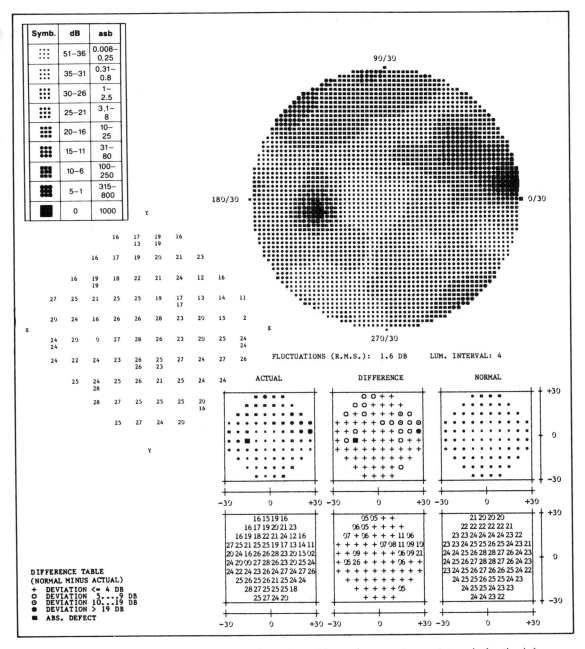

Figure 6–15. *Octopus grey scale, value table, and comparison printmode for the left eye program 32. Examination 1: 8/26/1980.*

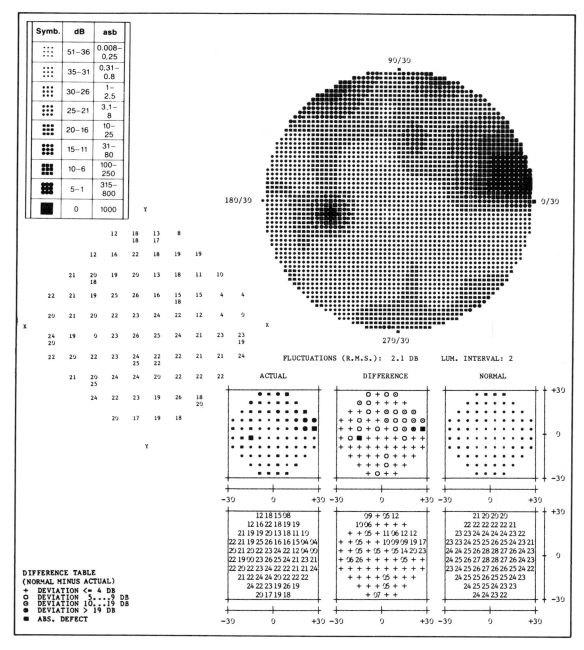

Figure 6–16. *Octopus grey scale, value table, and comparison printmode for the left eye program 32. Examination 2: 7/14/1981.*

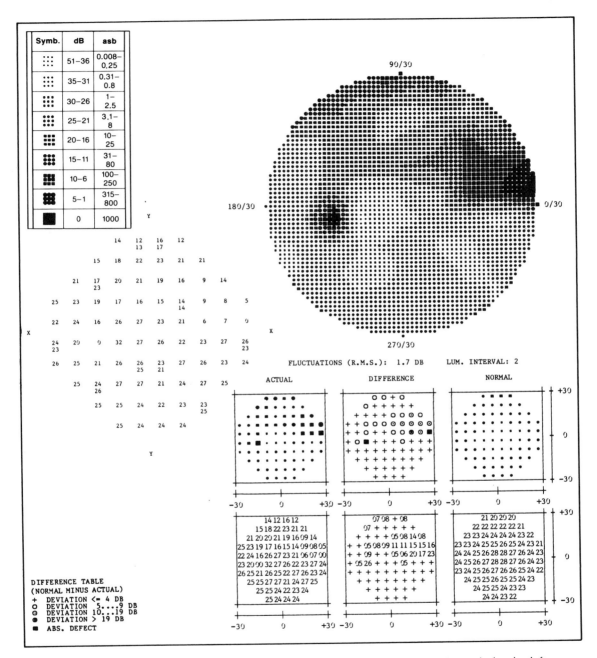

Figure 6–17. *Octopus grey scale, value table, and comparison printmode for the left eye program 32. Examination 3: 4/8/1982.*

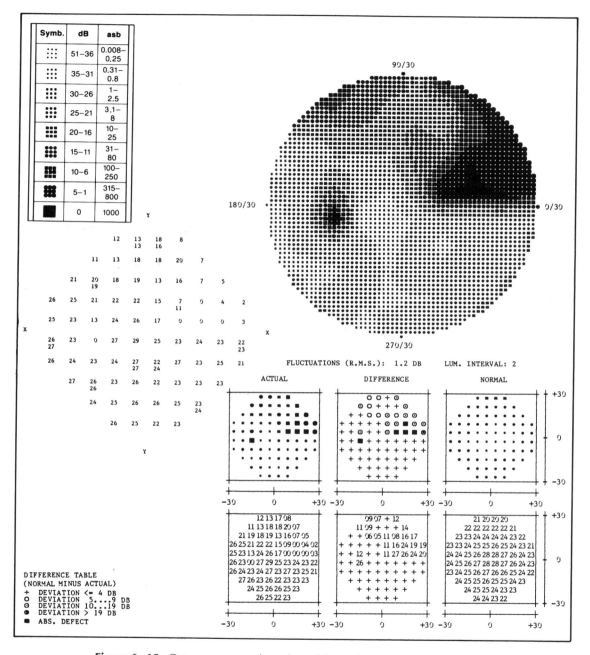

Figure 6–18. *Octopus grey scale, value table, and comparison printmode for the left eye program 32. Examination 4: 10/19/1982.*

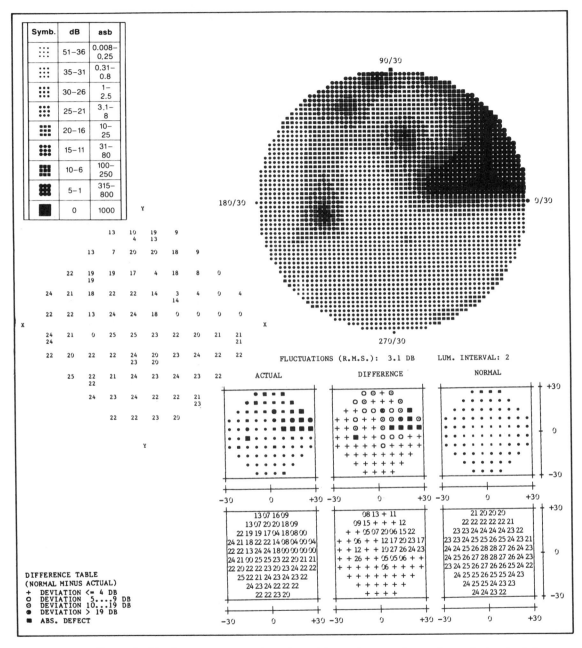

Figure 6–19. *Octopus grey scale, value table, and comparison printmode for the left eye program 32. Examination 5: 3/22/1983.*

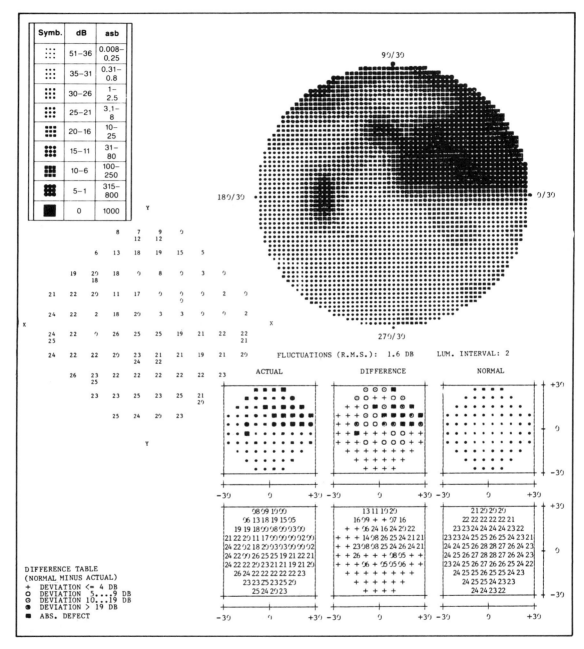

Figure 6–20. *Octopus grey scale, value table, and comparison printmode for the left eye program 32. Examination 6: 2/21/1984.*

	EX1	EX2	EX3	EX4	EX5	EX6	SUMMARY
DATE OF EXAM : DAY	26.08	07.14	04.08	10.19	03.22	02.21	
YEAR	1980	1981	1982	1982	1983	1984	
PROGRAM / EXAMINATION	32/01	32/03	32/05	32/06	32/07	32/09	
PUPIL SIZE (MM)	4	3	4	4	5	5	
TOTAL LOSS (WHOLE FIELD)	148	252	236	370	322	524	308 ± 53
MEAN LOSS (PER TEST LOC)							
WHOLE FIELD	2.0	3.4	3.2	5.0	4.3	7.1	4.2 ± 0.7
QUADRANT UPPER NASAL	5.2	9.7	9.6	15.0	14.5	19.6	12.2 ± 2.1
LOWER NASAL	0.6	0.8	0.3	1.2	0.0	1.5	0.7 ± 0.2
UPPER TEMP.	1.9	2.2	2.4	3.5	2.6	6.5	3.2 ± 0.7
LOWER TEMP.	0.3	0.7	0.3	0.0	0.0	0.3	0.3 ± 0.1
ECCENTRICITY 0 - 10	0.6	1.7	3.0	5.4	4.1	9.3	4.0 ± 1.3
10 - 20	2.1	3.8	4.0	6.3	5.3	10.1	5.3 ± 1.1
20 - 30	2.4	3.7	2.9	4.4	4.0	5.3	3.8 ± 0.4
MEAN SENSITIVITY							
WHOLE FIELD (N: 24.1)	21.8	19.1	20.7	17.8	19.2	16.0	19.1 ± 0.8
QUAD.UPP.NAS.(N: 23.4)	17.6	13.1	13.6	7.9	8.5	3.7	10.7 ± 2.0
LOW.NAS.(N: 24.4)	23.8	21.6	24.1	22.1	23.5	21.6	22.8 ± 0.5
UPP.TMP.(N: 23.5)	20.9	19.9	20.1	18.7	19.9	15.8	19.2 ± 0.7
LOW.TMP.(N: 25.1)	25.1	22.1	25.1	22.8	25.4	23.4	24.0 ± 0.6
ECC. 0 - 10 (N: 26.9)	25.1	23.1	23.5	20.0	21.5	16.7	21.6 ± 1.2
10 - 20 (N: 24.9)	22.0	19.8	20.2	17.4	18.5	13.8	18.6 ± 1.2
20 - 30 (N: 23.0)	20.9	17.8	20.1	17.3	18.9	16.8	18.6 ± 0.7
NO. OF DISTURBED POINTS	19	26	23	27	22	34	25 ± 2
R.M.S. FLUCTUATION	1.6	2.1	1.7	3.1	1.2	1.6	1.9
TOTAL FLUCTUATION							3.1

Figure 6–21. Octopus DELTA printout (series mode) showing summary statistics for the examinations in Figures 6–15 through 6–20. Pupil size has been added to machine printout.

The first statistic of interest is the "RMS fluctuation." As explained earlier, this statistic provides an estimate of measurement (short-term) error. A simple overview of the RMS values for this patient is sufficient to confirm that the fluctuation is generally around 2 dB (1.97 dB) and documents that the examinations are similar with respect to short-term error.

Total fluctuation, on the bottom line of Figure 6–21, provides an estimate of threshold variation that includes both short-term and long-term variations. That is, total fluctuation is an estimate of how much all thresholds on all examinations differed from each other. Notice that the total fluctuation (3.1 dB) is larger than the average RMS (fluctuation (1.97 dB). This implies that the long-term changes suspected from the grey scales are due in part to physiologic causes rather than short-term measurement error.

The set of numbers labeled "mean sensitivity" provides overall averages of field results (see the "Mean Sensitivity" section). If the values for each of the four field quadrants were plotted over time, the reader would readily see that the defect changed more in the two upper quadrants than in the two lower quadrants, and most in the upper nasal quadrant. This type of analysis allows the clinician to identify most active and most stable regions of the field.

The top set of statistics provides the "Loss Summaries." As explained earlier in this chapter, loss statistics (as defined for the Octopus) compare each observed value with an expected value based on a population average sensitivity corrected by age. An example of two "loss matrices" is shown in Table 6–6. In fact, the two examinations dated 7/14/81 and 2/21/84 correspond to the second and sixth columns on Figure 6–21 as well as Figures 6–16 and 6–20. Total loss is the sum of all loss scores greater than 4.0 (excluding two points in the blind spot area). Therefore total loss is determined by adding the values greater than four in the loss matrices shown in Table 6–6 or Figures 6–16 and 6–20. The total loss (dB) for each of the six examinations is shown in the row labeled "total loss (whole field)" in Figure 6–21. In general for this patient, field loss has accelerated from 148 dB (examination 1) to 524 dB (examination 6).

Mean loss (per test location) indicates the average loss score for either the whole field or for each of several subsections of the field. If average loss is plotted over time for each of the four field quadrants it can be seen that the increase in loss is greatest in the upper nasal quadrant and minimal in the lower temporal quadrant. As in the case of the sensitivity statistics, the loss statistics document the qualitative impression from the grey scales.

Although Octopus is to date the only automated field testing device that compares multiple fields over time, the user can easily calculate similar values to describe the dynamic status of any set of fields over some time for any machine. It must be kept in mind, however, that each field index is associated with some error that must be taken into account along with the index. Quantification of a field or group of fields provides invaluable (and previously unattainable) field information. However, field indices can do no more than provide documentation for making a clinical decision.

References

1. Bebie H, Fankhauser F, Spahr J: Static perimetry accuracy and fluctuation. Acta Ophthalmol 54:339–348, 1976.
2. Visual Field Atlas, ed 2. Schlieron, Switzerland, Interzeag AG, 1978, p 28.
3. Bebie H, Fankhauser F: Program DELTA (Handbook for operation and application of the Octopus DELTA program) Schlieron, Switzerland, Interzeag AG, 1981.
4. Snedecor GW, Cochran WC: Statistical Methods, ed 7. Iowa State University Press, Ames, Iowa, 1981.

7

How to Read a Visual Field Report

Much information is given in an automated visual field report, the printout of a visual field examination provides information on the type of equipment used, testing strategies, areas of normal and abnormal responses, and estimates of reliability. Depending on the methods used and output formats, much of this information can be confusing or even misleading. Often this information is given in a form that is unfamiliar to many practitioners. Therefore, it is important when approaching the visual field report from an automated or manual machine to have an organized method of reading the field to be able to extract and utilize this information. The physician must know the limitations of the testing method, the testing conditions, and any other factors that would affect the outcome of the visual field report. The visual field must be read in the context of previous visual field examinations done on that patient and in the context of the patient's other medical findings.

WANDER—A Systematic Approach

Rather than wandering aimlessly through reams of confusing data, we propose that the reader use a mnemonic WANDER to look at visual field reports in an organized fashion asking the following questions:

1. **W** *What* was done?
2. **A** How *accurate* are the results?
3. **N** Is the field *normal* or abnormal?
4. **D** If the field is abnormal, what kind of *defects* are present?

5. **E** *Evaluate* the visual field results and ask the question: "What disease processes are suggested by the defects that are present?"
6. **R** *Reevaluate* the visual field in terms of previous visual field examinations performed on the patient (DELTA analysis) and in the context of the patient's overall medical condition asking the question: "What conclusions can be drawn?"

QUESTION 1

WHAT Was Done?

It is important to know everything possible about the visual field testing situation. Was the visual field performed by a manual machine or an automated machine? If manual, which manual method was used, and if automated, which automated machine was used? Which software program was used and which options were used in that software program? Which areas of the visual field were tested and which areas were not tested? How intensely was each area tested (how many test spots) and were some areas tested more intensely than other areas? Was a lens correction used and what was the size of the pupil when the test was done?

All of these factors are very important. Standardization is certainly necessary for comparison. Changes in pupil size can cause changes in the appearance of the visual field and a small pupil can accentuate the effect of cataractous changes. If a lens correction is necessary and it was not used, the resulting visual field will be less accurate. If areas of the visual field are studied with a great number of spots, the results will obviously be more accurate in those areas. If a pure suprathreshold strategy is used, there will be no information concerning the depth of a defect; the breadth measured will be only the breadth to that particular testing intensity. If only the central field is tested, no conclusions will be able to be drawn about the peripheral field. Likewise, if only the right half of the visual field is tested, no conclusions can be drawn concerning the left half of the visual field.

QUESTION 2

How ACCURATE Are the Results?

It is most important to know the accuracy of the results of the visual field test. In manual visual field examinations, there should be a comment by the technician. The technician should note the patient's mental state, level of alertness, regions of inconsistent responses, and the ability or inability of the patient to maintain fixation.

In an automated visual field test, different information, depending on the machine and the software program, is provided that can be used to gauge accuracy. Commonly the number of fixation losses is noted; the higher the number, the more inaccurate the field. If information was thrown out that was obtained during the period of presumed fixation loss, however, the field results will be more accurate.

The root mean square (RMS) value indicates how consistent the responses were in a threshold examination at specific points. False-positive and false-negative ratings are good gauges of the consistency of a patient's responses.

A high RMS value, a large number of fixation losses, a large number of false-positive responses, and/or a large number of false-negative responses would indicate that the field results are somewhat inaccurate. Conversely, a low RMS value, a low number of fixation losses, a low number of false-positives, and/or a low number of false-negatives would indicate a more reliable visual field examination. A thorough discussion of the use of reliability factors is presented in Chapter 6.

QUESTION 3

Is the Field NORMAL or Abnormal?

Some visual field testing software will compare the patient's responses to preestablished "normal" results. Other software leaves this task to the examiner. If the software compares test results with "normals" and the logic used by the software is acceptable to the examiner, then the software's measurement of deviation from normal can be used.

Reference documentation for software can be consulted when "normal" information is not automatically provided. For example, the documentation for some suprathreshold or threshold-related software will indicate the testing intensities that most normal patients should be able to see. If the patient has diffuse difficulty at these intensity levels, then there is overall depression. If the patient has localized difficulty only, then a defect is indicated in that particular area.

QUESTION 4

If the Field Is Abnormal, What Kind of DEFECTS Are Present?

The question "What form did the visual field defects take?" should be asked after the field test has been performed on both eyes. Were the defects in the central portion of the field, the arcuate area, or the periphery? Were the defects on the right side of the visual field or the left side of the visual field? Were the defects shallow or were they deep? Were similar defects present in the both eyes?

Defects found should be classified as central, cecocentral, arcuate, peripheral, or combined. Defects should be classified further as to whether they are superior or inferior and whether they are right or left. After a description is given for each eye, the defects should be evaluated in a binocular fashion to determine if the defects are homonymous, if they are bitemporal, or if they are binasal.

Sensitivity statistics and loss statistics, if provided, can also be used to differentiate and define localized and generalized loss. These are discussed in Chapter 6.

QUESTION 5

The EVALUATION of Visual Field Defects

On the basis of the description of the visual field defects, what disease processes are suggested? At this point the field defects have to be categorized.

Defects pointing to the blind spot imply optic nerve or retinal vascular disease. Defects pointing to the macula imply macular, chiasmal, or postchiasmal disease. Homonymous defects frequently imply neurologic disease.

If the patient is being evaluated for glaucoma or if glaucoma is being considered, are classic glaucomatous defects such as an enlarged blind spot, a nasal step, central or arcuate area defects or constriction noted? If the patient is being evaluated for a neurologic defect, is the defect present in both eyes, is it right sided, left sided, bitemporal, binasal, located superiorly, or located inferiorly? How congruous are the defects?

The examiner should ask himself or herself if the pattern of field loss is most suggestive of neurologic, glaucomatous, or retinal disease. The presence of opacities in the media, miotic pupils, or uncorrected refractive errors must be ruled out.

QUESTION 6

REEVALUATION of the Visual Fields

The visual field should be evaluated in the context of previous visual field examinations done on the same patient and in the context of the patient's medical signs and symptoms. For example, a patient with a headache who is shown to have a bitemporal visual field defect needs to be evaluated for the presence of a tumor in the area of the chiasm. A patient who has an afferent pupillary defect accompanied by an ipsilateral visual field defect needs to be worked up for optic nerve disease. A patient who is being followed for elevated intraocular pressure, who has had previously normal visual fields to the same testing strategy, and who now has visual field defects, needs to be evaluated for the onset of glaucoma.

It is also important to evaluate the visual field in the context of the patient's present medical findings and the patient's past medical history. In evaluating a visual field from one point in time to the next, automated techniques can yield extremely valuable and accurate information.

The examiner needs to be careful in evaluating a change in the visual fields if a new testing method shows apparent changes. For example, a patient with glaucoma who has had stable tangent screen examinations might now be examined with an automated device and found to have additional, previously unrecorded, visual field defects. He or she might not have new defects, however. These defects might have gone undetected by the previous visual field testing strategy. It is important, therefore, when evaluating changes in the visual field, to repeat the previous method of testing the visual field prior to using a new method.

Using W A N D E R

When using WANDER to evaluate a visual field, the strengths and weaknesses of a particular visual field testing strategy can immediately be noted. Some visual field testing strategies do not enable measurements of accuracy to be made. Strategies that test more areas of the visual field and test them more intensely will obviously give more complete reports than strategies that only test a small area of the field or test it superficially. DELTA examination methods, which facilitate the automated comparison of data from one examination to the next, allow for more accurate comparisons to be made. These must be interpreted, however, with caution.

Each type of automated visual field examination provides valuable data. It is necessary to be careful not to over read or under read the field reports. Having an organized method of asking the important questions each time a field is examined helps to guard against misreading fields. It also helps to extract both the information present and the information not present that might be obtained by a different approach to study that particular field such as repeating the field or using additional testing strategies.

The following examples demonstrate how WANDER is used for evaluating different types of automated field reports.

EXAMPLE 1

1. W   What Was Done?
The patient had a Dicon AP 2000 two-zone stepped suprathreshold visual field performed on the left eye (Fig. 7–1). Standard settings (31.5 asb background illumination, 0.4-second stimulus duration, and 1.0-second stimulus interval) were used. The starting intensity was 100 asb. A Heijl-Krakau fixation monitoring technique was used.

2. A   Was the Field Accurate?
The patient had six fixation losses, however, all points tested during periods of possible fixation loss were retested. Because the test could be completed without having to turn the fixation monitor from normal to off, the field can be presumed to be accurate. The Dicon two-zone program does not measure an RMS and does not have catch trials, however, the Heijl-Krakau fixation monitoring system is a type of catch trial.

3. N   Was the Field Normal?
The field was not normal; there were many missed points. If the field were normal there would be only a few scattered missed points.

4. D   What Defects Are Present?
There was mild loss in the superior arcuate area and denser loss in the inferior

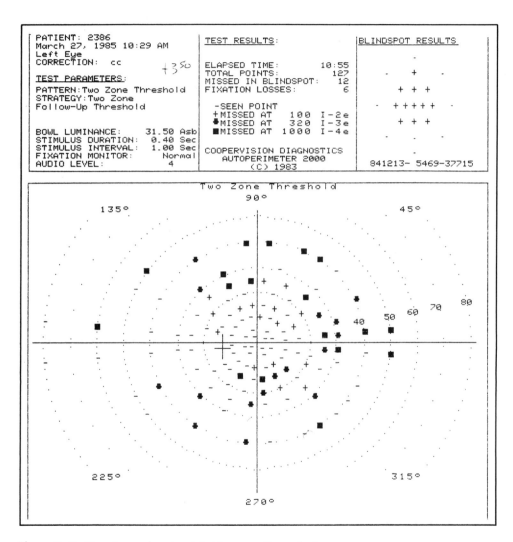

Figure 7–1. *How to read a visual field report: Example 1.*

arcuate area. There is also some peripheral loss (constriction) especially supero-nasally, with the formation of a superior nasal step.

5. E Evaluation of Visual Field Defects
Arcuate area loss, a nasal step, and peripheral constriction are all characteristic of glaucomatous visual field loss.

6. R Reevaluation of the Visual Fields
The patient is a glaucoma patient who has been under treatment with topical medications. The IOP has been stable at 17. Examination of the disc shows glaucomatous cupping that had not changed from previous examinations. Comparison of this visual field examination with previous studies shows no evidence of change (improvement or worsening). Therefore, it can be concluded that the field shows unchanging glaucomatous visual field loss and that the patient's glaucoma is under control in this eye.

EXAMPLE 2

1. W What Was Done?
A central 30-degree field study was performed on each eye on a Fieldmaster model 200 (Fig. 7–2). Program 4 (which tests all spots inside 30 degrees) was used. Test spots were white, their intensity was set at 44 asb, they had a 0.8-second duration, and there was a 0.9-second interval. The Fieldmaster 200 uses a suprathreshold strategy, so only one test spot intensity was used, but missed spots were automatically rechecked. Background intensity was 31.5 asb. The Synemed mosaic monitor was used and was set at −2.

2. A Was the Field Accurate?
There were no specific accuracy measurements. If fixation had been lost, the study could not have been completed, however, because the mosaic monitor was used and not turned off. Therefore, the results are probably accurate.

3. N Was the Field Normal?
The field is not normal. Many spots were missed by each eye.

4. D What Defects Are Present?
A right-sided field loss is seen in the right eye and a left-sided field loss is seen in the left eye.

5. E Evaluation of Visual Field Defects
A superior Chamlin step is seen in each eye. Furthermore, the loss is bitemporal. Therefore, the patient has a superior bitemporal hemianopsia.

6. R Reevaluation of the Visual Fields
The pateint had a visual field study because of slightly decreased, visual acuity (20/30 o.u.) and headaches. A bitemporal hemianopsia is suggestive of a lesion in the area of the optic chiasm.

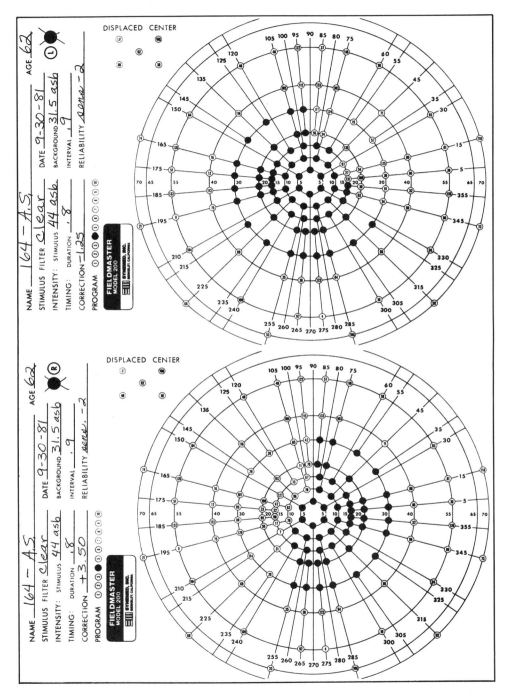

Figure 7–2. How to read a visual field report: Example 2.

8

The Visual Field in Glaucoma

It is essential to have exacting visual field studies to properly manage most glaucoma patients. Due to the new technology introduced in visual field testing, the ability of automated devices to pick up subtle visual field defects and to monitor these defects is unsurpassed. Perhaps the greatest potential for automated visual field testing lies in the diagnosis and management of the glaucoma patient.

The study of the visual field in the glaucoma patient can be divided into two phases—first, detection and second, assessment. In the detection phase we are dealing with the glaucoma suspect, the patient with an abnormal looking disk or an elevated intraocular pressure who might have glaucoma. If a visual field defect characteristic of glaucoma is found during this phase, the patient's field testing enters the assessment phase.

In the assessment phase the exact depth and breadth of each visual field defect is outlined. The defects are then studied from one examination to the next to determine whether or not the visual field is changing. A stable, unchanging visual field is usually regarded as an indication of adequate therapy. Recent studies have suggested, however, that the field of some glaucoma patients will improve slightly if the pressure is adequately treated,[1] although this still remains controversial.

Both examination of the fundus and examination of the visual field are important in the glaucoma patient. Whether changes can be noticed first in the visual field or in the appearance of the nerve head in glaucoma has long been debated. However, it is unusual for changes in the appearance of the nerve head to be appreciated without a corresponding change in the patient's visual field if the field examination is sufficiently rigorous. Furthermore, the normal variations of the disk make it difficult to decide whether some disks are pathologic or not, especially if the abnormalities are subtle. Therefore, a change in the appearance of the disk is more important than the initial appearance of the disk. Perhaps, as more exacting computerized video ophthalmoscopes are developed, disk changes will be discernible before visual field changes. With the present state of the art, however, visual field changes usually are the best and the most sensitive method of detecting glaucomatous damage.

The Nerve Fiber Bundle Defect

The basic form of visual field loss in glaucoma is the nerve fiber bundle defect. Such a defect follows the outlines of the nerve fiber bundles as they emerge from the optic nerve head. As a general rule, all glaucomatous field defects can be considered to point toward the optic nerve head or lie within nerve fiber bundles pointing toward the optic nerve head.

The nerve fiber bundle defect can take many forms. A scotoma may follow any nerve fiber bundle or group of bundles. It can arch very close to fixation or it can be away from fixation. Theoretically, it can even be wedge-shaped if it involves the nasal nerve fiber bundles. It may begin at the blind spot and extend for all or part of the nerve fiber bundle or it may be isolated within the nerve fiber bundle. It can look like a ring scotoma if both upper and lower nerve fiber bundles are affected, however, usually a step-like difference in the superior and inferior portions of the ring can be revealed with careful study. Usually a nerve fiber defect bundle will present as either (1) a nasal step, (2) a small scotoma in the arcuate Bjerrum area, (3) an enlargement of the blind spot, (4) a full arcuate scotoma, (5) peripheral depression, (6) central depression, or (7) generalized depression.

Visual Field Depression and Blind Spot Enlargement

It has long been recognized that an early sign of glaucoma is generalized depression of the visual field. Depression can involve the entire visual field or can be confined to just the peripheral or central fields (Fig. 8–1).

Peripheral depression is commonly seen in glaucomatous visual fields. It presents first in the nasal quadrants. If the nasal depression has a clear-cut delineation on the horizontal, a peripheral nasal step will be formed. The depression can occur either supranasally or infranasally, but is more common superiorly. Some investigators have found these types of peripheral loss to be the presenting visual field defect in many glaucoma patients. Eventually the peripheral depression coalesces with loss in the arcuate areas.

Enlargement of the blind spot frequently accompanies peripheral depression. Often this can be seen as baring of the blind spot superiorly, inferiorly, or both superiorly and inferiorly (Fig. 8–2). Baring of the blind spot means that the size of the blind spot has enlarged and, that to appropriate test objects, there is selective constriction of the visual field in the area of the blind spot.

Although baring of the blind spot can be one of the earliest changes that is seen in glaucoma, a false baring of the blind spot can be seen in normal patients. It has been shown by Drance,[2] and also by Aulhorn and Harms,[3] that the area surrounding the blind spot has a flat slope. Therefore test spots, if appropriately chosen, can be made to bare the blind spot in almost any patient. A target that formerly did not bare the blind spot can subsequently be shown to bare the blind spot from extraneous factors that affect visual field results such as miosis, an uncorrected refractive error, a lens opacity, or aging.

Other nonglaucomatous lesions can cause blind spot enlargement. These include papilledema, peripapillary atrophy, optic nerve drusen, tilted discs, colombomata, and myelinated nerve fibers.

Arcuate Area Defects

Many investigators have reported that the most common early visual defect in eyes with open-angle glaucoma is a paracentral scotoma in the arcuate area (between 10 and 25 degrees). It usually first presents as an isolated defect separated from the blind spot (Fig. 8–3). Later it can connect to the blind spot forming an arcuate scotoma (Figs. 8–4, 8–5, and 8–6).

The arcuate scotoma classically starts at the blind spot and extends in an arcuate fashion to the horizontal meridian on the other side of fixation (Fig. 8–7). It tends to form a band that is wider when it reaches the opposite horizontal meridian than it is when it starts. It is located in the area between 10 and 20 degrees from fixation, conforms to the anatomic nerve fiber bundle, and ends as a nasal step (Fig. 8–8). These defects can occur both above and below the horizontal. They can be symmetrical or asymmetrical. As they become more advanced they tend to extend into the periphery (Figs. 8–9, 8–10, and 8–12) and/or the center (Figs. 8–11, 8–13, and 8–14).

The presence of this type of defect has been known for many years. It was first described in 1856 by Von Graefe[4] and was later studied by Bjerrum in 1889.[5] Roenne was the first to call attention to the nasal step feature of this defect.[6]

Other names that have been used to describe the arcuate scotoma are Bjerrum scotoma, comet scotoma, and scimitar scotoma. When scotomas connect to the blind spot and extend both above and below the midline, a crescent-shaped defect is formed which has been called Seidel's scotoma (Figs. 8–5 and 8–8).

The presence of an arcuate scotoma in a visual field is not pathognomonic for glaucoma although the vast majority of such defects are caused by glaucoma. Other diseases that will produce similar appearing defects are summarized in Table 8–1.

TABLE 8-1. NONGLAUCOMATOUS CAUSES OF ARCUATE SCOTOMAS

A. Lesions of the disk
   1. juxtapapillary choroiditis
   2. myopia
   3. colobomas and pits of the optic nerve head
   4. drusen on the optic nerve
   5. papillaedema with increased intracranal pressure
   6. optic atrophy secondary to papillaedema
   7. papillitis
   8. a retinal arterial plaque on the disk
   9. papillaedema from malignant hypertension
   10. occlusion of a branch of the central retinal artery

B. Lesions of the anterior nerve
   1. ischemic optic neuropathy
   2. occlusion of the carotid or ophthalmic arteries
   3. branch retinal artery occlusion
   4. cerebral arteritis
   5. retrobulbar neuritis
   6. electric shock
   7. exophthalmos
   8. postpapilledema optic atrophy
   9. congenital optic nerve dysplasia

C. Lesions in the posterior nerve and chiasm
   1. meningiomas at the optic foramen and the dorsum sellae
   2. pituitary adenoma
   3. opticochiasmatic arachnoiditis

The Progression of Glaucomatous Visual Field Defects

Early glaucomatous visual field loss has certain important characteristics. Loss in the arcuate area tends to occur first superiorly (Fig. 8–16). Early on scotomas tend to be rather round, elongating as they become more advanced. As they enlarge, small scotomas tend to coalesce, extend peripherally, and extend centrally (Fig. 8–15). Paracentral scotomas as isolated defects, nasal steps, and peripheral depression are all seen commonly (Figs. 8–17 and 8–18). The most important factor affecting the progression of visual field loss in glaucoma is the extent of preexisting field loss. Therefore, the greater the amount of field loss, the more religiously a patient needs to be followed.

As visual field loss in glaucoma becomes more advanced, certain areas of the visual field tend to be the last to disappear. A tiny central area of vision usually remains. Visual acuity may remain at 20/20 in this small remaining central field even if the field defect is within a degree or two of fixation. The remaining central field tends to be oval in shape. The longest diameter is horizontal and it extends over the centrocecal area, often with a very small nasal step. The margins of this remaining visual field tend to be steep (Fig. 8–19). When the remaining visual field is lost, it is usually lost first on the nasal side. When the final central island of the visual field is lost, the loss tends to be sudden. A small island of temperoperipheral field also tends to remain (Fig. 8–21). This frequently persists even after the central visual field is lost. (Fig. 8–20). In some patients, all or most of the central field is lost while a relatively large portion of the peripheral field still remains (Fig. 8–22).

Angioscotomas in Glaucoma

The angioscotoma pattern has been noted by Evans to alter in the development of glaucoma.[7] Using his technique, very early widening and intensification of the angioscotomas and coalescence of the angioscotomas are seen to occur. Traditionally these have been demonstrated on a tangent screen at a distance of 2 m with a 1-mm test stimulus. The technique is difficult and time consuming. Therefore, clinicians usually do not look for angioscotomas, but rather rely on other defects in the field to diagnose and follow glaucoma patients.

Low-Tension Glaucoma

Low-tension glaucoma is an entity in which typical changes of glaucoma in the optic nerve and visual field occur despite an apparently "normal" intraocular pressure. It should be remembered that the progression of glaucoma is not due to a magic intraocular pressure level being exceeded; progression is due to the intraocular pressure level that a particular patient can safely tolerate being exceeded. Patients with low-tension glaucoma, therefore, can be considered to be patients who have a very low threshold for damage from elevated intraocular pressure (Fig. 8–23).

The paradox of glaucoma with a low intraocular pressure has inspired much research. Most researchers have felt that the pattern of visual field loss is identical in glaucoma with increased intraocular pressure and in low-tension glaucoma. Some have described the visual field defects in low tension glaucoma as being denser and closer to fixation. Recently, it has been suggested that scotomas in the low-tension group have a steeper slope, are closer to fixation, and are of greater depth.[8,9] These differences suggest that glaucomatous changes at higher intraocular pressure levels are mediated on a more mechanical basis and glaucomatous changes at lower intraocular pressure levels are mediated on a more vascular basis.

The Pathogenesis of Visual Field Loss in Glaucoma

The generally accepted etiology of visual field defects in glaucoma is that they are the result of diminished blood flow in the anterior optic nerve head in the region of the lamina cribrosa, the arterial circle of Zinn-Haller, or the peripapillary choroidal circulation. Increased intraocular pressure sufficient to overcome the normal arterial pressure in these arterioles can cause local hypoxia. A similar situation can be caused by decreased blood pressure in the ophthalmic artery. Obstruction to flow in the carotid artery from stenosis, occlusion, or arteriosclerotic plaques can lead to similar problems as can arterial insufficiency from embolic phenomenon. The sudden appearance of visual field defects of the nerve fiber bundle type similar to those seen in glaucoma have been reported after the rapid lowering of systemic blood pressure. Similar defects have been temporarily produced in patients with carotid insufficiency after the intraocular pressure is artificially increased with an ophthalmodynamometer.

Often a change in the visual field in a glaucoma patient, even a patient thought to be under good control, is accompanied by a small nerve fiber layer hemorrhage adjacent to the disk in the corresponding nerve fiber bundle. This hemorrhage is felt to be due to an acute ischemic change in the nerve head and will usually go on to lead to increased glaucomatous disk cupping and atrophy after it resolves. This tends to support the vascular ischemia theory of glaucomatous visual field loss. Certainly as our visual field techniques improve and become more exacting, and our ability to study the circulation of the eye and changes in cupping also improve, the correlation of these studies will lead to a better understanding of the pathogenesis of glaucomatous visual field loss.

The Visual Field in the Diagnosis and Management of Glaucoma

The visual field is vitally important in making the diagnosis of glaucoma, especially in cases where that diagnosis is questionable. Visual field loss needs to be evaluated in the light of other clinical findings, including optic disk cupping, nerve fiber layer atrophy, increased intraocular pressure, decreased facility of aqueous outflow, gonioscopic evidence of changes in the angle of the anterior chamber, color vision testing, and history. It is important to rule out other causes of visual field loss that could complicate evaluation of the field (Figs. 8–24 and 8–25).

Treatment in glaucoma should aim at least to maintain the visual field. Improvement in the visual field has been noted recently in successfully treated patients (Fig. 8–26).[1] This phenomenon, although not dramatic, has been rediscovered many times through history. With automated techniques the significance of this phenomenon should become more apparent in the near future.

It is important to use the same visual field testing plan from one visit to the next in a glaucoma patient. This enables subtle changes and trends to be recognized at the earliest possible stage. When a new technique is used, the old technique should also be repeated at least on the first follow-up examination. If there are any questionable changes, the old technique should be repeated on subsequent examinations, too. This allows for an orderly transition and insures that the recognition of a change will not be delayed because of confusion in interpreting results from different testing methods. Failure to adhere to this can cause needless loss of field (Fig. 8–27).

The principle of orderly transition is important regardless of whether a practitioner is converting from one form of manual visual field testing to another, from manual visual field testing to automated visual field testing, from automated visual field testing on one type of machine to automated visual field testing on another type of machine, or from one automated visual field testing software program on a particular machine to a different software program on the same machine.

When the diagnosis of glaucoma has been established, attention should be placed on evaluating visual fields for change. Ideally, this is done with a DELTA or automated program. It can be done manually, however. All visual field defects should be examined for an increase in depth or breadth. All new visual field defects should be noted. All areas of increased constriction or decreased threshold should be noted (Figs. 8–28, 8–29, and 8–30).

Examiners should be careful not to "over read" a new defect. It has been shown that the reliability of visual field measurements in glaucoma patients is decreased in those areas of the visual field affected by the glaucoma.[10] There is a similar but not as severe variability in glaucoma suspect patients. Therefore, even more important than a change from one examination to the next is the confirmation of that change or the confirmation of a trend on subsequent examinations.

Changes in the field can require an alteration in the method of therapy for the patient. Whenever the field changes are questionable or are not accompanied by other changes in clinical signs, the visual field should be repeated after a suitable period of several days or weeks.

It should always be remembered that visual field testing is subjective and not objective. Even though automated machines decrease the number of variables that have to be dealt with in testing technique, the patient's ability to respond can vary from one examination to another due to fatigue, general state of health, anxiety, and drug therapy.

Changes in the patient's eye findings, such as progression of corneal disease, progression of cataract, or the appearance of new vitreous floaters should be ruled out as a cause of the change in the visual field. Pupil size should always be noted when visual field testing is performed as a decrease in the size of the pupillary aperture can lead to increased field loss. This loss is not due to the progression of disease, but rather due to the optical effects of changes in the eye. The value of visual field testing should never be underestimated in glaucoma. It is conceivable, although certainly not desirable, that most glaucoma patients could be managed on the basis of visual field tests alone. The goal in glaucoma therapy should be maintainance of an intraocular pressure low enough to prevent further visual field loss rather than the maintainance of an arbitrary "low" intraocular pressure.

As progress is made in the development of other parameters for following glaucoma and glaucoma-suspect patients, changes in these parameters will be able to be correlated with the progression of visual field changes. Color vision testing and the determination of contrast sensitivity, both subjective tests, hold promise as valuable adjuncts to visual field testing. It has been theorized that a decrease in color perception and a decrease in contrast sensitivity precedes a visual field disturbance. Computer enhanced analysis of the optic disk and the nerve fiber layer of the retina will become an important objective means of following glaucoma patients. Objective tests have a distinct advantage over subjective tests in that they are not affected by intangible factors such as the patient's alertness or ability to sit through an exhausting examination such as visual field testing.

At our present state of knowledge, however, these other tests can only be considered as adjunct tests and cannot replace the visual field examination. Too little is known about the normal changes that take place in contrast sensitivity and color vision perception as a patient ages and the changes that take place in the early stages of glaucoma. Likewise, normal changes in the optic nerve and the nerve fiber layer need to be characterized before pathologic changes from early glaucoma can be separated out.

SPECIAL NOTE CONCERNING THE VISUAL FIELD ILLUSTRATIONS WHICH FOLLOW:

The visual field report from most automated machines is large and requires a full page for adequate presentation of each eye. Also, when examining the visual field of one eye it is useful to be able to view the visual field of the contralateral eye simultaneously. Therefore, we have endeavored, as much as possible, to keep visual field pairs on facing pages with the right eye on the right-hand side and the left eye on the left-hand side. This has necessitated some reordering of the in-text illustration callouts, but we hope that the benefits of being able to study both fields simultaneously will outweigh any inconvenience caused by the ordering.

References

1. Hirsch J, Caprioli J, Sears M: Serial computer directed perimetry of glaucomatous visual fields. Presented at American Academy of Ophthalmology, Chicago, Nov 1983.
2. Drance SM, Wheeler C, Pattulo M: The use of static perimetry in the early detection of glaucoma. Can J Ophthalmol 2:249, 1967.
3. Aulhorn E, Harms H: Early visual field defects in glaucoma, in Glaucoma Symposium, Turzing Castle, 1966, Basel, S. Karger AG, 1967.
4. von Graefe A: Examination of the visual field in amblyopic disease, in Lebensohn

JE (ed): An Anthology of Ophthalmic Classics. Baltimore, Williams & Wilkins, 1969, pp 62–68.

5. Bjerrum JP: An addition to the general examination of the field of vision, in Lebensohn JE (ed): An Anthology of Ophthalmology Classics. Baltimore, Williams & Williams, 1969, pp 74–80.

6. Roenne: Ueber das Gesichtfeld bein Glaukom. Klin Monatsbl f Augenheilk 47:12, 1909.

7. Evans JN: An Introduction to Clinical Scotometry. New Haven, Yale University Press, 1938.

8. Caprioli J, Spaeth G: Comparison of visual field defects in the low-tension glaucomas with those in the high-tension glaucomas. Am J Ophthalmol 97:730–737, 1984.

9. Hitchings RA, Anderton SA: A comparative study of visual field defects seen in patients with low-tension glaucoma and chronic simple glaucoma. Br J Ophthalmol 67:818–821, 1983.

10. Flammer J, Drance SM, Fankhauser F, Augustiny L: Differential light threshold in automated static perimetry. Arch Ophthalmol 102:876–879, 1984.

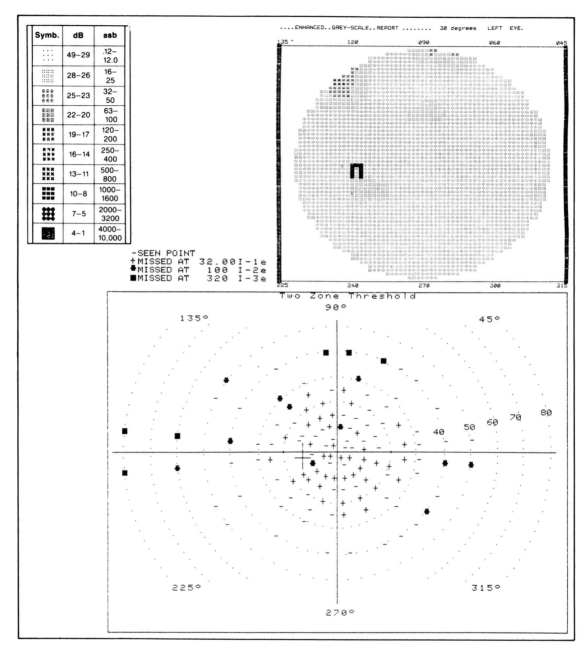

Figure 8–1. *Fifty-two-year-old woman with open-angle glaucoma. Visual fields were tested on a Dicon AP 2000 using the two-zone software with a starting intensity of 32 asb.* **A**. *Left eye shows mild peripheral constriction, distinct central depression, and very distinct inferior arcuate scotoma. (continued)*

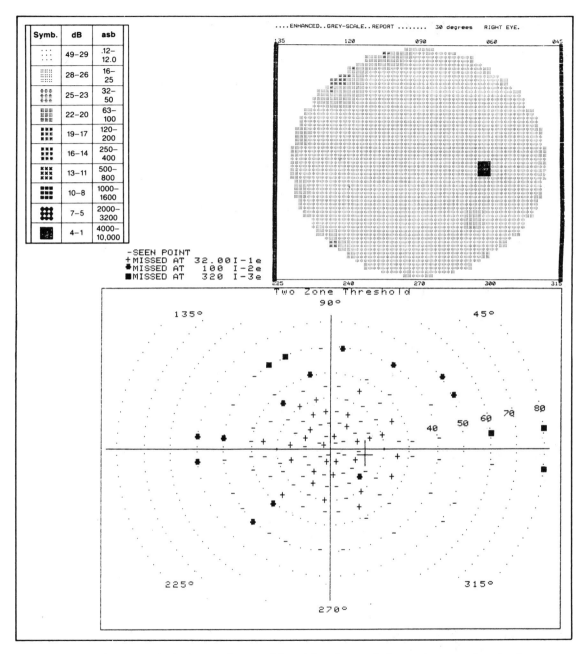

Figure 8–1B. Right eye shows mild peripheral constriction and scattered spots of depression in the central and arcuate areas.

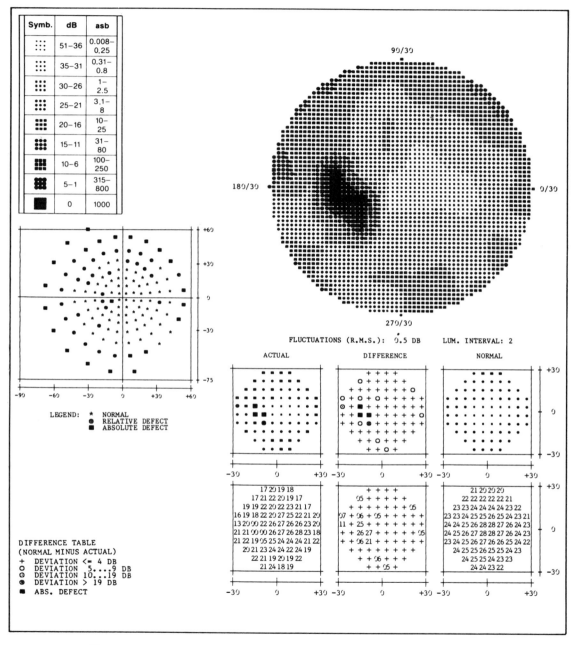

Symb.	dB	asb
:::	51–36	0.008–0.25
:::	35–31	0.31–0.8
:::	30–26	1–2.5
:::	25–21	3.1–8
:::	20–16	10–25
:::	15–11	31–80
:::	10–6	100–250
:::	5–1	315–800
■	0	1000

LEGEND: ★   NORMAL
          ⊙   RELATIVE DEFECT
          ■   ABSOLUTE DEFECT

FLUCTUATIONS (R.M.S.): 0.5 DB   LUM. INTERVAL: 2

ACTUAL   DIFFERENCE   NORMAL

DIFFERENCE TABLE
(NORMAL MINUS ACTUAL)
+   DEVIATION <= 4 DB
○   DEVIATION 5...9 DB
⊙   DEVIATION 10...19 DB
●   DEVIATION > 19 DB
■   ABS. DEFECT

Figure 8–2. *Seventy-five-year-old woman with open-angle glaucoma. The patient was examined on an Octopus 201 using the full-field screening program 7 (in boxes to the left) and the more rigorous diagnostic program 32. **A.** Examination of left eye shows an enlargement of the blind spot. This can be seen on the screening field but is more rigorously evaluated by program 32. (continued)*

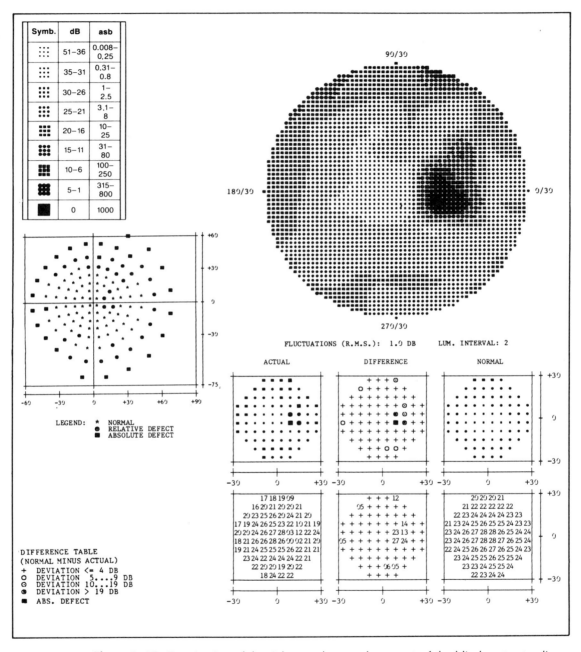

Figure 8–2B. *Examination of the right eye shows enlargement of the blind spot extending into the lower central field. This can be seen in the screening program but is more rigorously shown by program 32.*

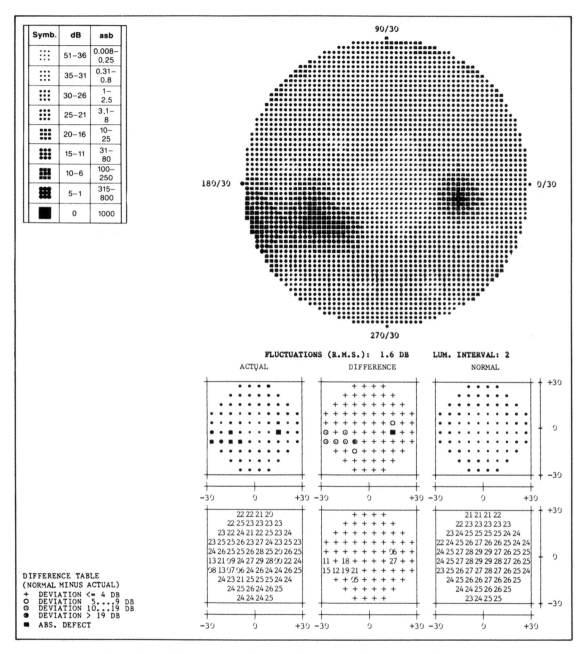

Figure 8–3. Fifty-five-year-old man with open-angle glaucoma. Visual field examination of the right eye was performed on an Octopus 201 using program 32. The blind spot is normal and there is no depression. However, there is an early inferior nasal arcuate scotoma that has produced a subtle nasal step.

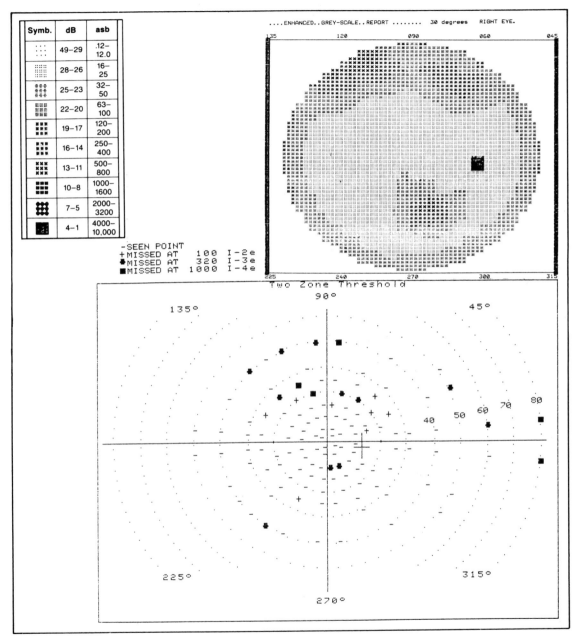

Figure 8–4. Sixty-year-old man with open-angle glaucoma. Visual field was performed on a Dicon AP 2000 with the two-zone software program. Starting intensity was 100 asb. Examination of the right eye shows a small inferior arcuate scotoma and a larger superior arcuate scotoma.

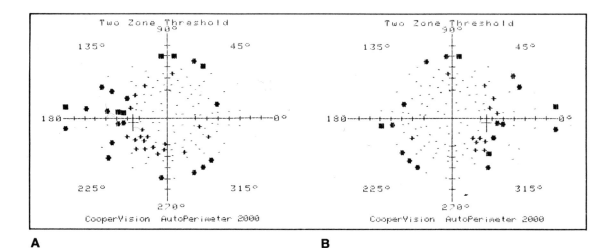

Figure 8–5. Forty-four-year-old woman with open-angle glaucoma. Patient was examined on a Dicon AP 2000 using the two-zone software with a starting intensity of 100 asb. **A.** Right eye shows enlargement of the blind spot with superior and inferior arcuate scotomas extending from it and forming a Seidel's scotoma. Peripheral constriction is greater inferiorly than superiorly with the formation of a peripheral nasal step. **B.** Left eye shows enlargement of and baring of the blind spot superiorly and inferiorly. Arcuate loss is present and adherent to the blind spot with inferior loss greater than superior.

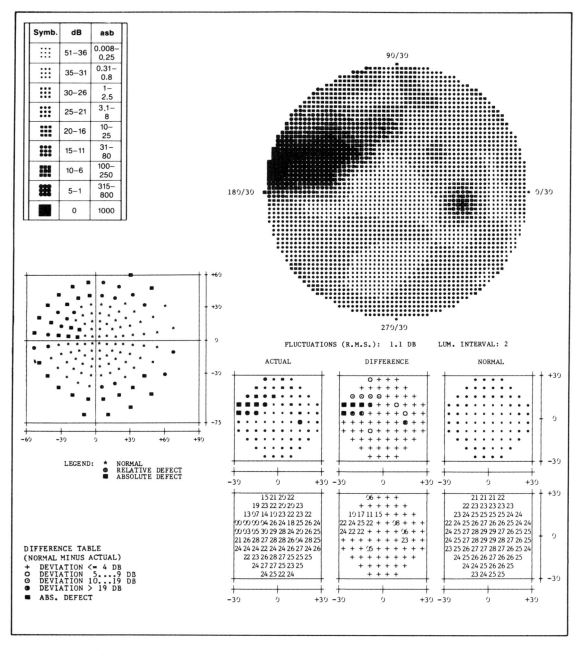

Figure 8–6. Fifty-five-year-old woman with open-angle glaucoma. Visual field examination was performed with an Octopus 201 using full-field screening program 7 and diagnostic central 30-degree program 32. Program 7 (in box to left) shows nasal step and peripheral constriction, especially superonasally. Program 32 shows loss in the superior arcuate area. This loss is subtle temporally and more obvious nasally. A classic nasal step can also be seen. Because program 32 only tested the central 30 degrees, the peripheral loss, which is seen in program 7, is not appreciated.

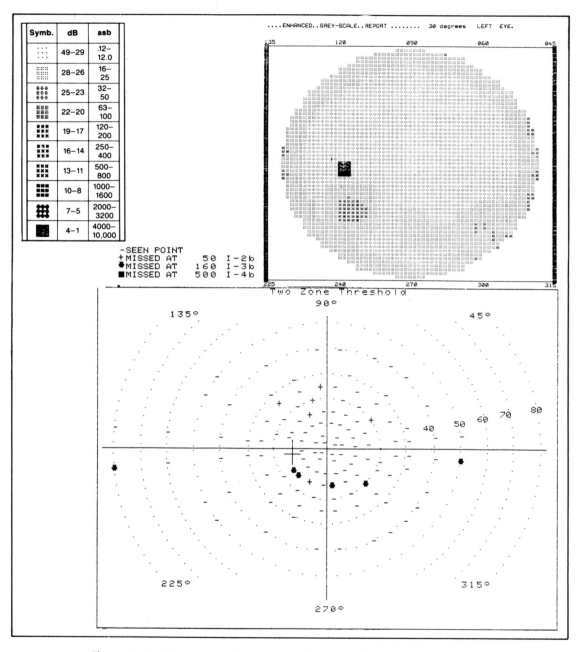

Figure 8–7. Fifty-six-year-old woman with open-angle glaucoma and early visual field loss in the left eye. Visual field examination was performed on the Dicon AP 2000 using the two-zone method with a starting intensity of 50 asb. Visual field examination of the right eye was unremarkable. Visual field examination of the left eye shows loss in the superior arcuate area and several scotomas within the inferior arcuate area. The inferior arcuate scotomas are still isolated from each other and have not coalesced into a complete arcuate scotoma.

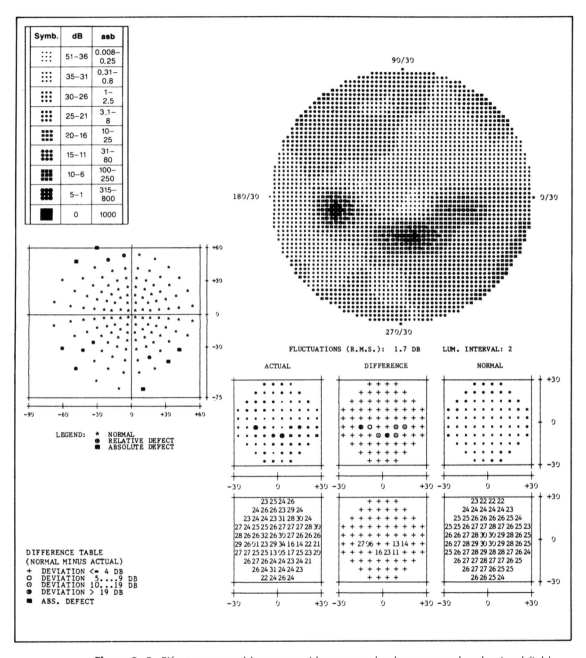

Figure 8–8. *Fifty-two-year-old woman with open-angle glaucoma and early visual field loss. Two examinations were performed on the Octopus 201—screening program 7 (box to left) and diagnostic program 32. Examination of the left eye with the screening program did not reveal any abnormalities. Program 32, however, revealed a classic early inferior arcuate scotoma. Examination of the right eye was unremarkable to both programs.*

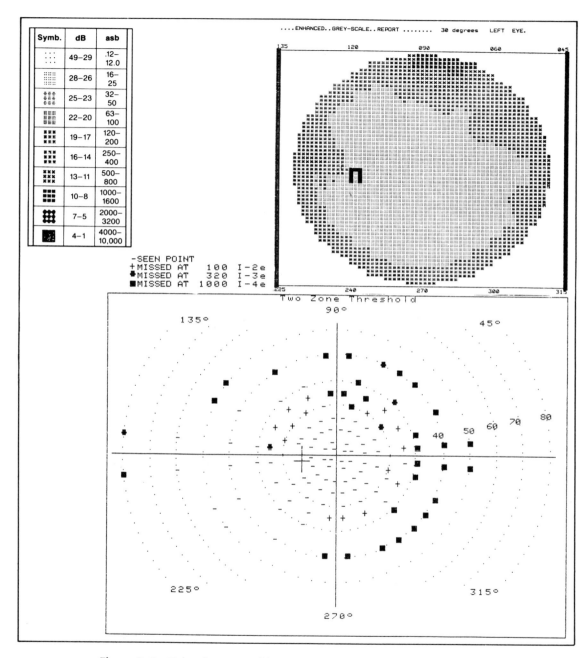

Figure 8–9. *Eighty-four-year-old woman with open-angle glaucoma. Examination was performed on the Dicon AP 2000 using two-zone stepped threshold strategy with a starting intensity of 100 asb o.u.* **A.** *Examination of the left eye shows peripheral constriction, which is greatest superiorly and inferonasally. (continued)*

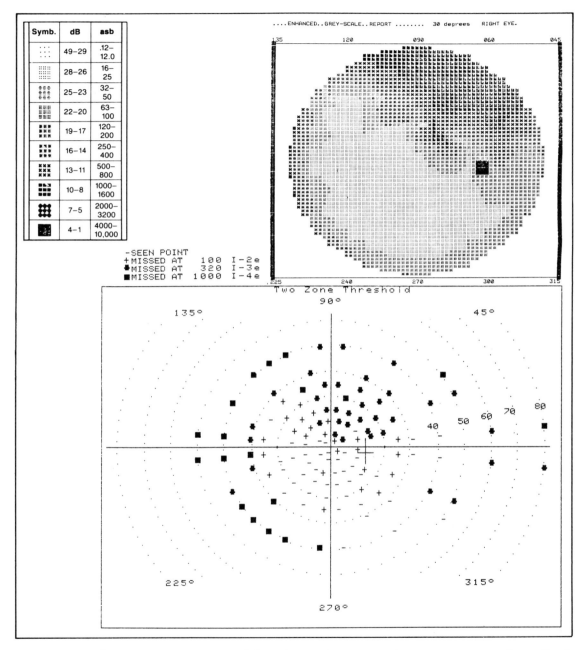

Symb.	dB	asb
⠿	49–29	.12–12.0
▦	28–26	16–25
✚	25–23	32–50
▦	22–20	63–100
▦	19–17	120–200
▦	16–14	250–400
✖	13–11	500–800
▦	10–8	1000–1600
✖	7–5	2000–3200
■	4–1	4000–10,000

....ENHANCED..GREY-SCALE..REPORT .... 30 degrees   RIGHT EYE.

–SEEN POINT
+MISSED AT   100 I–2e
✦MISSED AT   320 I–3e
■MISSED AT 1000 I–4e

Two Zone Threshold

Figure 8–9B. Examination of the right eye shows a superior arcuate scotoma. Generalized peripheral constriction can also be seen.

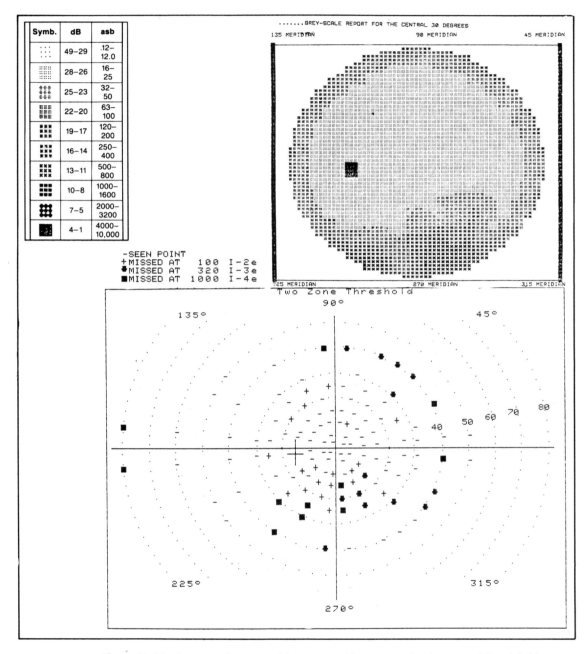

Symb.	dB	asb
::: :::	49–29	.12–12.0
::::: :::::	28–26	16–25
::: ::: :::	25–23	32–50
::: ::: :::	22–20	63–100
::: :::	19–17	120–200
::: :::	16–14	250–400
::: ::: :::	13–11	500–800
:::	10–8	1000–1600
:::	7–5	2000–3200
■	4–1	4000–10,000

Figure 8–10. *Seventy-nine-year-old woman with open-angle glaucoma. Visual fields were tested on a Dicon AP 2000 using the two-zone threshold software strategy with a starting intensity of 100 asb o.u.* **A.** *Examination of the left eye shows an inferior arcuate scotoma and peripheral constriction. (continued)*

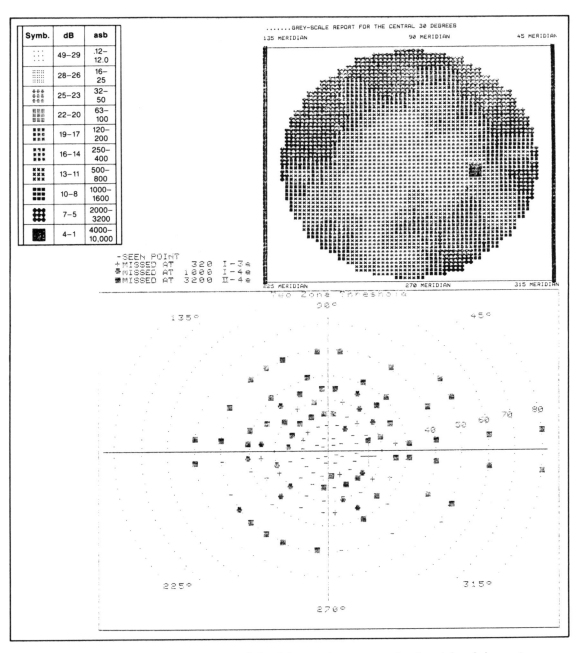

Figure 8–10B. *Examination of the right eye shows generalized peripheral depression. There are superior and inferior arcuate scotomas, denser superiorly, which extend into the periphery.*

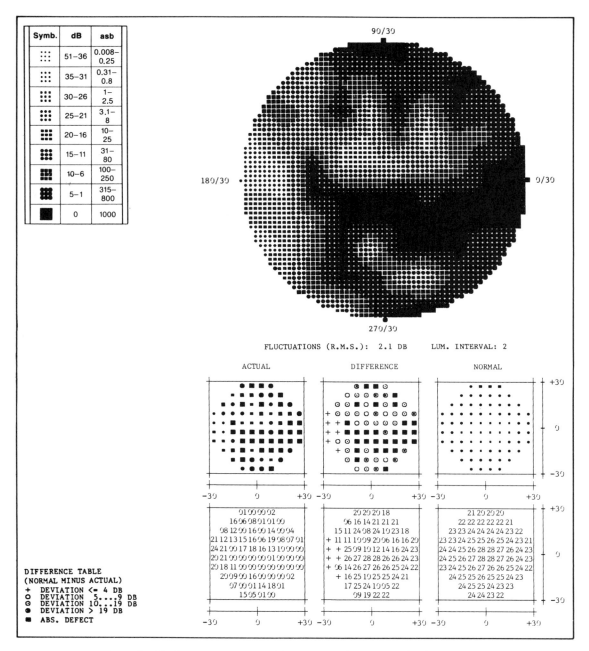

Figure 8–11. *Seventy-two-year-old woman with open-angle glaucoma. Patient was tested on an Octopus 201 using program 32. **A**. Left eye shows moderately advanced loss. There is generalized superior field depression and dense inferior central and arcuate loss. (continued)*

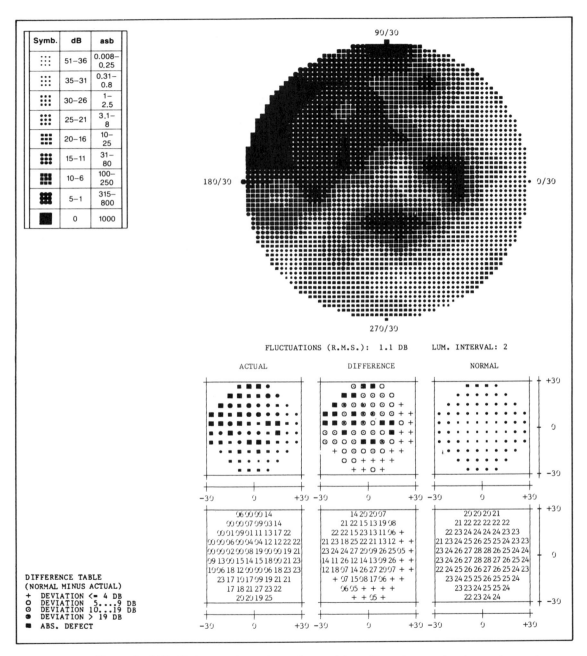

Symb.	dB	asb
⋮⋮⋮	51–36	0.008–0.25
⋮⋮⋮	35–31	0.31–0.8
⋮⋮⋮	30–26	1–2.5
⋮⋮⋮	25–21	3.1–8
⋮⋮⋮	20–16	10–25
⋮⋮⋮	15–11	31–80
⋮⋮⋮	10–6	100–250
⋮⋮⋮	5–1	315–800
■	0	1000

90/30

180/30

0/30

270/30

FLUCTUATIONS (R.M.S.): 1.1 DB   LUM. INTERVAL: 2

ACTUAL   DIFFERENCE   NORMAL

DIFFERENCE TABLE
(NORMAL MINUS ACTUAL)
+   DEVIATION <= 4 DB
O   DEVIATION 5...9 DB
⊙   DEVIATION 10...19 DB
●   DEVIATION > 19 DB
■   ABS. DEFECT

```
        06 00 00 14                      14 20 20 07                      20 20 20 21
      00 00 07 09 03 14                21 22 15 13 19 08              21 22 22 22 22 22
   00 01 09 01 11 13 17 22           22 22 15 23 13 11 06 +         22 23 24 24 24 24 23
 00 00 06 00 04 12 12 22 22        21 23 18 25 22 21 13 12 +  +    21 23 24 25 26 25 25 24 23 23
 00 00 02 00 08 19 00 00 19 21     23 24 24 27 20 09 26 25 05 +    23 24 26 27 28 28 26 25 24 24
 09 13 09 15 14 15 18 00 21 23     14 11 26 12 14 13 09 26 +  +    23 24 26 27 28 28 27 26 25 24
 19 06 18 12 00 00 06 18 23 23     12 18 07 14 26 27 20 07 +  +    22 24 25 26 26 27 26 25 24 23
    23 17 19 17 09 19 21 21           + 07 15 08 17 06 +  +           23 24 25 25 26 25 25 24
      17 18 21 27 23 22                 06 05 + + + +              23 23 24 25 25 24
        20 20 19 25                       + + 05 +                   22 23 24 24
```

Figure 8–11B. *Right eye shows less advanced loss. There is superior depression and arcuate loss densest nasally resulting in a dense nasal step. Inferior arcuate area shows dense scotomata surrounded by arcuate area depression.*

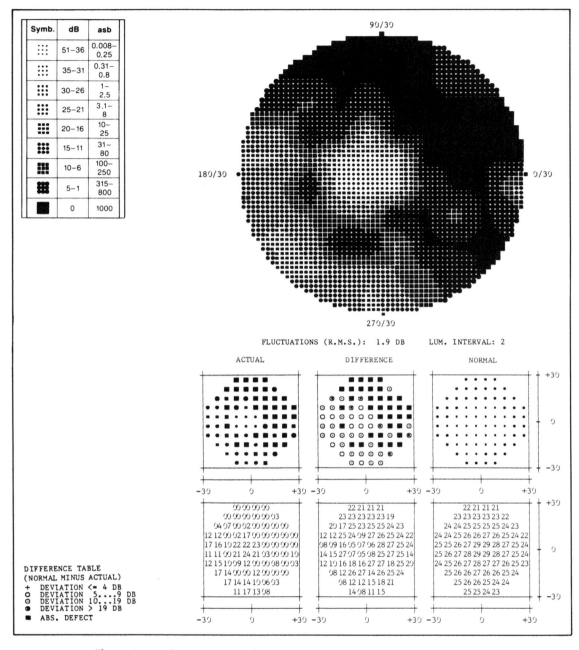

Figure 8–12. *Sixty-two-year-old woman with open-angle glaucoma. Octopus 201 examination was performed on the left eye using program 32. Generalized depression can be seen in the entire field. A large superior arcuate scotoma and a smaller inferior arcuate scotoma are seen to connect with the blind spot forming Seidel's scotoma, which has broken into the periphery superiorly. The coalescence of scotomas within the arcuate area form a complete arcuate scotoma as demonstrated by the varying intensity of the defects within the inferior arcuate area.*

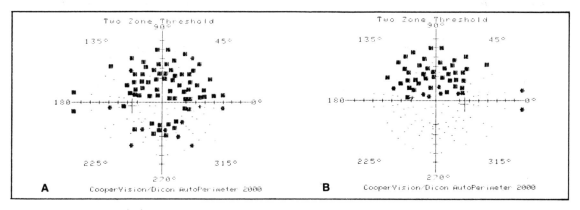

Figure 8–13. Seventy-six-year-old woman with open-angle glaucoma. Visual fields were examined with a Dicon AP 2000 using the two-zone software strategy with a starting intensity of 250 asb. **A**. Examination of the left eye shows dense superior loss but also shows an inferior arcuate scotoma. **B**. Examination of the right eye shows dense superior loss.

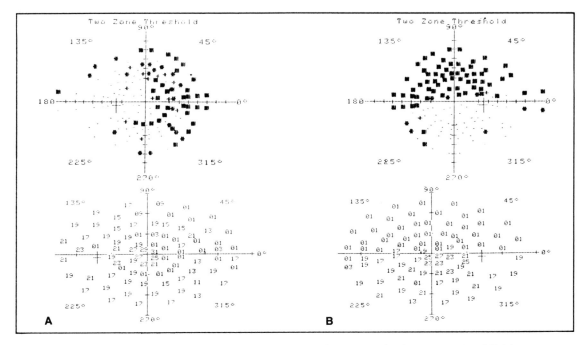

Figure 8–14. Sixty-four-year-old woman with open-angle glaucoma. Visual fields were performed on a Dicon AP 2000 using the two-zone threshold software strategy and also the numeric strategy. The two-zone program tests both the peripheral and central fields. The numeric strategy tests only the central 30 degrees. **A**. Examination of the left eye shows severe nasal constriction with loss of most of the superior nasal quadrant and much of the inferior nasal quadrant. Broad superior and narrow inferior arcuate scotomas are also present. These are demonstrated equally well by both strategies. **B**. Examination of the right eye shows complete loss of the superior visual field with inferior nasal constriction. This is demonstrated equally well by both strategies.

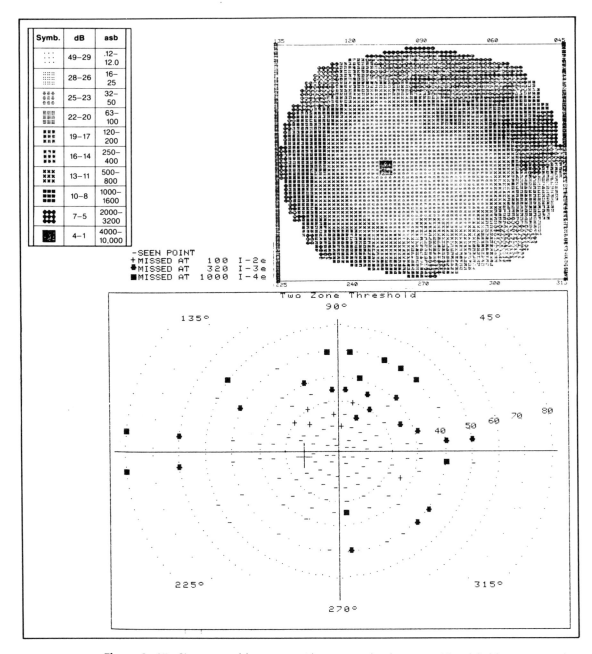

Figure 8–15. Sixty-year-old woman with open-angle glaucoma. Visual fields were tested on the Dicon AP 2000 using the two-zone threshold software strategy with a starting intensity at 100 asb o.u. **A.** Examination of the left eye shows scattered scotomas within the superior arcuate area extending into the periphery superotemporally. There is also some generalized peripheral constriction o.u. (continued)

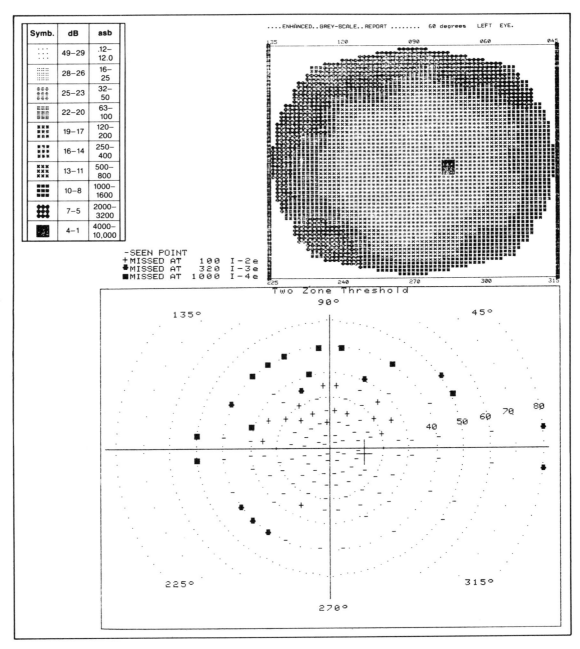

Figure 8–15B. *Examination of the right eye shows a superior arcuate scotoma forming a nasal step. In addition there is peripheral loss greatest superiorly.*

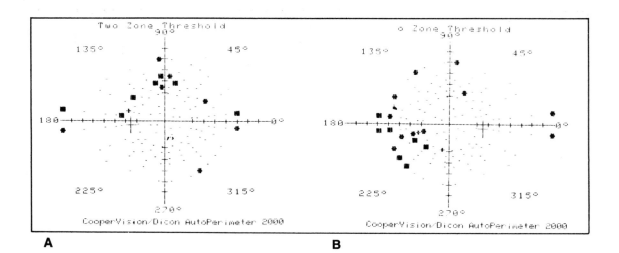

A B

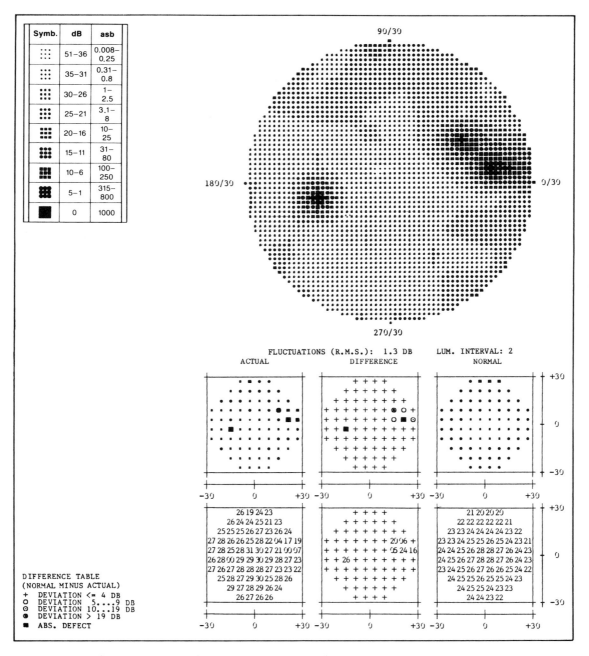

Figure 8–17. Sixty-four-year-old woman with open-angle glaucoma. Examination was performed on the Octopus 201 using program 32. Examination of the left eye shows a normal blind spot and no overall depression. A superior nasal arcuate scotoma, which is forming a nasal step, can be appreciated. Visual field examination of the right eye was unremarkable.

166

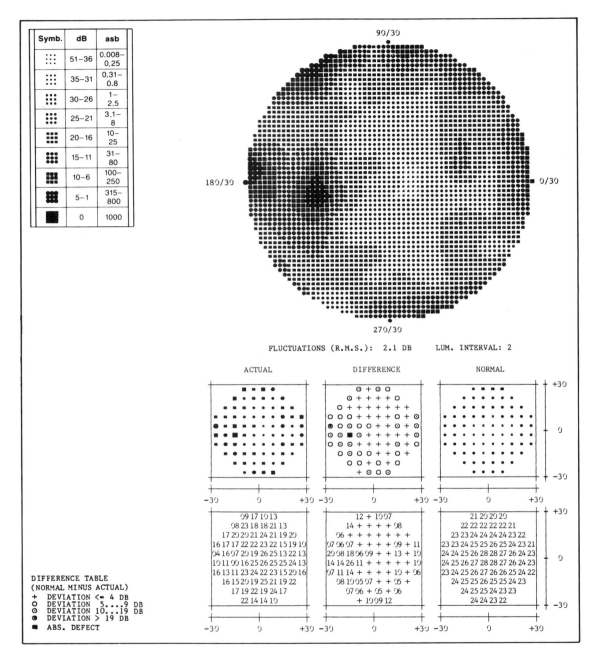

Figure 8–18. *Seventy-year-old man with open-angle glaucoma examined with the Octopus 201 using program 32.* **A.** *Examination of the left eye shows an enlargement of the blind spot extending into the superior and inferior arcuate areas. (continued)*

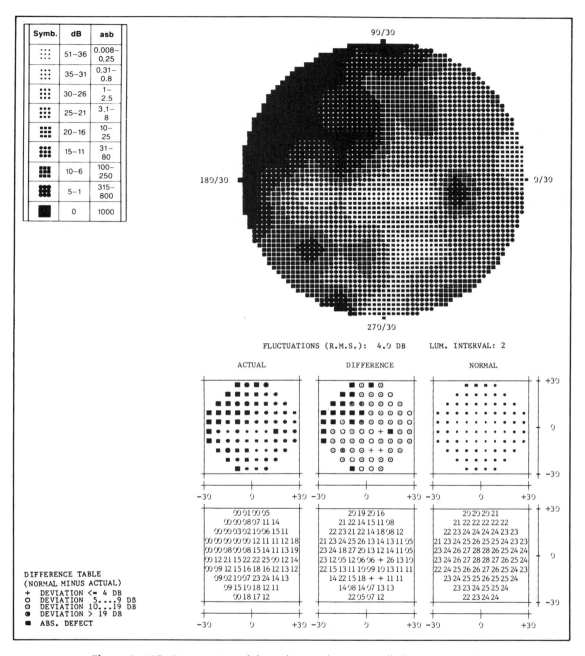

Figure 8–18B. Examination of the right eye shows overall depression with greatest loss in the superior nasal quadrant.

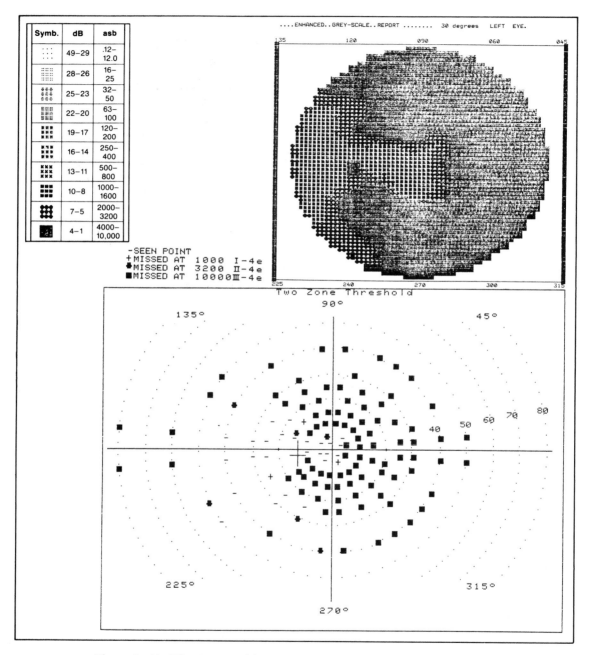

Figure 8–19. Fifty-six-year-old woman with advanced open-angle glaucoma in the left eye. Visual fields were studied with the Dicon AP 2000 using the two-zone threshold software strategy. The initial testing intensity was 1000 asb. Large arcuate scotomas extending into the periphery are present. Only a small 5-degree island of central field and a temporal island of field remain.

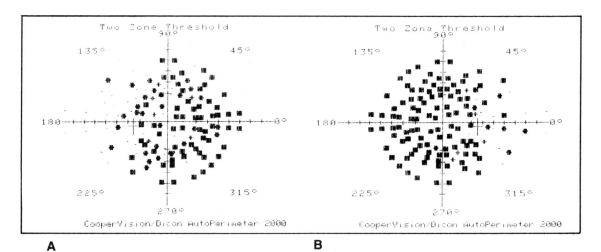

A   **B**

Figure 8–20. *Seventy-nine-year-old woman with advanced open-angle glaucoma. Most of the visual field is lost.* ***A.*** *A large peripheral field persists in the left eye with a tiny island of central field also remaining.* ***B.*** *Only a tiny island of peripheral field remains in the right eye.*

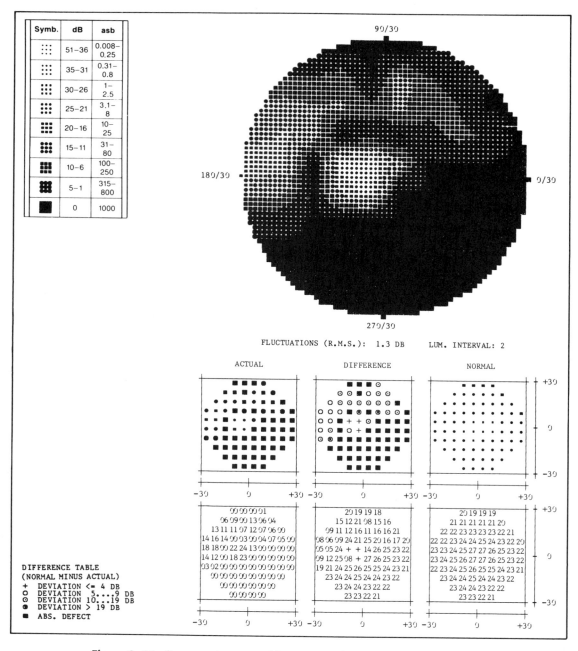

Figure 8–21. *Seventy-nine-year-old woman with open-angle glaucoma. Visual fields were examined on the Octopus 201 using program 32. **A.** Examination of the left eye shows advanced loss. There is almost complete loss of the inferior field. An island of central field remains but is depressed. A superior arcuate scotoma is densest near fixation with less loss at greater eccentricities. (continued)*

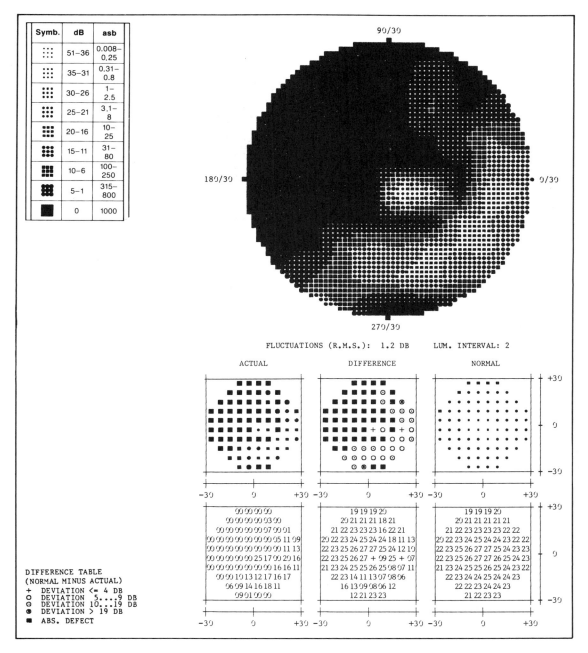

Figure 8–21B. *Examination of the right eye shows dense nasal loss and dense superior loss. Remaining, but depressed field, is seen inferiorly, superotemporally, and a small island can be seen centrally.*

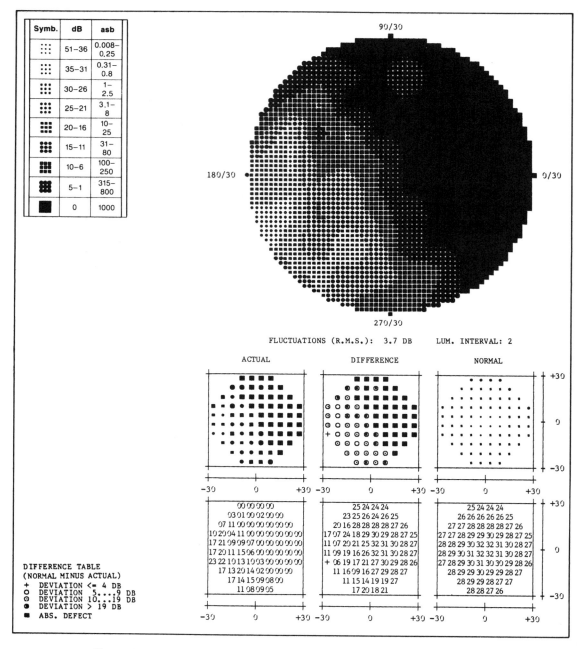

Symb.	dB	asb
⋮⋮⋮	51–36	0.008–0.25
⋮⋮⋮	35–31	0.31–0.8
⋮⋮⋮	30–26	1–2.5
⋮⋮⋮	25–21	3.1–8
▦	20–16	10–25
▦	15–11	31–80
▦	10–6	100–250
▦	5–1	315–800
■	0	1000

90/30

180/30   0/30

270/30

FLUCTUATIONS (R.M.S.): 3.7 DB   LUM. INTERVAL: 2

ACTUAL   DIFFERENCE   NORMAL

DIFFERENCE TABLE
(NORMAL MINUS ACTUAL)
+ DEVIATION <= 4 DB
o DEVIATION 5....9 DB
☉ DEVIATION 10...19 DB
● DEVIATION > 19 DB
■ ABS. DEFECT

ACTUAL
```
          00 00 00 00
        03 01 00 02 00 00
     07 11 00 00 00 00 00 00
  10 20 04 11 00 00 00 00 00 00
  17 21 09 09 07 00 00 00 00 00
  17 20 11 15 06 00 00 00 00 00
  23 22 10 13 10 03 00 00 00 00
     17 13 20 14 02 00 00 00
     17 14 15 09 08 00
        11 08 09 05
```

DIFFERENCE
```
          25 24 24 24
        23 25 26 24 26 25
     20 16 28 28 28 27 26
  17 07 24 18 29 30 29 28 27 25
  11 07 20 21 25 32 31 30 28 27
  11 09 19 16 26 32 31 30 28 27
  + 06 19 17 21 27 30 29 28 26
     11 16 09 16 27 29 28 27
     11 15 14 19 19 27
        17 20 18 21
```

NORMAL
```
          25 24 24 24
        26 26 26 26 26 25
     27 27 28 28 28 28 27 26
  27 27 28 29 29 30 29 28 27 25
  28 28 29 30 32 32 31 30 28 27
  28 29 30 31 32 32 31 30 28 27
  27 28 29 30 31 30 30 29 28 26
     28 29 29 30 29 28 27
     28 29 29 28 27 27
        28 28 27 26
```

Figure 8–22. Twenty-eight-year-old woman with severe open-angle glaucoma. Visual fields were examined by both the Octopus 201 using program 32 and the Dicon AP 2000 using the two-zone threshold software strategy with a starting intensity of 1000 asb o.u. **A.** Octopus 201 examination of the left eye shows generalized depression and loss of most of the nasal field. (continued)

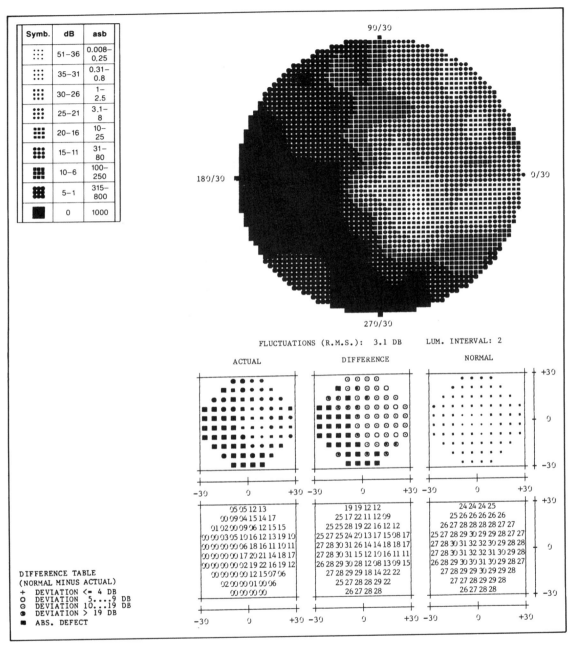

Symb.	dB	asb
⠿	51–36	0.008–0.25
⠿	35–31	0.31–0.8
⠿	30–26	1–2.5
⠿	25–21	3.1–8
⠿	20–16	10–25
⠿	15–11	31–80
⠿	10–6	100–250
⠿	5–1	315–800
■	0	1000

90/30

180/30   0/30

270/30

FLUCTUATIONS (R.M.S.): 3.1 DB   LUM. INTERVAL: 2

ACTUAL   DIFFERENCE   NORMAL

DIFFERENCE TABLE
(NORMAL MINUS ACTUAL)
+   DEVIATION <= 4 DB
○   DEVIATION 5....9 DB
◎   DEVIATION 10...19 DB
◕   DEVIATION > 19 DB
■   ABS. DEFECT

ACTUAL:
```
            05 05 12 13
         00 09 04 15 14 17
      01 02 00 09 06 12 15 15
   00 00 00 03 05 10 16 12 13 19 19
   00 00 00 00 06 18 16 11 10 11
   00 00 00 00 17 20 21 14 18 17
   00 00 00 00 02 19 22 16 19 12
      00 00 00 00 12 15 07 06
         02 00 00 01 00 06
            00 00 00 00
```

DIFFERENCE:
```
            19 19 12 12
         25 17 22 11 12 09
      25 25 28 19 22 16 12 12
   25 27 25 24 20 13 17 15 08 17
   27 28 30 31 26 14 14 18 18 17
   27 28 30 31 15 12 10 16 11 11
   26 28 29 30 28 12 08 13 09 15
      27 28 29 29 18 14 22 22
         25 27 28 28 29 22
            26 27 28 28
```

NORMAL:
```
            24 24 24 25
         25 26 26 26 26 26
      26 27 28 28 28 28 27 27
   25 27 28 29 30 29 29 28 27 27
   27 28 30 31 32 32 30 29 28 28
   27 28 30 31 32 32 31 30 29 28
   26 28 29 30 30 31 30 29 28 27
      27 28 29 29 30 29 29 28
         27 27 28 29 29 28
            26 27 28 28
```

Figure 8–22B. *The Octopus 201 examination of the right eye shows generalized depression, loss of most of the nasal field, especially inferonasally. (continued)*

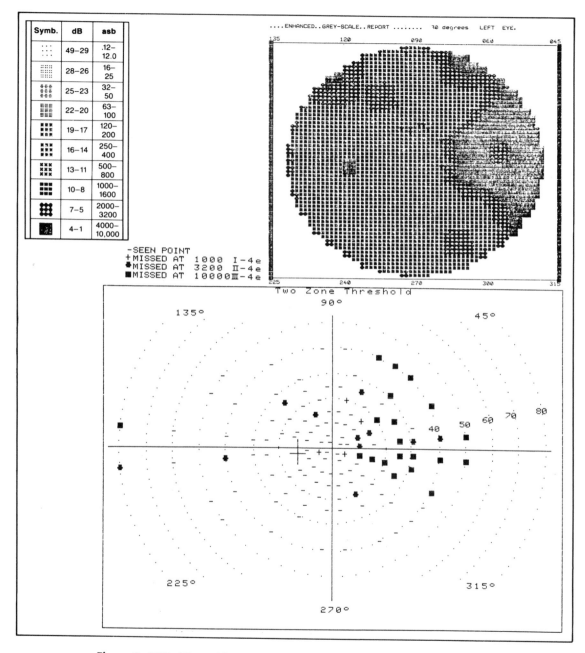

Figure 8–22C. Dicon AP 2000 examination of the left eye confirms the findings found on the Octopus examination. Enlargement of the blind spot and extension of that into the central field is also clearly demonstrated. (continued)

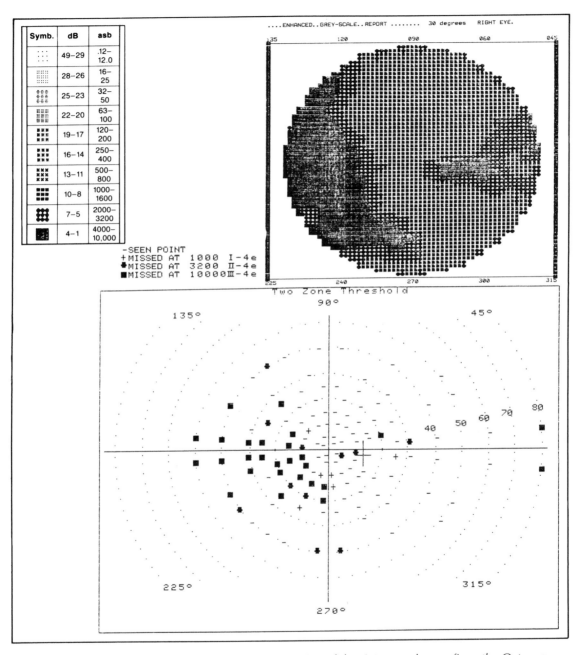

Figure 8–22D. *Dicon AP 2000 examination of the right eye also confirms the Octopus 201 examination. The large extent of inferior loss with a dense inferior arcuate scotoma as seen on the Octopus examination is also seen on the Dicon examination.*

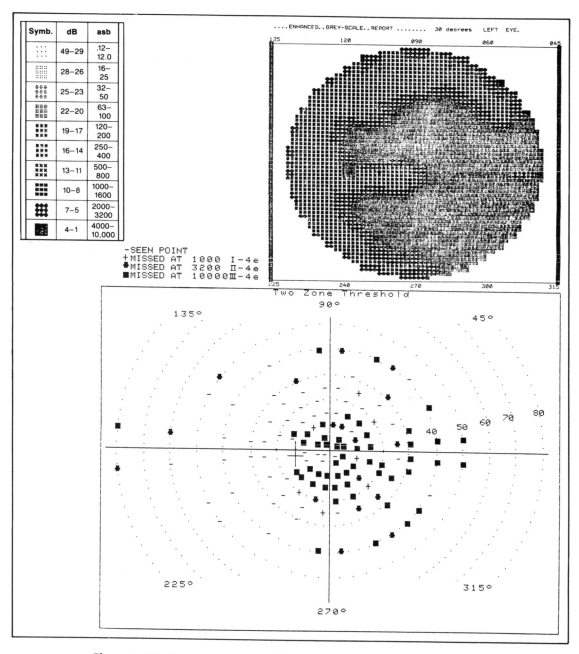

Symb.	dB	asb
∴	49–29	.12–12.0
⠿	28–26	16–25
✢	25–23	32–50
▦	22–20	63–100
▩	19–17	120–200
▩	16–14	250–400
▩	13–11	500–800
▦	10–8	1000–1600
✿	7–5	2000–3200
▣	4–1	4000–10,000

....ENHANCED..GREY-SCALE..REPORT .... 30 degrees LEFT EYE.

-SEEN POINT
+MISSED AT 1000 I-4e
✦MISSED AT 3200 II-4e
■MISSED AT 10000 III-4e

Two Zone Threshold

Figure 8–23. Seventy-seven-year-old woman with low tension glaucoma. Visual field studies were performed on a Dicon AP 2000 using the two-zone testing strategy. Starting intensity was 1000 asb in the left eye and 100 asb in the right eye. **A.** A severe glaucomatous loss is seen in the left visual field. Superior and inferior arcuate and central loss is seen. This loss is close to fixation, is deep, and has steep borders. Nasally the loss has broken into the periphery. (continued)

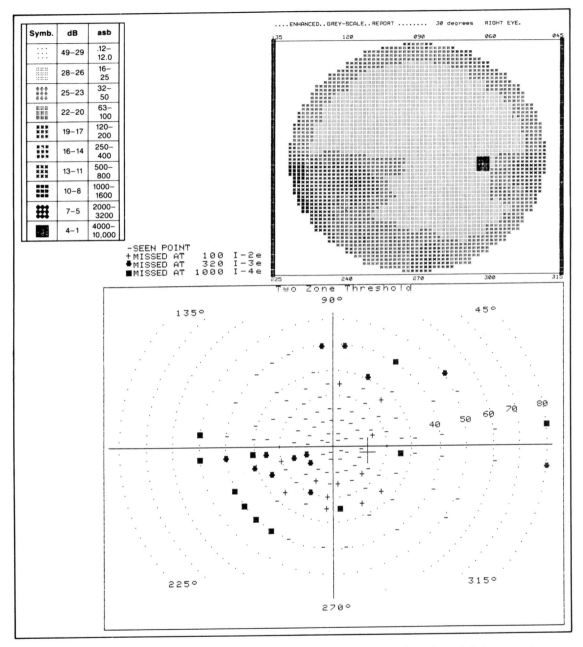

Figure 8–23B. *Field loss is not as severe in the right eye. There is an inferior arcuate scotoma that has broken into the periphery nasally with the formation of a dense nasal step.*

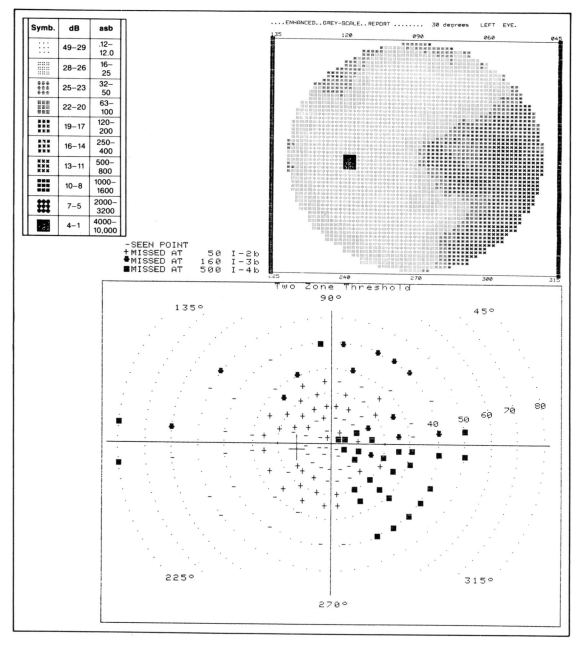

Symb.	dB	asb
⋮⋮⋮	49–29	.12–12.0
⦂⦂⦂⦂	28–26	16–25
✤✤✤	25–23	32–50
▦▦▦	22–20	63–100
■■■	19–17	120–200
■■■	16–14	250–400
✖✖✖	13–11	500–800
■■■	10–8	1000–1600
✿	7–5	2000–3200
▓	4–1	4000–10,000

```
....ENHANCED..GREY-SCALE..REPORT .........  30 degrees   LEFT EYE.
```

```
-SEEN POINT
+MISSED AT      50  I-2b
✦MISSED AT     160  I-3b
■MISSED AT     500  I-4b
```

Two Zone Threshold

Figure 8–24A. Sixty-six-year-old hypertensive female with open-angle glaucoma and history of cerebral vascular accident. Visual fields were performed on a Dicon AP 2000 using the two-zone threshold software strategy starting at 50 asb o.u. Visual field defects are present from two distinct causes. The cerebral vascular accident has caused a right inferior homonymous quadrantanopia. The glaucoma has caused a mild superior arcuate scotoma. (continued)

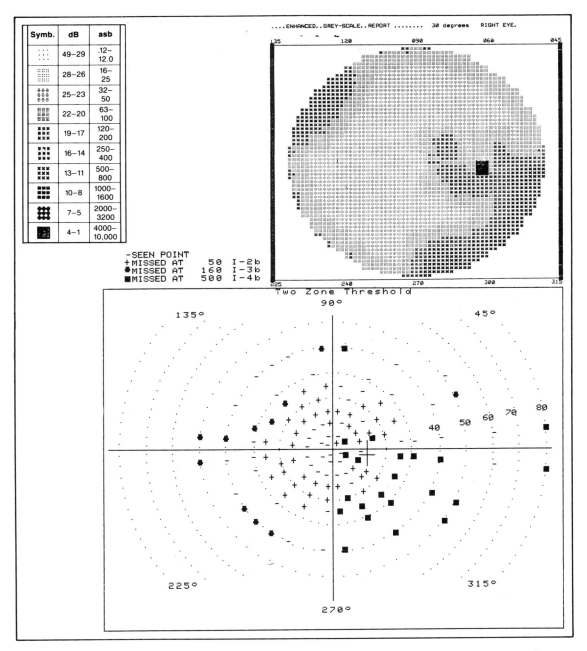

Figure 8–24B. Sixty-six-year-old hypertensive female with open angle glaucoma and a history of a cerebral vascular accident. A right inferior homonymous quadrantanopsia is present from the cerebral vascular accident. The glaucoma has caused some nasal constriction in the right eye and superior arcuate scotomas o.u.

180

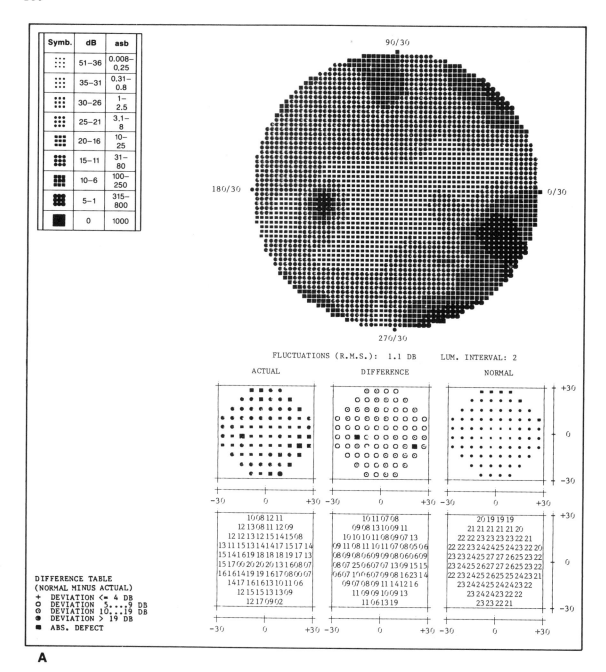

Figure 8–25A. Eighty-six-year-old man with ocular hypertension. Patient was followed at regular intervals with an Octopus 201 using program 32.

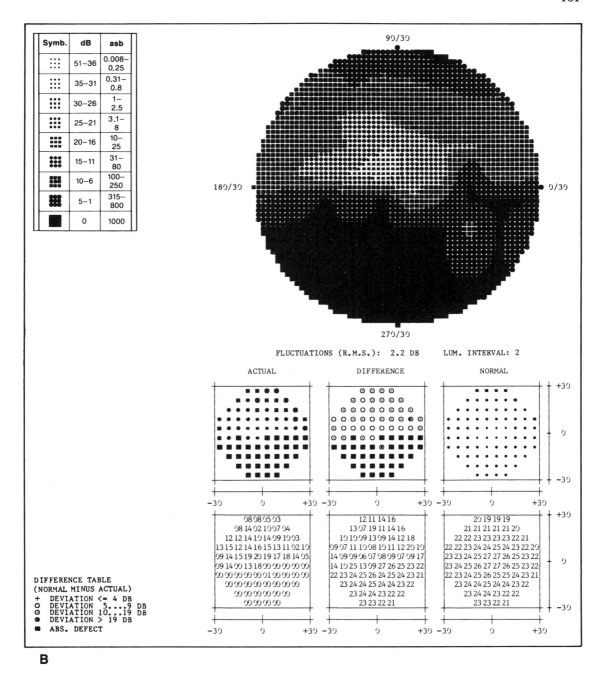

Symb.	dB	asb
⋮⋮⋮	51–36	0.008–0.25
⋮⋮⋮	35–31	0.31–0.8
⋮⋮⋮	30–26	1–2.5
⦂⦂⦂	25–21	3.1–8
▦	20–16	10–25
▦	15–11	31–80
▦	10–6	100–250
▦	5–1	315–800
■	0	1000

90/30

180/30

0/30

270/30

FLUCTUATIONS (R.M.S.): 2.2 DB   LUM. INTERVAL: 2

ACTUAL   DIFFERENCE   NORMAL

DIFFERENCE TABLE
(NORMAL MINUS ACTUAL)
+   DEVIATION <= 4 DB
○   DEVIATION 5...9 DB
⊙   DEVIATION 10...19 DB
●   DEVIATION > 19 DB
■   ABS. DEFECT

```
        98 08 05 03                  12 11 14 16                20 19 19 19
      08 14 02 10 07 04            13 07 19 11 14 16          21 21 21 21 20
    12 12 14 19 14 09 10 03       10 10 09 13 09 14 12 18     22 22 23 23 23 23 22 21
  13 15 12 14 16 15 13 11 02 10  09 07 11 10 08 10 11 12 20 10 22 22 23 24 24 25 24 23 22 20
  09 14 15 19 20 19 17 18 14 05  14 09 09 06 07 08 09 07 09 17 23 23 24 27 27 26 25 23 22
  09 14 00 13 18 00 00 00 00 00  14 10 25 13 09 27 26 25 23 22 23 24 25 26 27 27 26 25 23 22
  00 00 00 00 00 00 01 00 00 00  22 23 24 25 26 24 25 24 23 21 22 23 24 25 26 25 25 24 23 21
    00 00 00 00 00 00 00 00      23 24 24 24 24 23 22       23 24 24 24 24 23 22
      00 00 00 00 00 00          23 24 24 23 22 22          23 24 24 23 22 22
        00 00 00 00              23 23 22 21                23 23 22 21
```

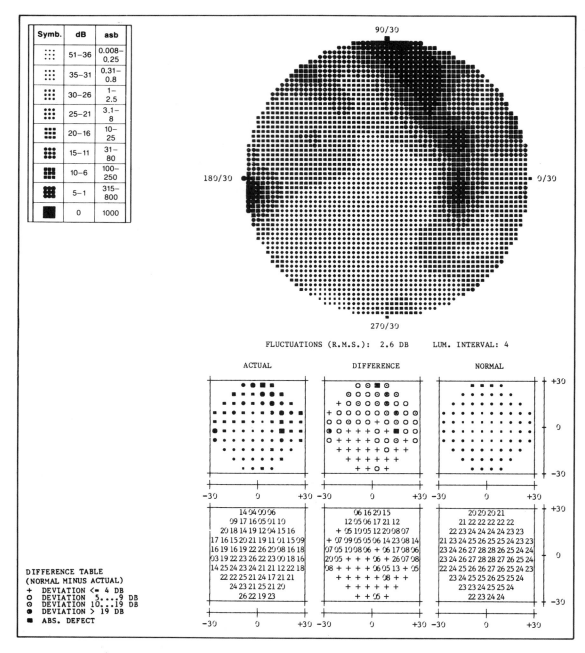

Symb.	dB	asb
⫶⫶⫶	51–36	0.008–0.25
⫶⫶⫶	35–31	0.31–0.8
▪▪▪	30–26	1–2.5
▪▪▪	25–21	3.1–8
▪▪▪	20–16	10–25
▪▪▪	15–11	31–80
▪▪▪	10–6	100–250
▦	5–1	315–800
■	0	1000

90/30

180/30

0/30

270/30

FLUCTUATIONS (R.M.S.): 2.6 DB   LUM. INTERVAL: 4

ACTUAL   DIFFERENCE   NORMAL

DIFFERENCE TABLE
(NORMAL MINUS ACTUAL)
+   DEVIATION <= 4 DB
o   DEVIATION 5...9 DB
⊙   DEVIATION 10...19 DB
●   DEVIATION > 19 DB
■   ABS. DEFECT

```
          14 04 00 06                    06 16 20 15                  20 20 20 21
       09 17 16 05 01 10              12 05 06 17 21 12            21 22 22 22 22 22
     20 18 14 19 12 04 15 16        +  05 10 05 12 20 08 07      21 23 24 24 24 23 23
   17 16 15 20 21 19 11 01 15 09   +  07 09 05 05 06 14 23 08 14  21 23 24 25 26 25 25 24 23 23
   16 19 16 19 22 26 20 08 16 18      07 05 10 08 06 + 06 17 08 06  23 24 26 27 28 28 26 25 24 24
   03 19 22 23 26 22 23 00 18 16    20 05 + + + 06 + 26 07 98    23 24 26 27 28 28 27 26 25 24
   14 25 24 23 24 21 21 12 22 18    08 + + + + 06 05 13 + 05    22 24 25 26 26 27 26 25 24 23
     22 22 25 21 24 17 21 21          + + + + + 08 + +          23 24 25 25 26 25 25 24
      24 23 21 25 21 20                + + + + + +              23 23 24 25 25 24
        26 22 19 23                     + 05 +                  22 23 24 24
```

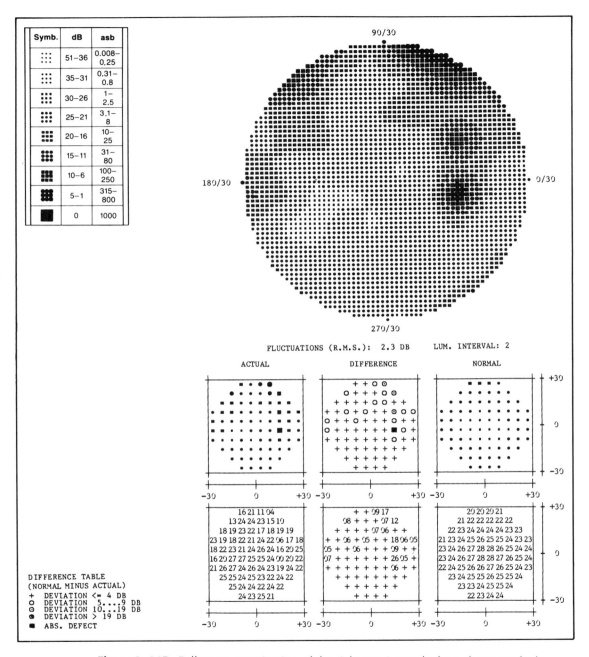

Figure 8–26B. Follow-up examination of the right eye 8 months later shows marked improvement. There is less enlargement of the blind spot, disappearance of most of the superior arcuate scotoma, and disappearance of the nasal step. (continued)

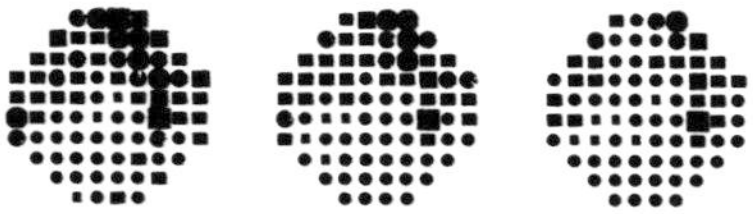

Figure 8–26C. Series mode
Delta analysis of the right eye
including an intermediate
examination at 4 months shows
improvement of the visual field.
Reliability is confirmed by the
low RMS fluctuation readings on
each examination. The number
of disturbed points dropped from
46 to 31 to 17. Total field loss
dropped from 440 to 278 to 135.
Mean sensitivity improved
slightly in the lower quadrants
but improved markedly in the
upper quadrants. Mean loss per
test location improved markedly
in all quadrants. (continued)

	EX1	EX2	EX3	SUMMARY
DATE OF EXAM : DAY	09.27	01.25	05.23	
YEAR	1983	1984	1984	
PROGRAM / EXAMINATION	32/01	32/03	32/05	
TOTAL LOSS (WHOLE FIELD)	440	278	135	284 ± 88
MEAN LOSS (PER TEST LOC)				
WHOLE FIELD	5.9	3.8	1.8	3.8 ± 1.2
QUADRANT UPPER NASAL	6.7	3.8	1.6	4.0 ± 1.5
LOWER NASAL	1.7	0.9	0.4	1.0 ± 0.4
UPPER TEMP.	12.1	9.2	4.8	8.7 ± 2.1
LOWER TEMP.	3.5	1.3	0.6	1.8 ± 0.9
ECCENTRICITY 0 – 10	3.6	2.5	0.9	2.3 ± 0.8
10 – 20	7.4	4.7	2.4	4.8 ± 1.5
20 – 30	6.0	3.7	1.8	3.8 ± 1.2
MEAN SENSITIVITY				
WHOLE FIELD (N: 24.1)	17.4	19.3	21.3	19.3 ± 1.1
QUAD.UPP.NAS.(N: 23.4)	16.4	18.1	20.6	18.3 ± 1.2
LOW.NAS.(N: 24.4)	21.5	23.3	24.1	23.0 ± 0.8
UPP.TMP.(N: 23.5)	11.3	13.7	17.7	14.2 ± 1.8
LOW.TMP.(N: 25.1)	20.2	22.2	22.7	21.7 ± 0.8
ECC. 0 – 10 (N: 26.9)	22.2	22.7	24.3	23.0 ± 0.6
10 – 20 (N: 24.9)	16.7	19.3	21.4	19.1 ± 1.3
20 – 30 (N: 23.0)	16.4	18.5	20.4	18.4 ± 1.2
NO. OF DISTURBED POINTS	46	31	17	31 ± 8
R.M.S. FLUCTUATION	2.6	1.9	2.3	2.3
TOTAL FLUCTUATION				3.0

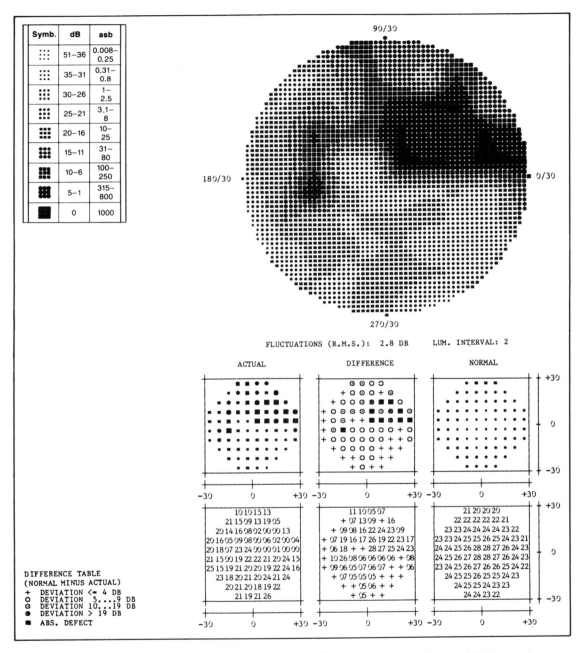

Symb.	dB	asb
⠿	51–36	0.008–0.25
⠿	35–31	0.31–0.8
⠿	30–26	1–2.5
⠿	25–21	3.1–8
⠿	20–16	10–25
⠿	15–11	31–80
⠿	10–6	100–250
⠿	5–1	315–800
■	0	1000

90/30

180/30

0/30

270/30

FLUCTUATIONS (R.M.S.): 2.8 DB   LUM. INTERVAL: 2

ACTUAL   DIFFERENCE   NORMAL

DIFFERENCE TABLE
(NORMAL MINUS ACTUAL)
+ DEVIATION <= 4 DB
○ DEVIATION 5...9 DB
⊙ DEVIATION 10...19 DB
● DEVIATION > 19 DB
■ ABS. DEFECT

Figure 8–26D. *Initial examination of the left eye shows more advanced field loss than was seen in the right eye. The blind spot is enlarged. There is generalized inferior central and arcuate depression. There is a superior arcuate scotoma, densest nasally ending in a sharp nasal step. (continued)*

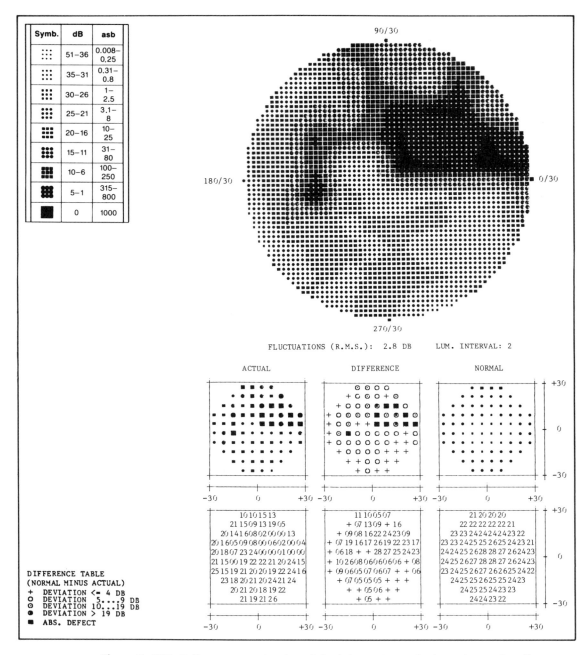

Figure 8–26E. *Follow-up examination of the left eye 8 months later shows virtually no change in the visual field. (continued)*

	EX1	EX2	EX3	SUMMARY
DATE OF EXAM : DAY	09.27	01.25	05.23	
YEAR	1983	1984	1984	
PROGRAM / EXAMINATION	32/01	32/03	32/05	
TOTAL LOSS (WHOLE FIELD)	640	723	622	661 ± 31
MEAN LOSS (PER TEST LOC)				
WHOLE FIELD	8.6	9.8	8.4	8.9 ± 0.4
QUADRANT UPPER NASAL	18.3	17.9	18.4	18.2 ± 0.1
LOWER NASAL	3.5	6.2	2.9	4.2 ± 1.0
UPPER TEMP.	9.2	9.3	7.7	8.7 ± 0.5
LOWER TEMP.	3.3	5.4	4.3	4.3 ± 0.6
ECCENTRICITY 0 - 10	11.6	13.6	11.4	12.2 ± 0.7
10 - 20	12.0	13.2	11.7	12.3 ± 0.5
20 - 30	6.5	7.3	6.3	6.7 ± 0.3
MEAN SENSITIVITY				
WHOLE FIELD (N: 24.1)	14.6	13.9	15.1	14.5 ± 0.3
QUAD.UPP.NAS.(N: 23.4)	4.9	5.5	4.9	5.1 ± 0.2
LOW.NAS.(N: 24.4)	19.8	17.7	20.9	19.5 ± 0.9
UPP.TMP.(N: 23.5)	13.4	14.0	14.8	14.1 ± 0.4
LOW.TMP.(N: 25.1)	20.6	18.7	20.0	19.8 ± 0.6
ECC. 0 - 10 (N: 26.9)	14.7	13.0	14.9	14.2 ± 0.6
10 - 20 (N: 24.9)	12.1	11.6	13.1	12.2 ± 0.4
20 - 30 (N: 23.0)	15.6	15.2	16.0	15.6 ± 0.2
NO. OF DISTURBED POINTS	49	59	51	53 ± 3
R.M.S. FLUCTUATION	4.6	2.1	2.8	3.2
TOTAL FLUCTUATION				2.5

Figure 8–26F. Series mode Delta examination of the left eye including an intermediate examination performed at 4 months shows stability of the visual field loss. Delta analysis shows transiently increased difficulty in the lower nasal area at the intermediate examination, but this is back to baseline by the third examination.

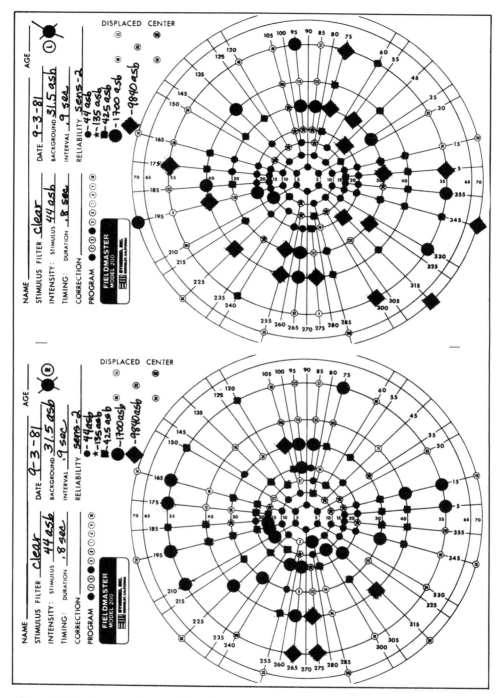

Figure 8–27. *Seventy-six-year-old aphakic male with open-angle glaucoma. The patient was seen by several physicians over a period of 3 years. Visual fields were performed on various devices.* **A.** *Initial examination in 1981 was performed on a Fieldmaster 200. Central field examinations were performed at 44 asb and 135 asb. Full-field examination was performed at 425 asb, 1700 asb, and 9840 asb. Although five sheets of paper were produced for each eye, these are summarized on one report for each eye. (continued)*

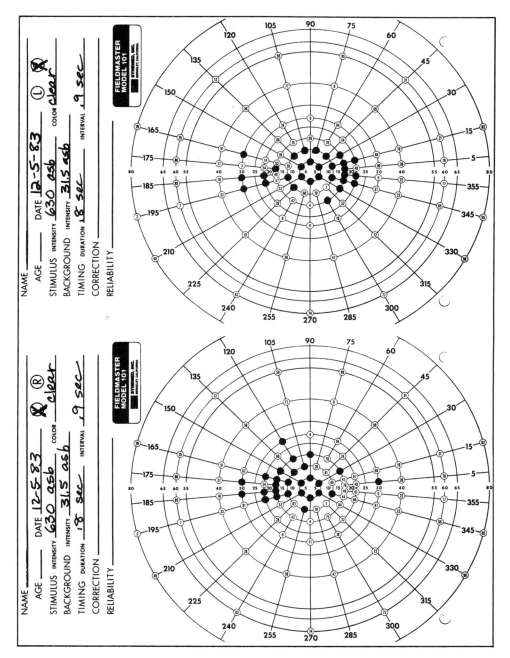

Figure 8–27B. *A second examination was performed 2 years later on a Fieldmaster 101. Only one intensity, 630 asb, was tested. Although little information is produced, because only one intensity was used, it could be concluded that the field had worsened. The fields to 630 asb were more constricted than the corresponding fields to 135 asb performed 2 years earlier. It was concluded that IOP has not been under adequate control. The patient was referred for further evaluation. (continued)*

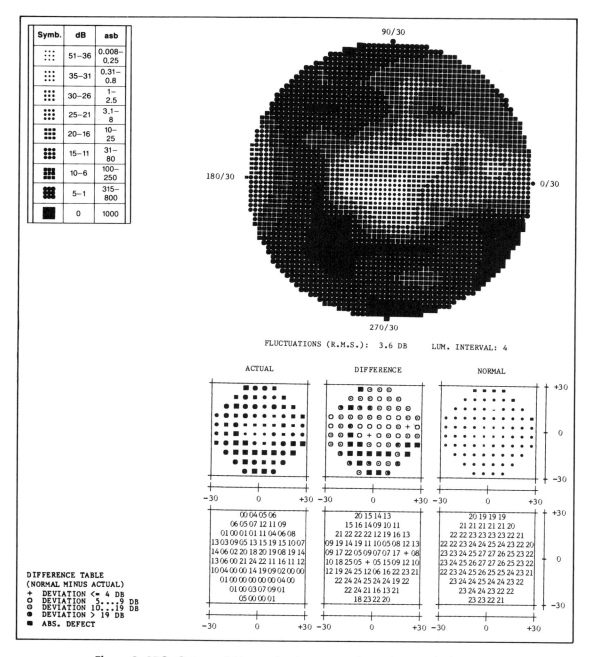

Symb.	dB	asb
⁙	51–36	0.008–0.25
⁙	35–31	0.31–0.8
⁙	30–26	1–2.5
⁙	25–21	3.1–8
▦	20–16	10–25
▦	15–11	31–80
▦	10–6	100–250
▦	5–1	315–800
■	0	1000

FLUCTUATIONS (R.M.S.): 3.6 DB   LUM. INTERVAL: 4

ACTUAL   DIFFERENCE   NORMAL

DIFFERENCE TABLE
(NORMAL MINUS ACTUAL)
+ DEVIATION <= 4 DB
○ DEVIATION 5...9 DB
◉ DEVIATION 10...19 DB
● DEVIATION > 19 DB
■ ABS. DEFECT

```
        00 04 05 06
       06 05 07 12 11 09
    01 00 01 01 11 04 06 08
  13 03 09 05 13 15 19 15 10 07
  14 06 02 20 18 20 19 08 19 14
  13 06 00 21 24 22 11 16 11 12
  10 04 00 00 14 19 09 02 00 00
    01 00 00 00 00 00 04 00
       01 00 03 07 09 01
        05 00 00 01
```

```
        20 15 14 13
       15 16 14 09 10 11
    21 22 22 22 12 19 16 13
  09 19 14 19 11 10 05 08 12 13
  09 17 22 05 09 07 07 17 + 08
  10 18 25 05 + 05 15 09 12 10
  12 19 24 25 12 06 16 22 23 21
    22 24 24 25 24 24 19 22
       22 24 21 16 13 21
        18 23 22 20
```

```
        20 19 19 19
       21 21 21 21 21 20
    22 22 23 23 23 23 22 21
  22 22 23 24 24 25 24 23 22 20
  23 23 24 25 27 27 26 25 23 22
  23 24 25 26 27 27 26 25 24 22
  22 23 24 25 26 25 25 24 23 21
    23 24 24 25 24 24 23 22
       23 24 24 23 22 21
        23 23 22 21
```

Figure 8–27C. *Octopus 201 examination was performed 3 months later using program 32. Left eye shows advanced glaucomatous field and is well documented. (continued)*

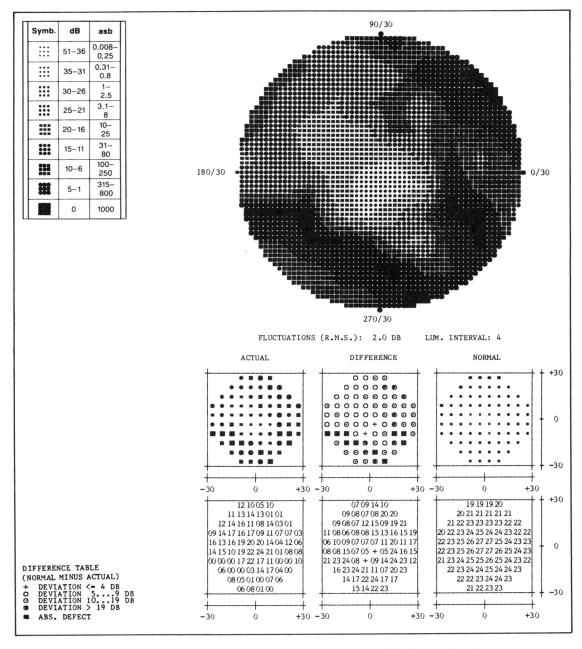

Symb.	dB	asb
:::	51–36	0.008–0.25
:::	35–31	0.31–0.8
:::	30–26	1–2.5
:::	25–21	3.1–8
:::	20–16	10–25
:::	15–11	31–80
:::	10–6	100–250
:::	5–1	315–800
■	0	1000

90/30

180/30

0/30

270/30

FLUCTUATIONS (R.M.S.): 2.0 DB   LUM. INTERVAL: 4

ACTUAL   DIFFERENCE   NORMAL

DIFFERENCE TABLE
(NORMAL MINUS ACTUAL)
+ DEVIATION <= 4 DB
o DEVIATION 5....9 DB
⊙ DEVIATION 10...19 DB
● DEVIATION > 19 DB
■ ABS. DEFECT

ACTUAL:
```
        12 10 05 10
      11 13 14 13 01 01
    12 14 16 11 08 14 03 01
  09 14 17 16 17 09 11 07 07 03
  16 13 16 19 20 20 14 04 12 06
  14 15 10 19 22 24 21 01 08 08
  00 00 00 17 22 17 11 00 00 10
      06 00 00 03 14 17 04 00
        08 05 01 00 07 06
          06 08 01 00
```

DIFFERENCE:
```
        07 09 14 10
      09 08 07 08 20 20
    09 08 07 12 15 09 19 21
  11 08 06 08 08 15 13 16 15 19
  06 10 09 07 07 07 11 20 11 17
  08 08 15 07 05 + 05 24 16 15
  21 23 24 08 + 09 14 24 23 12
      16 23 24 21 11 07 20 23
        14 17 22 24 17 17
          15 14 22 23
```

NORMAL:
```
        19 19 19 20
      20 21 21 21 21 21
    21 22 23 23 23 23 22 22
  20 22 23 24 25 24 24 23 22 22
  22 23 25 26 27 27 25 24 23 23
  22 23 25 26 27 27 26 25 24 23
  21 23 24 25 26 25 24 23 22 22
      22 23 24 24 24 23
        22 22 23 24 24 23
          21 22 23 23
```

Figure 8–27D. *Octopus 201 program 32 examination of right eye also documents advanced glaucomatous field loss although not as severe as left eye. (Octopus exam courtesy of Elizabeth Hodapp, M.D.) (continued)*

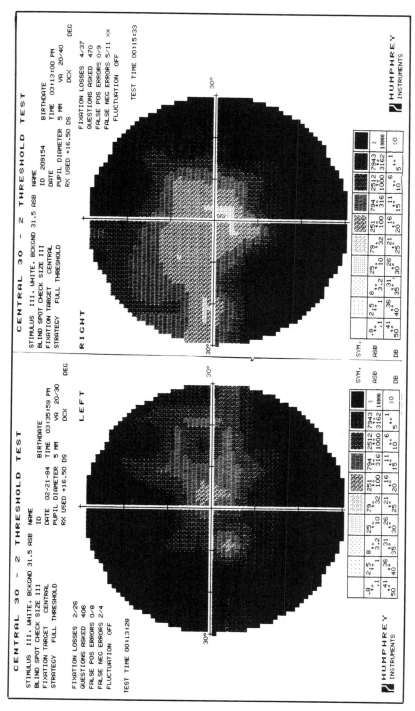

Figure 8–27E. Humphrey Visual Field Analyzer examination was performed simultaneously with the Octopus examinations shown in Figures 8–28 C and D. At the top are the grey scales. In the middle are the actual threshold values. At the bottom are the deviations from expected values. The field loss seen on the Octopus examination is confirmed. (Humphrey field examinations courtesy of Elizabeth Hodapp, M.D.) (continued)

Figure 8–27E. (continued)

Upper visual field plot:

LEFT · RIGHT

Left eye (upper):
```
              2    2   (↓)  <0                          4   (↕)  0    <0
        <0   <0   <0  (↓)  6    5                  (↓₁) 10  (↓₀) 0   <0   <0
   <0   <0    2    0    2   10   0  (8/6)      (9/11) 14 (10/15)(14/15)(11/7)(11/5) 9  <0
(6/4)(<0)  <0 (13/5) 4  6  (17/5)(14/10)(12/8) 3    14 (4/14) 16 (21/21)(16/18) 17 (19/17) 3 (1/0) <0
   <0   <0   0    6   10  (18/20)12   4  (14/10) 0   19 (29/15)18 (16/18)(16/14) 21 15  7 (1/1) 0
```
30° —————————————————————————— 30°   30° ——————————————————————————— 30°
```
   6   <0   <0   19   5   16  12  12  10  10        10  14   6  14  21  21  13  <0  <0  <0
  <0   <0   <0 (7/1) 5 (0/2)(13/3)<0 <0 <0          <0  <0  <0 (1/0)(16/20)(4/6)(9/7)<0 <0 <0
       <0   <0   <0   <0  <0  <0  <0  <0                  <0  <0  <0  <0  <0  <0  <0
            <0   <0   <0  <0  <0  <0
```

NO.   = THRESHOLD IN DB   NO.   = THRESHOLD IN DB
(NO.) = 2ND/3RD TIME   (NO.) = 2ND/3RD TIME

Lower visual field plot:

LEFT · RIGHT
```
            15   16   18   17                          13   6   18   17
       18   19   19   19   13   13                  8   9   12   19   19   18
   18   19   19   21   19   11   19   12          8   5   8   6   12  16  10  18
12 19 21 14 19  17  10  9  9  14         °  10  5  °  6  6  °  18  19  17
18 19 21 17 15  6  11  17  7  18         °  °  °  6  9  °  8  14  18  18
```
30° ——————————————————————————— 30°   30° ——————————————————————————— 30°
```
12 19 21 ° 20  9  11  9  9  8           8  5  15  9  °  °  10  21  19  18
17 19 21 18 18  22  13  21  19  17      17  19  21  22  5  18  14  21  19  17
   18   19   21   21  21  21  19  18         18  19  21  21  21  21  19  18
        18   19   19   19   19   18              18  19  19  19  19  18
             17   18   18   17                         17  18  18  17
```

° = WITHIN 4 DB OF EXPECTED   ° = WITHIN 4 DB OF EXPECTED
NO. = DEFECT DEPTH IN DB   NO. = DEFECT DEPTH IN DB
26 DB ×× = CENTRAL REF LEVEL   26 DB ×× = CENTRAL REF LEVEL

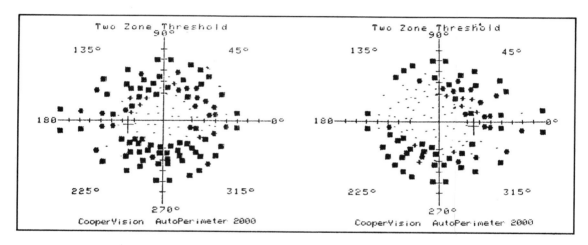

Figure 8–27F. Dicon AP 2000 examination was performed 4 months later using the two-zone stepped suprathreshold testing strategy. The Octopus and Humphrey examinations are confirmed. The patient is currently being tested with the Dicon AP 2000. Visual field examinations have been stable with the IOP under good control.

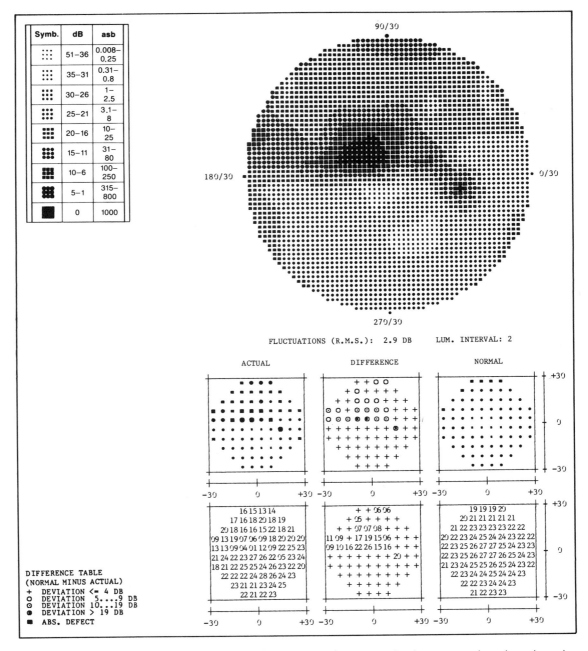

Figure 8–28. *Eighty-one-year-old woman with open-angle glaucoma and moderately early visual field loss. The patient was followed on the Octopus 201 using program 32. All studies are of the right eye. **A.** First examination shows loss in superior central and superior arcuate areas only. (continued)*

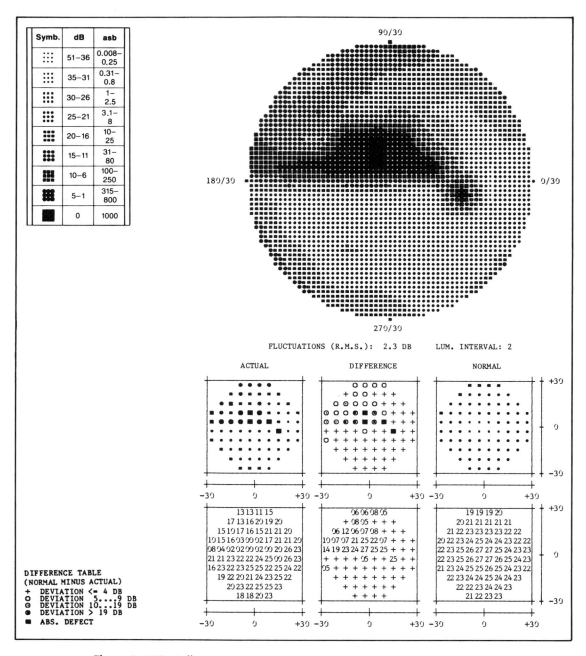

Figure 8–28B. *Follow-up examination 6 months later shows deepening of the arcuate defects. The inferior half of the visual field are the deepening of the superior arcuate defect. Inferior half of the visual field remains normal. (continued)*

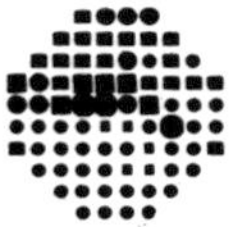

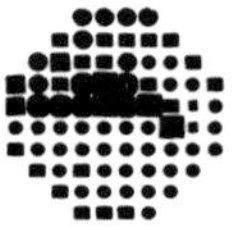

Figure 8–28C. *Series mode Delta examination confirms increase in loss. The number of disturbed points increased from 19 to 27. The total loss increased from 230 to 343. Most of the increased loss occurred in the upper nasal quadrant with considerable increased loss also in the upper temporal quadrant. (continued)*

	EX1	EX2	SUMMARY
DATE OF EXAM : DAY	08.10	02.20	
YEAR	1983	1984	
PROGRAM / EXAMINATION	32/04	32/06	
TOTAL LOSS (WHOLE FIELD)	230	343	286 ± 56
MEAN LOSS (PER TEST LOC)			
WHOLE FIELD	3.1	4.6	3.9 ± 0.8
QUADRANT UPPER NASAL	8.3	12.3	10.3 ± 2.0
LOWER NASAL	0.0	0.5	0.3 ± 0.3
UPPER TEMP.	4.0	5.6	4.8 ± 0.8
LOWER TEMP.	0.0	0.0	0.0 ± 0.0
ECCENTRICITY 0 - 10	9.4	12.8	11.1 ± 1.7
10 - 20	3.4	4.4	3.9 ± 0.5
20 - 30	1.3	2.5	1.9 ± 0.6
MEAN SENSITIVITY			
WHOLE FIELD (N: 23.1)	19.1	17.7	18.4 ± 0.7
QUAD.UPP.NAS.(N: 22.4)	12.9	10.0	11.5 ± 1.5
LOW.NAS.(N: 23.4)	22.4	21.1	21.8 ± 0.7
UPP.TMP.(N: 22.5)	17.6	16.3	16.9 ± 0.6
LOW.TMP.(N: 24.1)	23.8	23.7	23.7 ± 0.1
ECC. 0 - 10 (N: 25.9)	15.7	12.4	14.0 ± 1.6
10 - 20 (N: 23.9)	20.0	18.4	19.2 ± 0.8
20 - 30 (N: 22.0)	19.7	18.9	19.3 ± 0.4
NO. OF DISTURBED POINTS	19	27	23 ± 4
R.M.S. FLUCTUATION	2.9	2.3	2.6
TOTAL FLUCTUATION			2.2

Figure 8–28D. *Change printout of Delta examination shows uniform minimal loss in inferior half of the field but results are still within the "normal" range. In the superior half, especially in the central and nasal arcuate areas, significant change can be noted. T-test shows alteration for both the whole field and the pathologic areas. (continued)*

```
            - 3.  - 2.  - 2    1

       0:  - 3  - 2.   0:   1:   1:

   - 5.  - 8.   1     0    0  - 1:   3:  - 1:

 1    2  - 3.  - 4   - 6  - 7  - 1   1:   1:   0:

- 5  - 9  - 7  - 2  - 1  -10  - 9        1:   0:

 0:  - 3:   1:  - 1:  - 5.  - 2:   3:        3:  - 1:

- 2.   2:   0:  - 2:   0:   1:  - 4:   2:   2:   2:

    - 3:   0:  - 2:  - 3:  - 4:  - 3:   1:  - 1:

       - 3:   2:   1:   2:   1:  - 2:

          - 4:  - 3:  - 2:   0:
```

DIFFERENCE TABLE : MEAN B MINUS MEAN A (NEGATIVE VALUES: DECREASED SENSITIVITY)
0-0 ALL RESULTS ZERO   ◇ LOW NORMAL VALUES
DOTS INDICATE THAT SOME (.) OR ALL (:) RESULTS ARE IN NORMAL RANGE (FULLY VALID)
CONFIDENCE INTERVAL FOR MEAN DIFFERENCE / T-TEST
(1) PATHOL. AREA (UNDOTTED)   - 3.2 ± 1.9 (T-TEST: ALTERATION IS INDICATED)
(2) WHOLE FIELD   - 1.4 ± 0.7 (T-TEST: ALTERATION IS INDICATED)

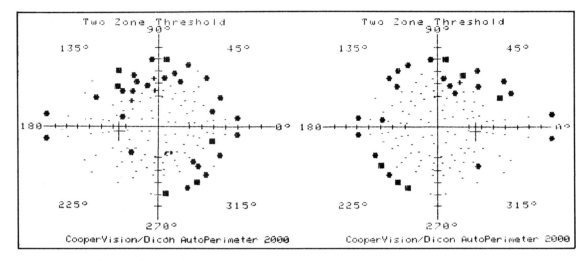

Figure 8–29. *Thirty-nine-year-old man with pigmentary glaucoma. Examinations were performed on the Dicon AP 2000 using the two-zone threshold program with a starting intensity of 32 asb.* **A.** *First examination shows field loss in the superior arcuate area of the right eye and the superior and inferior arcuate areas of the left eye with an enlargement of the left blind spot. (continued)*

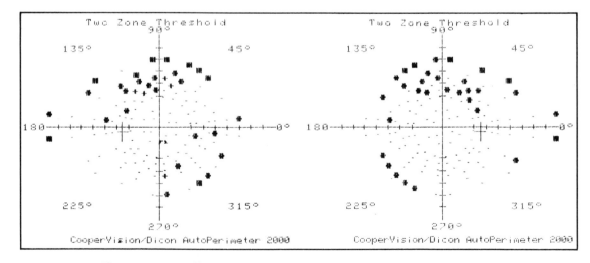

Figure 8–29B. *Follow-up examination performed 6 months later shows an enlargement of the superior arcuate scotoma of the right eye, which is now contiguous with the blind spot. This change was confirmed on a subsequent examination.*

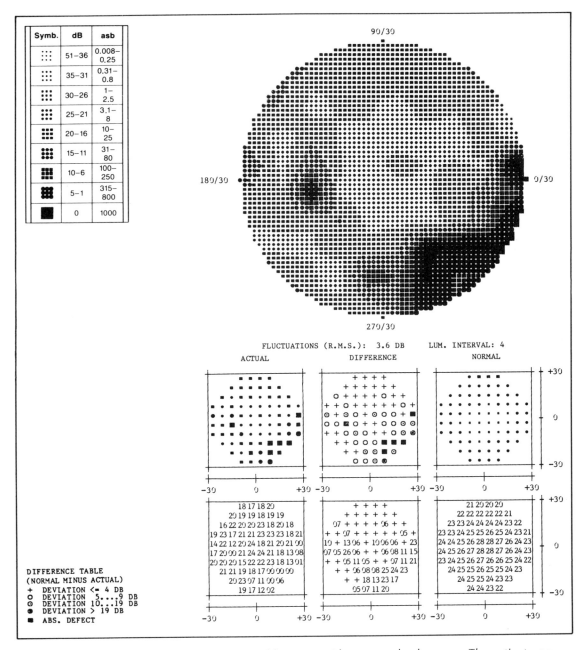

Figure 8–30. *Seventy-two-year-old woman with open-angle glaucoma. The patient was followed on an Octopus 201 using program 32 and examined four times over a 2-year period.* **A.** *First examination of left eye reveals generalized inferior field depression with a dense inferonasal arcuate scotoma. (continued)*

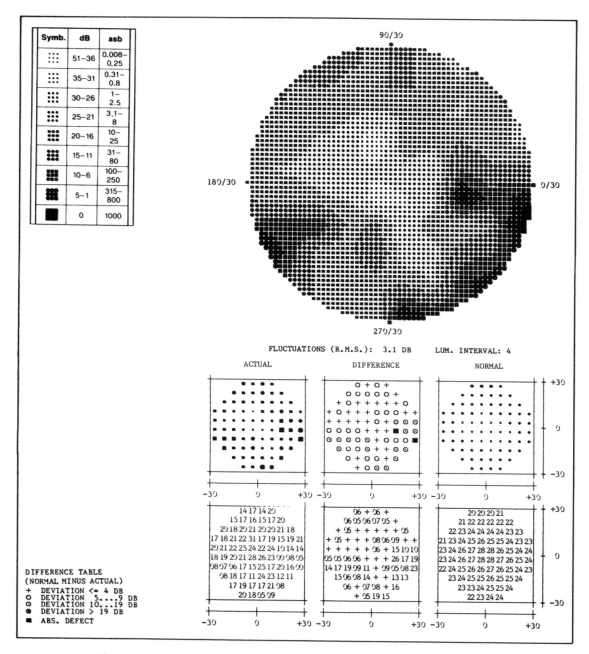

Symb.	dB	asb
⦂⦂⦂	51–36	0.008–0.25
⦂⦂⦂	35–31	0.31–0.8
⦂⦂⦂	30–26	1–2.5
⦂⦂⦂	25–21	3.1–8
⦂⦂⦂	20–16	10–25
⦂⦂⦂	15–11	31–80
⦂⦂⦂	10–6	100–250
⦂⦂⦂	5–1	315–800
■	0	1000

FLUCTUATIONS (R.M.S.): 3.1 DB   LUM. INTERVAL: 4

ACTUAL   DIFFERENCE   NORMAL

DIFFERENCE TABLE
(NORMAL MINUS ACTUAL)
+   DEVIATION <= 4 DB
o   DEVIATION 5...9 DB
⊙   DEVIATION 10...19 DB
●   DEVIATION > 19 DB
■   ABS. DEFECT

Figure 8–30B. *Fourth examination of left eye shows depression now involving the superior field. There is also an enlargement in the size of the inferonasal arcuate scotoma. (continued)*

	EX1	EX2	EX3	EX4	SUMMARY
DATE OF EXAM : DAY	07.16	03.22	10.25	05.29	
YEAR	1982	1983	1983	1984	
PROGRAM / EXAMINATION	32/01	32/02	32/03	32/05	
TOTAL LOSS (WHOLE FIELD)	412	474	455	615	489 ± 43
MEAN LOSS (PER TEST LOC)					
WHOLE FIELD	5.6	6.4	6.1	8.3	6.6 ± 0.6
QUADRANT UPPER NASAL	2.9	3.1	1.1	4.1	2.8 ± 0.6
LOWER NASAL	12.8	14.8	16.3	17.2	15.3 ± 1.0
UPPER TEMP.	1.7	3.8	2.3	5.4	3.3 ± 0.8
LOWER TEMP.	4.6	3.6	4.6	6.3	4.8 ± 0.6
ECCENTRICITY 0 - 10	3.3	4.5	3.4	7.1	4.6 ± 0.9
10 - 20	5.4	6.4	6.6	8.7	6.8 ± 0.7
20 - 30	6.3	6.9	6.7	8.5	7.1 ± 0.5
MEAN SENSITIVITY					
WHOLE FIELD (N: 24.1)	17.1	16.5	16.4	15.0	16.2 ± 0.4
QUAD.UPP.NAS.(N: 23.4)	19.0	18.5	19.8	18.2	18.9 ± 0.3
LOW.NAS.(N: 24.4)	11.0	9.4	7.8	7.2	8.8 ± 0.9
UPP.TMP.(N: 23.5)	19.6	18.4	19.0	17.2	18.5 ± 0.5
LOW.TMP.(N: 25.1)	19.1	20.0	19.1	17.8	19.0 ± 0.4
ECC. 0 - 10 (N: 26.9)	21.8	21.8	21.5	19.8	21.2 ± 0.5
10 - 20 (N: 24.9)	18.5	17.5	17.3	15.7	17.2 ± 0.6
20 - 30 (N: 23.0)	15.3	14.6	14.6	13.5	14.5 ± 0.4
NO. OF DISTURBED POINTS	37	46	39	58	45 ± 5
R.M.S. FLUCTUATION	3.6	1.2	1.2	1.2	1.8
TOTAL FLUCTUATION					2.2

Figure 8–30C. Delta analysis of the left eye examination, including two intermediate examinations, shows total loss increased greatly between examinations 1 and 2, decreased slightly between examinations 2 and 3, but increased greatly again between examinations 3 and 4. Mean loss in the lower nasal quadrant increased steadily with each successive examination. The lower nasal quadrant was clearly getting worse faster than the whole field in general. *(continued)*

202

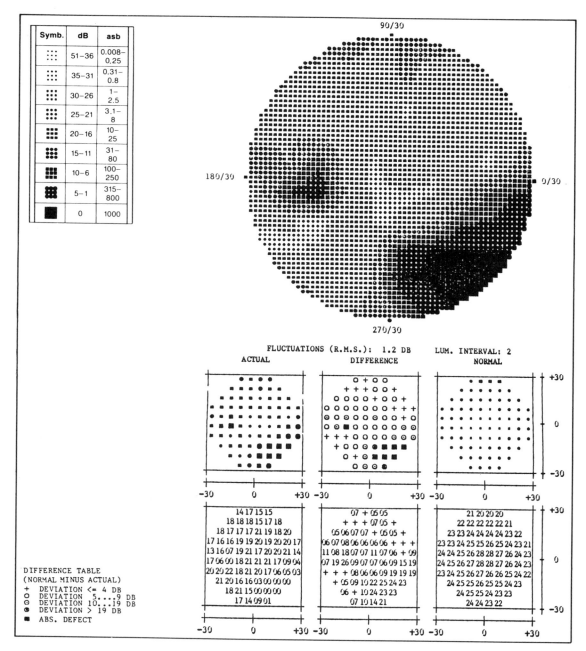

Figure 8–30D. *First examination of the right eye reveals moderately early glaucomatous loss. Inferior and superior arcuate loss is seen greater inferiorly with the formation of a nasal step. (continued)*

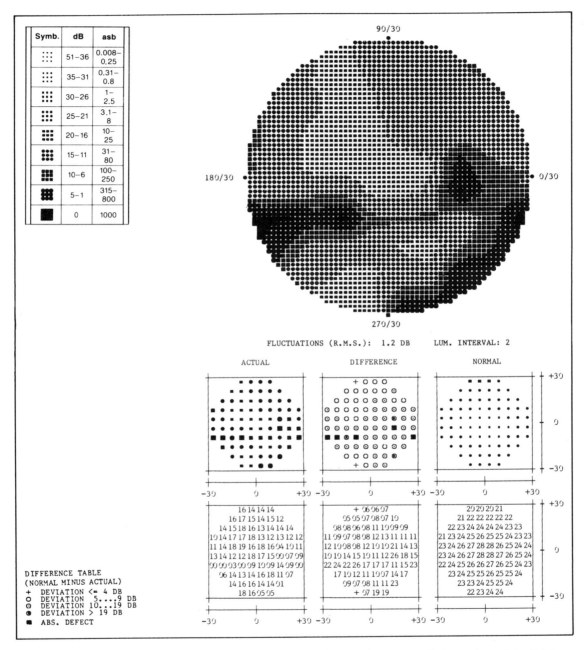

Symb.	dB	asb
⋮⋮⋮	51–36	0.008–0.25
⋮⋮⋮	35–31	0.31–0.8
⋮⋮⋮	30–26	1–2.5
⋮⋮⋮	25–21	3.1–8
▪▪▪	20–16	10–25
●●●	15–11	31–80
■■■	10–6	100–250
▓	5–1	315–800
■	0	1000

90/30

180/30

0/30

270/30

FLUCTUATIONS (R.M.S.): 1.2 DB   LUM. INTERVAL: 2

ACTUAL   DIFFERENCE   NORMAL

DIFFERENCE TABLE
(NORMAL MINUS ACTUAL)
+   DEVIATION <= 4 DB
o   DEVIATION 5...9 DB
⊙   DEVIATION 10...19 DB
◉   DEVIATION > 19 DB
■   ABS. DEFECT

```
      16 14 14 14                    +  06 06 07                 20 20 20 21
     16 17 15 14 15 12              05 05 07 08 07 10            21 22 22 22 22 22
    14 15 18 16 13 14 14 14        08 08 06 08 11 10 09 09      22 23 24 24 24 24 23 23
  10 14 17 17 18 13 12 13 12 12   11 09 07 08 08 12 13 11 11 11  21 23 24 25 26 25 24 24 23 23
  11 14 18 19 16 18 16 04 10 11   12 10 08 08 12 10 12 21 14 13  23 24 26 27 28 28 26 25 24 24
  13 14 12 12 18 17 15 09 07 09   10 10 14 15 10 11 12 26 18 15  23 24 26 27 28 28 27 26 25 24
  00 09 03 00 09 10 09 14 09 00   22 24 22 26 17 17 17 11 15 23  22 24 25 26 26 27 26 25 24 23
     06 14 13 14 16 18 11 07       17 10 12 11 19 07 14 17        23 24 25 26 25 25 24
     14 16 16 14 14 01             09 07 08 11 11 23              23 23 24 25 25 24
      18 16 05 05                   +  07 19 19                   22 23 24 24
```

	EX1	EX2	EX3	EX4	SUMMARY
DATE OF EXAM : DAY	07.16	03.22	10.25	05.29	
YEAR	1982	1983	1983	1984	
PROGRAM / EXAMINATION	32/01	32/02	32/03	32/05	
TOTAL LOSS (WHOLE FIELD)	423	670	721	849	665 ± 89
MEAN LOSS (PER TEST LOC)					
WHOLE FIELD	5.7	9.1	9.7	11.5	9.0 ± 1.2
QUADRANT UPPER NASAL	1.7	5.0	5.9	7.7	5.1 ± 1.2
LOWER NASAL	8.1	10.9	10.4	13.2	10.7 ± 1.1
UPPER TEMP.	4.0	8.7	10.2	10.1	8.2 ± 1.5
LOWER TEMP.	9.2	11.7	12.6	15.0	12.1 ± 1.2
ECCENTRICITY 0 - 10	2.6	7.1	9.1	11.8	7.6 ± 1.9
10 - 20	4.7	9.4	9.3	11.8	8.8 ± 1.5
20 - 30	7.0	9.5	10.1	11.3	9.4 ± 0.9
MEAN SENSITIVITY					
WHOLE FIELD (N: 24.1)	17.3	14.6	14.1	12.5	14.6 ± 1.0
QUAD.UPP.NAS.(N: 23.4)	19.9	17.7	16.9	15.5	17.5 ± 0.9
LOW.NAS.(N: 24.4)	16.0	13.2	13.7	10.9	13.5 ± 1.0
UPP.TMP.(N: 23.5)	18.3	14.6	13.3	13.4	14.9 ± 1.2
LOW.TMP.(N: 25.1)	15.0	12.9	12.4	10.1	12.6 ± 1.0
ECC. 0 - 10 (N: 26.9)	23.4	19.4	17.8	15.1	18.9 ± 1.7
10 - 20 (N: 24.9)	18.6	15.1	15.4	13.2	15.6 ± 1.1
20 - 30 (N: 23.0)	15.2	13.1	12.6	11.5	13.1 ± 0.8
NO. OF DISTURBED POINTS	44	65	70	72	63 ± 6
R.M.S. FLUCTUATION	3.1	2.4	1.9	1.2	2.1
TOTAL FLUCTUATION					2.9

Figure 8–30F. Delta program analysis of the right eye including two intermediate examinations shows steady progressive loss. Mean loss increased from 423 to 627 to 721 to 849. Number of disturbed points increased from 44 to 65 to 70 to 72. Steady progressive loss is seen in all quadrants and eccentricities.

9

The Visual Field in Neurologic Disease

The patient with a neurologic problem can be a very difficult visual field patient. Often the patient is ill or has difficulty responding. Frequently the patient is frightened. Usually he or she has never had a visual field examination before. The patient occasionally is confined to bed or has limitations on movement. The patient is often very tired from having gone through a large battery of tests. Because of these limitations, the method of visual field testing has to be tailored to each patient. Often simplicity in the technique of field testing is necessary to obtain any information at all. The luxury of being able to do a sophisticated analysis of the patient's entire visual field is not always present.

When approaching the neuroophthalmic patient, it is wise to start with as simple a procedure as possible. The patient's symptoms often suggest the possibility of certain defects. These areas should be tested early on in the visual field testing process. For the detection phase of the visual field examination, adequate information can often be obtained by simple confrontation tests, but the qualitative and quantitative phases of visual field testing usually require more sophisticated equipment.

Testing Strategy in the Neuroophthalmic Patient

A testing strategy is important in a neuroophthalmic patient regardless of the method utilized. The examiner should have an idea of what type of defect he or she expects. Careful study of either side of the midline must be made to ascertain the presence or absence of a Chamlin step (a defect of one side of the visual field that comes up to but does not cross the vertical meridian). A subtle hemianopsic defect is often detectable only as a small Chamlin step. The areas of the blind spot and the fixation must be examined carefully as retinal vascular defects tend to originate in the blind spot and optic nerve defects tend to originate at fixation.

Gun barrel fields, or severe constriction, can result from a variety of diseases. A junctional scotoma consists of a central scotoma with a contralateral upper temporal defect. Small central scotomas can be found most easily with an Amsler grid. Bitemporal hemianopsias can be upper and/or lower. Binasal defects are also possible.

Multiple types of homonymous hemianopsias can be present and these can be either congruous or incongruous. Incongruous defects tend to be due to more anteriorly placed lesions and congruous defects tend to be due to more posteriorly placed lesions. Temporal and occipital lobe lesions affect the superior visual field more so than the inferior field and parietal lobe lesions affect the inferior field more than the superior field. Hemianopsias can either split fixation or spare fixation and can be confined to the paracentral field.

The Visual Pathway

Visual stimuli are collected by the eyes and then transmitted to the posterior portion of the brain. Nerve fibers involved in vision remain precisely organized over their entire course through the brain and, therefore, cerebral lesions often interrupt the visual pathway. Depending on the site of the lesion, different types of field defects can be generated (Fig. 9–1).

Visual stimuli are focused by the anterior optical portion of the eyes onto the retina where they are received and processed by the rods and the cones. They are then transmitted to the optic nerves, which are composed of the axons of the retinal ganglion cells. The axons continue in the chiasm and optic tracts ending in the lateral geniculate bodies. There is a hemidecusation of the fibers in the chiasm so that the fibers from the left half of each retina (representing the right half of the visual field of each eye) end in the left lateral geniculate body and the fibers from the right half of each retina (representing the left half of the visual field of each eye) end in the right lateral geniculate body. The final visual neurons originate in the lateral geniculate bodies and form the geniculocalcarine tracts (or optic radiations). These fibers are first directed down and forward, they then bend backward in a sharp loop and pass through the temporal lobe sweeping around the anterior aspect of the temporal horn of the lateral ventricles and finally end in the posterior occipital cortex. The most anterior inferior fibers form Meyer's loop, which passes around the tip of the temporal ventricular horn. Meyer's loop contains the inferior retinal fibers representing the most superior portions of the visual field. All fibers end in area 17 of the occipital cortex. Visual information is then integrated in areas 18 and 19.

Lesions of the visual pathway create different visual field defects depending

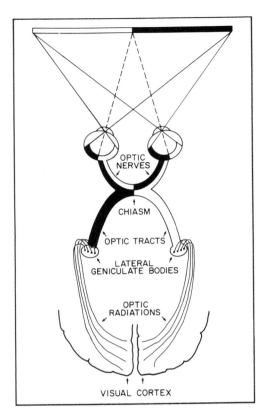

Figure 9–1. *The visual pathway.*

on their location. Lesions through the optic nerve anterior to the chiasm will only affect the ipsilateral eye. Lesions through the center of the chiasm affect the crossing fibers and therefore affect the temporal field of both eyes. Lesions of the optic tract beyond the chiasm but anterior to the lateral geniculate body affect the contralateral half of the visual field of each eye. Lesions through the optic radiation affect the contralateral halves of the visual field of both eyes. The pattern of loss in each eye becomes more congruous as the occipital cortex is approached.

The cuneus, the gyrus above the calcarine fissure in area 17, receives the fibers from the inferior half of the retina. Lesions through it affect the superior half of the contralateral field of each eye.

Types of Neurologic Visual Field Defects

HOMONYMOUS DEFECTS

Homonymous visual field defects usually are caused by lesions affecting one side of the brain. As a lesion becomes closer to the striate cortex, the field defect it creates becomes more congruous. Lesions present in the area of

Meyer's loop tend to give a pie-in-the-sky superior homonymous field defect, but this can occur in other lesions also. Accurate identification of the site of the lesion causing the defect usually cannot be made just on the pattern of the visual field loss. Figure 9–2 shows the effect of a right-sided hemispheric cerebrovascular accident on the visual fields. The entire left half of the visual field of each eye was lost.

ARCUATE SCOTOMAS

Arcuate scotomas, although usually caused by glaucoma, can be caused by juxtapapillary choroiditis, colobomata, optic nerve pits, papillitis, arteriosclerotic plaques in vessels coming off the disk, ischemic anterior optic neuropathy, temporal arteritis, retrobulbar neuritis, a meningioma of the optic foramen or dorsum sella, a pituitary adenoma, or opticochiasmal arachnoiditis. Most arcuate scotomas are caused by glaucoma, however.

BLIND SPOT ENLARGEMENT

Enlargement of the blind spot can be seen in papilledema, peripapillary atrophy, glaucoma, optic nerve head drusen, juxtapapillary choroiditis, myelination of the optic nerve head, a tilted disk, and colobomata.

CENTRAL VISUAL FIELD DEFECTS

Cecocentral defects can be caused by glaucoma, nutritional amblyopia, pernicious anemia optic neuritis, and Leber's optic atrophy.

The use of color in visual field testing is useful in detecting subtle central scotomas. The most effective color for such testing is red. When the test object is brought from an area of nonvision to an area of vision, the test object is first seen without recognition of the color and then with red recognition. Usually a 6- to 9-mm red test object is the most effective size on a tangent screen and a 3-mm test spot is the most effective size on a bowl-type field tester. Most automated devices do not test for color recognition.

Central defects can be seen as areas of haziness or absent vision on an Amsler grid. A subtle central defect, which can barely be appreciated on a standard white on black grid, can often be appreciated on a red on black grid. The Amsler grid is a valuable adjunct to full field testing.

THE CHAMLIN STEP

A Chamlin step is a peripheral defect on one side only of the 90-degree meridian. For a defect to qualify as a Chamlin step there must be a 10-degree difference from one side to another. If there is a small difference to white, a larger difference might be detectable to a red test object. Confirmation of the step is made in kinetic perimetry by moving the object over the vertical meridian. Confirmation in automated static field testing is best made by thresholding multiple corresponding points on either side of the vertical meridian.

GENERALIZED CONSTRICTION

Generalized constriction of the visual field can be due to many causes, including optic neuritis and toxic amblyopia. It can also be seen in retinitis pigmentosa, the late stages of glaucoma, optic lobe infarctions, quinine toxicity, syphilitic parineuritis, and chronic disk edema.

Peripheral constriction from optic nerve lesions is nonspecific and of little localizing value. Generalized constriction usually is associated with reduced contrast sensitivity. It can be likened to a sinking of the visual island and it often accompanies central defects, centrocecal defects, or arcuate defects. When present in the remaining nasal fields of patients with a bitemporal hemianopsia, it usually indicates impaired nerve conduction in the ipsilateral uncrossed, as well as crossed, fibers in the chiasm. When caused by chronic papilledema the defect is usually more severe nasally and also inferiorly.

GUN BARREL FIELDS

Highly constricted "gun barrel" visual fields of only 5 or 10 degrees in size can be caused by numerous conditions. These include glaucoma, retinitis pigmentosa, a bilateral occipital lobe infarction with macula sparing, a central retinal artery occlusion with a persistent cilioretinal artery, extensive chorioretinitis, hysteria, and malingering.

In such patients, glaucoma should be explored by the measurement of intraocular pressure, careful examination of the anterior segment, a careful history, and an optic nerve examination with close attention paid to the presence of glaucomatous cupping of the nerve. Retinitis pigmentosa usually presents with classic bone-spickling on retinal examination. Electrophysiologic tests are usually very helpful.

Bilateral occipital lobe infarctions with macular sparing, although exceedingly rare, result in visual fields of 5 degrees or less. Computerized tomographic scans can prove to be useful in such cases. The presence of a cilioretinal artery can be determined by careful examination of the posterior pole. Extensive chorioretinitis is apparent upon examination of the retina.

The Visual Field in Lesions of the Optic Nerve

When examining the visual field in patients with lesions affecting the optic nerves or the chiasm, it is important to detect the depth as well as the breadth of the defect. Lesions in this area usually effect the central visual field. A reduction in sensitivity to light and contrast in the center of the field is often accompanied by poor visual acuity, but often the visual field defects can still be plotted with great accuracy. The depth of the defect corresponds to the degree of impairment of visual function, whereas the size and the location of the defect does not give the full extent of visual loss.

Often a patient with minimal optic nerve disease or early optic nerve disease complains of a reduced brightness of objects and a reduced intensity of colors. The visual acuity is often normal, but visual field defects and depression in the central field can be found with appropriate visual field testing (Fig. 9–3).

Visual field defects from diseases of the optic nerve can be of several types. These include: (1) attitudinal or sector arcuate defects, (2) central scotomas, (3) cecocentral scotomas (defects encompassing both fixation and the blind spot), (4) paracentral scotomas and enlargement of the blind spot, and (5) generalized constriction.

Arcuate defects radiate from the blind spot, have sharp borders on the horizontal meridian, can be surrounded by retained vision on both sides, or extend to the periphery of the field. An altitudinal defect can be considered to be an arcuate defect that has extended into the periphery. Usually arcuate defects are the result of anterior optic nerve lesions, but can result from more proximal lesions. A monocular arcuate defect that radiates from the blind spot but stops at a sharp vertical border can signify a lesion at the junction of the optic nerve and the chiasm. Arcuate scotomas are usually vascular in etiology. Glaucoma, temporal arteritis, ischemic optic neuropathy, migraine, and collagen vascular diseases all have been shown to cause arcuate scotomas.

Central scotomas result from mass lesions pressing on the optic nerve or optic neuritis. Fibers from the central visual field area are more susceptible to damage than peripheral fibers. They are thinner and have less myelination, and therefore seem to be effected before peripheral fibers are effected.

Cecocentral field defects in diseases of the optic nerve are usually from toxic or nutritional amblyopias, demyelinating diseases, hereditary diseases such as Leber's optic neuropathy, inflammatory conditions of the optic nerve, or compression of the nerve. Axial optic nerve disease with peripheral sparing of the visual field is usually due to demyelinating disease. In contrast to this, if the central field is spared but the peripheral field is lost due to optic nerve disease, the most likely etiology is lues.

Cecocentral defects result because ganglion cell fibers from the peripapillary retina run with the macular projection through the center of the optic nerve. Therefore, lesions involving the axis of the optic nerve, such as demyelinating disease, produce a central scotoma and also an enlarged blind spot. This is often important in differentiating papilledema from optic neuritis. In optic neuritis a central visual field defect is seen. In early papilledema the size of the blind spot might increase, but the central vision and the central field remain normal.

If a lesion is situated near the junction of the optic nerve and the chiasm, a specific visual field defect known as a "junctional scotoma" will occur. A central scotoma is seen in one eye with a superotemporal field defect in the contralateral eye. The inferonasal fibers of the contralateral eye loop back for a short distance into the ipsilateral optic nerve forming von Willebrand's knee. The etiology of the contralateral superotemporal defect is an interruption of the fibers of von Willebrand's knee.

Although the anterior portion of the optic nerve can be examined with the ophthalmoscope, we are dependent on other means of examination for the posterior portion of the optic nerve. Specifically, we are limited to visual field examination, electrophysiologic tests, x-ray examination including computerized axial tomography and magnetic resonance imaging. Even when there is ophthalmoscopic evidence of optic nerve disease, the appearance is usually nonspecific, necessitating further testing. Other quick clinical tests that are of use in evaluating the optic nerve include color vision testing and the examination of pupillary function looking for an afferent pupillary defect or the Marcus-Gunn phenomenon. Because optic nerve defects usually cause central visual field defects, the Amsler grid is invaluable for examination of the very central portion of the visual field.

THE VISUAL FIELD IN PAPILLEDEMA

Generalized visual field constriction is often seen in optic nerve disease and usually it is the result of diffuse involvement of the optic nerve. This can be conceptualized as a sinking of the island of Traquair because the generalized constriction is always accompanied by a generalized loss of sensitivity throughout the remaining visual field.

Visual field defects in papilledema usually do not appear until after there is gross ophthalmoscopic evidence of nerve involvement. The first visual field defect to occur tends to be an enlargement of the blind spot. This can occur in even mild edema. The temporal portion of the disk is affected to a greater degree than the nasal portion due to the greater number of nerve fibers on the temporal side. The blind spot, although enlarging in all directions, tends to enlarge to a greater degree toward fixation.

Chronic papilledema can cause visual field defects that simulate those seen in glaucoma. Dense paracentral scotomas have been found in the arcuate areas as well as classic complete arcuate scotomas.

When papilledema is prolonged, secondary optic atrophy can occur. In such cases there is a generalized visual field depression and this tends to be most marked in the nasal field. Eventually there will be complete loss of the visual field. Although visual field loss from prolonged papilledema is felt to be irreversible, optic nerve head decompression has shown that in some patients there can be some return of visual function.

OPTIC NERVE ABNORMALITIES

Myelinated nerve fibers usually do not cause a visual field defect. When a defect is caused it is usually due to an interference of a nerve fiber bundle. The most frequent defect resembles that of an arcuate scotoma. Occasionally there is an irregular enlargement of the blind spot and very rarely there can be a paracecal scotoma if the myelinated nerve fibers extend for a considerable distance onto the retina. A visual field defect from myelinated nerve fibers can easily be correlated with the ophthalmoscopic picture.

A visual field defect from a coloboma also can be easily correlated with the ophthalmoscopic picture, although as exact a correlation usually cannot be made as can be made with myelinated nerve fibers. Often a large coloboma yields a small visual field defect and a small coloboma yields a large visual field defect. Defects from a coloboma can look like glaucomatous defects and, especially when there is a deeply cupped optic disk, differentiation can be difficult. As with myelinated nerve fibers, visual field defects from colobomata are nonprogressive.

A tremendous variation in field defects can be found in optic nerve hypoplasia. Often hypoplastic optic nerves can be associated with other central nervous system maldevelopment such as agenesis of the anterior commissure and malformation of the septum pellucidum and chiasm. Often hypoplastic optic nerves are bilateral, although the maldevelopment can be much worse in one eye than the other. The area of visual field loss corresponds to the area of optic nerve involvement with inferior loss being most common and temporal loss the least common.

Optic nerve head drusen can lead to extensive visual field loss. The drusen can take decades to develop and the visual field loss presentation parallels development of the drusen. Because a large portion of the body of the drusen tends to be buried in the nerve tissue, it is difficult to correlate ophthalmoscopic appearance with actual field loss. Visual field loss can take the form of blind spot enlargement, arcuate scotomas, and peripheral constriction. Visual field loss can be progressive, although the progression is usually slow. Loss of central vision tends to occur only if there is vascular damage at the disk margin.

Optic nerve pits are a common congenital abnormality. They can be associated with visual field loss, although visual field loss does not have to be present. Central visual field loss, if present, takes the form of an irregular scotoma with a sloped margin. Central field loss is usually present when there is an associated serous detachment of the macula. Blind spot enlargement also can be seen as can arcuate scotomas and paracentral scotomas.

OPTIC NERVE INFLAMMATORY DISORDERS

Optic neuritis can affect the anterior or posterior portions of the nerve. Usually a central scotoma is present and this can sometimes be accompanied by a generalized depression of the visual field. Often, however, the central scotoma can only be elicited using very small test spots or red test objects.

Lesions of the retrobulbar portion of the optic nerve often show no ophthalmoscopic evidence of their presence until late nerve head atrophy develops. Visual field involvement can be seen in a much earlier stage and for this reason, visual field examination is quite crucial in diagnosing and following these patients. Visual field defects can be central, paracentral, cecocentral, or peripheral depending on where the involvement is (Fig. 9–3).

Ischemic optic neuropathy is usually seen in elderly patients and tends to have an acute onset. Visual loss can be complete or partial and an edematous disk is always present. If there is a sectoral or altitudinal visual field defect, there is a corresponding localization of disk edema. As the edema recedes, an atrophic looking sector of the nerve head will persist.

Patients presenting with ischemic optic neuropathy need to be evaluated immediately for the possibility of temporal arteritis. Corticosteroid therapy is mandatory to prevent further visual loss, involvement of the other eye, or other systemic involvement if temporal arteritis is found.

OPTIC NERVE TRAUMA

Direct trauma to the optic nerve head can be either contusive or avulsive. If avulsive, the visual field defects correspond to the nerve fibers that were cut. Contusive injuries of the nerve head can also cause extensive visual field loss; often only a small island of peripheral field remains after a contusive injury.

MULTIPLE SCLEROSIS

Visual field defects in multiple sclerosis are quite common. The classic defect is a central scotoma, although arcuate, paracentral, or cecocentral scotomas are common. Visual field loss is often bilateral but can be unilateral. Often the scotomas are vague and even fleeting. In many patients exposure to heat causes an increase in the size and the depth of the scotoma. Clinically this can be investigated by testing the patient's visual field both before and immediately after a hot bath. A patient often gives a history of visual field defects being present after exposure to extreme heat.

Red test objects are very sensitive for picking up central scotomas in multiple sclerosis. Red-tipped matches are useful for bedside confrontation examination of the visual field. As the match tip is brought into the area of the field defect the red color will disappear, even though the tip of the match can still be seen without color.

Visual field examination of multiple sclerosis patients is important both for following the progression of the disease and as a baseline for future studies. Patterson and Heron[1] studied 54 patients with multiple sclerosis and found the visual fields to be abnormal in 94 percent of patients with definite multiple sclerosis. Three-quarters of the multiple sclerosis patients who had no history of documented visual symptoms showed visual field loss. The most common defect was an arcuate scotoma. Mienberg, Flammer, and Luden,[2] using automated perimetric techniques, studied 14 patients with definite but inactive multiple sclerosis. Most of these patients had visual field defects and the severity and the extent of the defects were unrelated to a history of optic neuritis. The defects could not be correlated with abnormalities in the visually evoked potentials.

LEBER'S OPTIC ATROPHY

Leber's optic atrophy presents with central visual field loss. Peripheral depression of the field can be seen in late stages. Onset is relatively acute, usually in late adolescent males. Patients are left with a large central scotoma.

OPTIC NERVE LESIONS IN SYPHILIS

Visual field loss in syphilis is dependent upon the area of the optic nerve that is affected. Syphilitic retrobulbar neuritis produces central scotomas. Initially the peripheral visual field is unaffected in these patients but, if untreated, it, too, will eventually be affected. Wedge-shaped areas of visual field loss pointing to fixation occurs and optic atrophy is usually present in these patients. The optic atrophy either corresponds to the sector of visual field lost or can affect the entire optic nerve. Often these visual field defects can give appearance of chiasmal or postchiasmal lesion defects.

A gradually contracting visual field with steep margins can also occur in syphilis due to peripheral inflammation of the nerve slowly advancing toward the center of the nerve. If the peripheral inflammation is localized, then localized sectors of visual field loss can be seen. Central vision can remain intact for long periods of time in these patients. If untreated, central vision, too, is eventually affected.

ORBITAL LESIONS

Lesions in the anterior and middle portions of the orbit usually do not cause visual field defects but lesions in the posterior orbit can cause visual field loss by compression of the optic nerve. Usually a central scotoma is produced that can involve an area up to 20 degrees around fixation. Greater field loss is seen in the portion opposite the direction of the pressure and often the loss assumes a quadrantic or hemianopic appearance. Therefore, pressure on the medial side of the nerve gives rise to a unilateral hemianopsic scotoma on the temporal side of fixation. The periphery, however, is usually spared unless there is optic atrophy or exophthalmos. When a tumor is present within the nerve tissue itself, such as an optic nerve glioma, the initial visual field loss is also usually central with steep margins.

FOSTER-KENNEDY SYNDROME

The Foster-Kennedy syndrome consists of optic atrophy in one eye with papilledema in the contralateral eye. It is usually caused by an olfactory roof meningioma, but also can be caused by frontal lobe tumors, ophthalmic artery aneurysms, arachnoid cysts, optic nerve gliomas, or cerebellar tumors with third ventricle dilation. There is a visual acuity loss with a central scotoma in the eye with the optic atrophy. Additional areas of field loss are usually present but vary greatly.

Lesions of the Chiasm

Visual field defects caused by lesions in the area of the chiasm are characterized by early involvement of central vision. There is invariably a bitemporal pattern with a sharp border on the superior vertical meridian (Fig. 9–4).

The pituitary gland is located below the chiasm and tumors in the area of the pituitary press on both the inferior chiasm and its blood supply. The blood supply comes from below and is particularly vulnerable to pressure exerted by such lesions. Central vision is impaired early on because about 90 percent of the ganglion cell fibers arise at the macula. Often a temporal hemianopsia can be seen in the central field but not in the peripheral field (Fig. 9–5). Small stimuli and red stimuli tend to be the best at bringing out these visual field defects. Rarely, bitemporal hemianopsias start in the inferotemporal visual field. This suggests a lesion above the chiasm.

Patients presenting with bitemporal hemianopsia need to be carefully evaluated for lesions in the chiasmal area. Radiologic examination, especially computerized axial tomography, is of paramount importance. Endocrinologic studies can detect pituitary dysfunction. Naturally, a careful neurologic examination needs to be performed.

When a tumor in the area of the chiasm, such as a pituitary adenoma, is removed, a recovery of visual function is often seen. Recovery takes place in the opposite order of progression of the visual field loss. This is graphically demonstrated in Figs. 9–4 and 9–6.

Patients usually are unaware of a bitemporal hemianopsia until the defect reaches an advanced stage. Because the macula is spared and the nasal field of one eye overlaps the defective field of the other eye, it is not surprising that the patient does not notice the defect. Frequently, however, patients sense a generalized blurriness to their vision without realizing that there is a defect in their visual field.

LOCALIZATION OF CHIASMAL LESIONS

Localization of a chiasmal lesion can often be made by the visual field defect. Defects caused by interruption of fibers in different areas of the chiasm give characteristic visual field defects. It is important to remember that because the chiasm is responsible to a large degree for macular areas of the retina, field defects resulting from chiasmal lesions are first noted on central field examinations rather than on peripheral field examinations. Very often a field defect can be evident as a central depression for red or with automated machines as a generalized central depression.

Lesions at the midline of the chiasm tend to yield bitemporal defects because the central portion of the chiasm is made up entirely of crossing fibers. When there is a lesion in the posterior portion of the chiasm at the beginning of one or both optic tracts, a homonymous hemianopsia can result. If this lesion compresses the inner side of the tract, a temporal field loss in the opposite field and a nasal field loss in the ipsilateral side result. If compression is from the lateral side, however, the field loss occurs in the nasal field on the ipsilateral side of the lesion followed by both temporal fields.

When a lesion is pressing on the chiasm from above, the bitemporal hemianopsia that results usually starts in the inferotemporal quadrant. Lesions leading to such defects include lesions from the anterior superior aspect including meningiomas of the olfactory groove, the tuberculum sella and the lesser wing of the sphenoid bone, frontal lobe gliomas, and frontal lobe meningiomas. Tumors pressing from the posterior superior aspect include craniopharyngiomas, third ventricle dilitation and rare tumors including cholesteatomas, osteomas, and osteochondromas. These tumors can also lead to a homonymous hemianopsia because of involvement of the optic tract.

When a chiasmal lesion is large enough, complete interruption of both the crossing and noncrossing fibers results in a defect that includes the temporal and nasal portions of the visual field. The usual progression is involvement of the superotemporal quadrant followed by the inferotemporal quadrant followed by the inferonasal quadrant and finally the superonasal quadrant.

Interruption of the optic nerve at the chiasm causes a junctional scotoma. Because the inferonasal fibers of the optic nerve dip into the contralateral optic nerve for 1 mm before entering the optic tract (von Willebrand's knee), lesions at the junction of the optic nerve and the chiasm also involve these fibers. Interruption yields a central scotoma in one eye with a superotemporal defect in the other eye.

When a lesion is affecting the posterior chiasm, such as enlargement of the third ventricle causing pressure on the posterior chiasm, a bitemporal hemianopsia totally confined to the central field is theoretically possible, but this is quite rare. Usually the defect involves the peripheral field also.

"False" bitemporal hemianopsias can be caused by third ventricle enlargement yielding compression of the posterior chiasm, such as in stenosis of the Sylvian aqueduct. Tilted optic disks show a peripheral hemianopsia that is nonprogressive. Characteristically there is a situs inversus with a tilting of the vertical axis of the disk obliquely.

If there is interruption of the macular crossing fibers, a paracentral homonymous defect occurs in the other eye with a temporal defect in the ipsilateral eye.

TUMORS AFFECTING THE CHIASM

Pituitary adenomas tend to be slow growing and frequently cause nearly symmetrical bitemporal defects. Other tumors, however, such as angiomas, meningiomas of the planum sphenoidum or sphenoid wing, or craniopharyngiomas can frequently affect only one optic nerve long before they involve the contralateral optic nerve. Examination of the 90-degree meridian is critical and very careful attention needs to be paid to both sides of this meridian.

Pituitary tumors usually demonstrate roentgenographic evidence of enlargement of the sella turcica. Eighty-five percent of craniopharyngiomas show suprasella calcification. Long-standing aneurysms show curvilinear calcifications, although an aneurysm of recent origin does not. A glioma of the chiasm can show a J-shaped sella turcica. Meningiomas of the sphenoid are also common causes of chiasmal defects.

Arcuate visual field defects can be caused by chromophobe adenomas of the pituitary gland. Although the way in which this visual field defect is produced is not completely understood, it has been speculated that it must be due to vascular changes in the optic nerve rather than in the chiasm, because the defects cross the midline. These field defects also tend not to be bitemporal. The occurrence of arcuate defects in patients with pituitary tumors is rare, however, this should be kept in mind when an arcuate defect is present that does not seem to be confirmed by ophthalmoscopic examination.

Chamlin has done extensive studies on visual field defects in patients with pituitary tumors. He has shown that the visual field defect seen at 90 degrees with a 1-mm white test object on a tangent screen at 2 m is the earliest defect to be seen from a lesion in the chiasm and it is also the last defect to disappear after the tumor is removed. Even when there is also a peripheral defect, the loss to the 1/2000 tangent screen field will also be at least as great and is usually much larger. Although a field with a colored test object can be useful for demonstrating such a field defect, following these defects is much more accurate with the 1/2000 white test object.

Based on his clinical observations Chamlin conceptualized the vertical distribution of peripheral, intermediate, and central fibers in the chiasm. By intermediate fibers he referred to the area between 10 and 25 degrees. He concluded that for early detection of chiasmal tumors, a tangent screen field with a 1-mm test object at 2 m carefully exploring the 90-degree meridian was indispensible.[3]

Careful examination of the 90-degree meridian can also be performed by the static techniques of automated field testing. Test spots should be presented at corresponding points on either side of the vertical meridian and not directly on it. Many automated devices have special neurologic testing patterns to look for a Chamlin step.

Lesions of the posterior chiasm can cause small central bitemporal hemianopsias, which can either split or spare the macula, but more commonly split the macula. After surgical removal of the tumor pressing on the chiasm, return of lost visual field can be seen. This usually occurs in the opposite progression of the original field loss.

It should be noted that when chiasmal tumors have been resected, patients need to be followed for recurrence of the lesion. Following the visual fields is as important as is computerized tomographic scanning. A progressive, renewed loss of the visual field does not necessarily mean that the tumor is recurring, however, loss can occur from a hemorrhage within the residual tumor causing a large, firm hematoma that presses on the chiasm.

In most cases of chiasmal area lesions, the visual field defects are not being caused by pressure on the chiasm as much as by vascular compression. Arterial ischemia and venous stasis lead to both edema and anoxia of the nerve. It is felt that this accounts for the distinct borders that are seen with field defects from chiasmal lesions. When the nerve is invaded by the tumor itself, the field defects seen tend to be quite irregular.

THE ROLE OF VISUALLY EVOKED RESPONSE TESTS IN CHIASMAL LESIONS

When a patient has a bitemporal hemianopsia from a chiasmal lesion, the visually evoked response test (VER) is usually abnormal if the visual field defect is severe. The correlation between the VER and the visual field is much better if a hemiretinal VER examination is performed. Under such circumstances the correlation tends to be good. Muller-Jensen and colleagues[4] have found that damage in the retinal nasal hemifield can be found prior to damage in the temporal retinal hemifield. Slight abnormalities are found in the amplitude and latency of the VER if the visual field defect is small and large abnormalities are found if the visual field defect is large.

DEMYELINATING DISEASE

Demyelinating disease has been noted to cause bitemporal visual field defects that would otherwise seem to indicate a mass lesion pressing on the chiasm. Systemic corticosteroid therapy is sometimes useful in treating these lesions. Neuroradiologic studies are important to rule out mass lesions. Magnetic resonance imaging techniques demonstrate the presence of demyelinating plaques, if present. The prognosis is usually good for a return of visual function and recovery.

VASCULAR LESIONS OF THE CHIASM

Because there is an intimate relationship between the chiasm and the basilar arteries of the brain in the circle of Willis, aneurysms in the circle of Willis cause chiasmal compression and result in visual field defects.

The most frequent aneurysm seen is that of the internal carotid artery, causing pressure on the lateral aspect of the chiasm. If the aneurysm is in the supraclinoid area, visual field loss is an early sign. If it is subclinoid in origin (within the cavernous sinus), ocular motor and trigeminal nerve involvement occurs first with visual field loss occurring later.

BINASAL FIELD DEFECTS

Binasal defects are most commonly due to glaucoma, optic nerve head drusen, or chronic elevated intracranial pressure. Compression of the chiasm by arteriosclerotic carotid arteries, however, can also cause binasal field defects. Binasal defects imply a bilateral involvement of the uncrossed portions of the arcuate bundles. Characteristically these defects lack sharp vertical borders.

Bilateral retinoschisis can also cause a field defect that looks like a binasal hemianopsia. Ophthalmoscopic examination allows for each differential with other lesions. There will be a sharp demarcation between the defect and the remainder of the field.

LESIONS OF THE POSTCHIASMAL VISUAL PATHWAYS

Visual field defects occurring behind the chiasm always yield homonymous hemianopsias. This is in contrast to lesions of the chiasm that yield bitemporal or, less commonly, binasal hemianopsias and lesions anterior to the chiasm that yield monocular visual field defects.

The visual pathway beyond the chiasm is divided into four parts: the optic tracts, the lateral geniculate body, the optic radiations, and the striate cortex of the occipital lobe. The optic tract is simply the continuation of the fibers of the optic nerve after they have traveled through the chiasm. An injury to any fiber within the tract yields destruction to that fiber from that point forward through the chiasm and the optic nerve to the ganglion cell layer of the retina. The lateral geniculate body is a true ganglion and is the end station of these neurons.

Due to the partial decussation of the nerve fibers of the visual pathway in the chiasm, the homonymous hemianopsia that is produced by a lesion on one side of the visual pathway is located in the contralateral visual field. When other signs and symptoms are absent, homonymous hemianopsias usually indicate a temporal or occipital lobe lesion. When a patient has a complete unawareness that the visual field defect exists, the lesion is usually in the parietal lobe. This is especially true if the hemianopsia is only elicited with simultaneous double stimulation to the right and left halves of the visual field.

Lesions anterior to the geniculate body occur within the fibers of the optic nerve; homonymous hemianopsias with associated optic atrophy usually imply the presence of a lesion in the geniculate body or the optic tract. The optic atrophy from such a lesion, however, is very slow in developing. The pupillomotor fibers travel with the optic nerve as far as the geniculate body, but do not travel into the optic radiations. Therefore an incongruity in the hemianopsic pupillary reactions theoretically would be valuable in localizing a homonymous hemianopsia to the geniculate body or anterior to it. This test is quite difficult to perform, however.

It should be noted that accurate identification of the site of the lesion in the retrochiasmal pathways on the basis of the visual field is the exception rather than the rule. Congruity alone is usually not sufficient for localization of any single lesion. Progressive lesions usually yield sloping borders, whereas acute lesions tend to have sharp borders. This does not refer to the anatomic borders along the vertical meridian, however, which are usually sharp. When there are areas of relative field loss, rather than absolute field loss, these areas tend to be the most likely to improve if the lesion is successfully treated.

Optic Tract Defects

Optic tract lesions cause incongruous homonymous hemianopsic field defects. Because the defect in one eye can be quite subtle, looking for a Chamlin step is very important when an optic tract defect is being considered (Fig. 9–7). As the optic tract fibers are grouped in a very small area, the most common result of an optic tract lesion is total destruction of the tract. If destruction of the optic tract is complete, a total homonymous hemianopsia is seen. When the interruption of the optic tract fibers is not complete, however, optic tract hemianopsias are very incongruous, and in fact hemianopsias caused by lesions of the optic tract or lateral geniculate body are the most incongruous of the postchiasmal defects.

Visual field defects of the optic tract usually start as quadrantanopias with macular sparing. They proceed to involve the entire half of the visual field and also to split the macula. They can be so incongruous that often a visual field defect in the less involved side is only seen after a very careful search for a Chamlin step.

Primary lesions of the optic tract are exceedingly rare, however, gliomas have been reported and the optic tract can be affected in multiple sclerosis. The most common lesions affecting the optic tract are tumors of adjacent structures and aneurysms of the posterior arteries of the circle of Willis, specifically the posterior communicating, the posterior cerebral, the internal carotid, and the middle cerebral arteries. The tract can be affected by tumors arising in the third ventricle, the pituitary, the basal ganglia, the transverse fissure, and the middle portion of the temporal lobe. Optic atrophy resulting from lesions of the optic tract may appear as early as 2 or 3 months after the optic tract injury.

LESIONS OF THE GENICULATE BODY

Lesions of the geniculate body are similar to those produced by the more posterior portions of the optic tract. In theory, a lesion of the medial aspect of the geniculate body would yield a homonymous lower quadrantanopia of the contralateral field, and a lesion of the lateral aspect of the geniculate would yield an upper quadrantanopia of the opposite field side.

Geniculate lesions are rarely suspected and therefore seldom diagnosed. Lesions of the geniculate should be suspected if the homonymous hemianopsia involves primarily the central visual field, sparing the peripheral field, as the geniculate body mainly represents macular fibers. Because the thalamus is in close approximation, hemianesthesia on the side of the hemianopsia is often associated.

LESIONS OF THE OPTIC RADIATIONS

From the geniculate body the visual pathway extends to the visual cortex. This pathway is known as the optic radiations or the geniculocalcarine pathway. It constitutes the third and fourth neurons in the visual pathway. Because they are the longest and most vulnerable portion of the visual pathway, with the exception of the chiasmal decussation, and because a wide area is occupied within the cerebral hemisphere, the pathway is subject to interruption at many points. This is what makes visual field testing in neurologic lesions of the parietal, temporal, and occipital lobes so valuable.

The optic radiation leaves the geniculate body and runs laterally through the retrolenticular portion of the internal capsule. This is done in a compact mass that is known as the optic peduncle. These fibers then fan out forming the medullary optic lamella. Fibers from the upper and lower retinal quadrants are separated with the macular fibers running in between. Fibers from the medial aspect of the geniculate coming from the upper retinal quadrant run in a dorsal manner in the optic lamella and in a straight course through the parietooccipital lobe. They then descend in a horizontal fan-like manner over the coil end of the calcarine fissure and enter the cortex in the dorsal portion of the striate area.

Fibers from the lateral side of the geniculate that have come from the lower retinal quadrants run in the ventral portion of the lamella. These run forward in the temporal lobe and form Meyer's temporal loop. They extend far forward, enveloping the temporal horn of the lateral ventricle and then pass along its body and around the posterior horn, finally ending in the ventral portion of the calcarine cortex. The macular fibers run from the dorsal part of the geniculate as a flat bundle between the dorsal and ventral fibers. They end in the posterior pole or the operculum of the occipital cortex.

Lesions in the most anterior portion of the optic radiation occur in the area of the internal capsule. They give rise to a homonymous hemianopsia of the contralateral side and are often associated with hemianesthesia or hemiplegia or both. The most common lesions affecting the internal capsule are vascular, in particular, hemorrhages of the branches of the middle cerebral artery. The onset is usually sudden. Tumors in this area are exceedingly rare.

Temporal Lobe Lesions

Temporal lobe defects usually produce incongruous hemianopsias in which there is an upper quadrantanopia with sloping margins. Lesions confined to the extreme anterior tip of temporal lobe do not tend to cause visual field defects. Temporal lobe defects are quite incongruous as opposed to occipital lobe defects, which tend to be very congruous visual field defects.

Uncinate fits can occur when the uncinate gyrus, located beneath the temporal lobe is involved by a lesion. In these fits the patient complains of abnormal smells or tastes with visual hallucinations of persons, animals, or known objects. In right-handed persons with tumors of the left temporal lobe, aphasia can occur.

The pattern of visual field loss in lesions of the temporal lobe has been quite controversial. Computerized axial tomography and angiography tend to be more valuable than visual field testing for localizing lesions within the temporal lobe. Because the tip of the temporal lobe contains no fibers of Meyer's loop, tumors in this area do not produce visual field defects until they become quite large. Formed visual hallucinations are highly suggestive of temporal lobe disease.

Parietal Lobe Lesions

Lesions of the parietal lobe tend to be accompanied by a lack of awareness by the patient of the field loss. This behavioral defect is quite characteristic of lesions of the parietal lobe and causes the extinction phenomenon. A patient is often able to see moving test object in either half of the visual field, but when two stationary test objects are simultaneously presented in the right and left fields, the object in the involved side of the field will be ignored. This is so even when the test objects are quite large.

The extinction phenomenon is a special sign of a parietal lobe lesion and can only be detected if both nasal and temporal fields are examined simultaneously. Another important sign of a parietal lobe lesion is a motor impersistence sign, in which a patient cannot maintain a willed motor act. Therefore, he or she often cannot maintain fixation and when there is simultaneous nasal and temporal field stimulation the patient looks toward the noninvolved side.

The most common field defect is an inferior homonymous quadrantanopia with some incongruity. Even when there is a hemianopsia, the densest part of the defect is below (Fig. 9–8).

When there is superior quadrant loss and parietal lobe disease, there is probably also temporal lobe involvement. Superior loss from involvement of the parietal lobe alone is exceedingly rare (Fig. 9–9).

Parietal lobe lesions are often associated with speech disorders or motor defects. There tends to be right to left confusion, finger agnosia, dyscrasia, or dyslexia. Asymmetric optikinetic nystagmus responses are always present in association with a homonymous hemianopsia due to a lesion of the parietal lobe.

Occipital Lobe Lesions

Lesions of the occipital lobe are hemianopsic lesions that are characterized most particularly by their congruity and steep margins. They can be exceedingly small, such as the small scotomas seen after small embolic lesions, or they can encompass the entire hemianopsic field. Fixation can be either split or spared (Fig. 9–10).

Occipital lesions are usually vascular in etiology. They are often characterized by normal opticokinetic nystagmus (OKN) responses as opposed to parietal lobe lesions, which have abnormal OKN responses, and they are often characterized by the Riddoch phenomenon.

In the Riddoch phenomenon, movement is able to be seen, but stationary objects cannot be seen. Although this was originally felt to be pathognomonic for an occipital lobe lesion, it has been described for lesions that affect almost any portion of the visual system.

A unilateral loss of the temporal crescent of field can be caused by lesions that affect the most anterior portion of the calcarine fissure. This area of the field is seen by one eye only. Conversely, if this area is spared, a patient may exhibit a homonymous hemianopsia with this crescent of visual field remaining. The presence of a temporal crescent defect or the retention of the temporal crescent of field in an otherwise hemianopsic defect is pathognomonic for a lesion of the occipital cortex.

Bender and Battersby[5] have described tumors of the occipital lobe that have produced scotomas in the macular fields. The scotomas were homonymous and surrounded by an extensive area of metamorphopsia and defective color vision. As the tumors enlarged, defects developed in the peripheral fields and these extended toward the center and eventually merged with the macular scotomas. After surgical removal of these lesions, the hemianopsias receded from the center toward the periphery.

Computerized tomographic scanning has proved to be an effective method of demonstrating areas of cerebral infarction in the occipital lobe. Studies have been done to correlate visual field defects with these tomographic lesions. To date these studies have supported the original 1916 work of Holmes and Lister[6] that proposed the clinical pathological correlations between areas of the occipital lobe and vision.

MACULAR SPARING

To test for macular sparing it is essential to maintain exact fixation. This is often exceedingly difficult and an effective method for determining the macula has been split or spared is by manually presenting three test objects simultaneously. The three objects are equally spaced, with the central object along the 180-degree meridian and the other two objects lined up at a 90-degree angle to that meridian.

Macular sparing can be explained in a number of ways. First, the macular area comprises a large portion of the occipital cortex, a greater portion than the peripheral projections comprise. Lesions can affect only peripheral field representation areas in the cortex. Second, there is a dual blood supply coming from both the middle and posterior cerebral circulations. It has been theorized that there is a crossed representation of the central 2 to 3 degrees of the macular area in some patients. This has been found in nonprimate animals.

It should be remembered that patients retain their normal visual acuity even if the macula is split. In such cases half the macular representation remains and the patient's previous visual acuity, even if 20/20 or better, is retained. True macular sparing is seen infrequently.

THE RIDDOCH PHENOMENON

The phenomenon of the visual extinction of stationary stimuli was first described by Riddoch in 1917.[7] He found patients who were able to perceive movement on the affected side, but could not appreciate stationary objects, or, if they did appreciate stationary objects, did so to a much lesser degree. All of his patients had occipital lobe lesions and he concluded that visual functions concerned with recognition of movement and recognition of stationary objects were dissociated from each other in the occipital cortex. The presence of this dissociation for a period of several months was felt to be a poor prognostic sign. If recovery did indeed occur, movement returned before the recognition of the stationary objects.

The Riddoch phenomenon has been described in nonoccipital lobe lesions. It has been described in other lesions, including an aneurysm of the internal carotid artery compressing the optic tract and a pituitary tumor.

CORTICAL BLINDNESS

Cortical blindness results from infarction of both occipital lobes. Sometimes a patient with cortical blindness will deny that he or she is blind.

When a central 2- to 3-degree field persists, it is due to macular sparing. It should be noted, however, that if the field is that constricted, a 20/200 letter cannot be seen and only smaller letters can be seen. A tip of the lobe, where macular projection is located, is spared in such patients. In fact, in 20 percent of the population this area has a secondary blood supply from the carotid arteries.

In cortical blindness there is loss of the reflex closure of the eyelids on sudden exposure to light or to danger, however, the pupillary reactions remain normal to both light and convergence. The optic nerve looks normal on ophthalmoscopic examination. Denial of visual loss, or Anton's syndrome, is highly characteristic of cortical blindness. In fact, patients who have lost half their visual field on a cortical basis often are unaware that they have lost half their field.

HOMONYMOUS HEMIANOPSIAS FROM NONOCCIPITAL LESIONS

Occipital homonymous hemianopsias can be caused by other lesions in the central nervous system due to a pressure effect. A frontal lobe tumor, for example, can cause displacement of the brain with a secondary compression of the posterior cerebral arteries. This cerebral arterial compression causes an occipital lobe field defect. Computed tomographic scanning, however, clearly shows both the tumor and the lesion created in the posterior cerebral circulation by the pressure of the tumor.

VASCULAR LESIONS

The most common vascular lesion affecting the occipital lobe is a thrombosis of the calcarine artery or one of the posterior cerebral arteries. This causes extensive damage resulting in a complete homonymous hemianopsia. If only small branches of the posterior cerebral artery are involved, sector defects, quadrantanopias, or scotomas can result. Because the macular portion of the occipital cortex is supplied in part by the middle cerebral artery, macular areas can often be spared.

VISUAL PHENOMENA ASSOCIATED WITH OCCIPITAL LESIONS

Specific visual phenomenon have been associated with lesions of the occipital cortex. These include visual hallucinations, cortical blindness, scintillating scotomas and hemianopsias of migraine, and light flashes and homonymous visual field defects associated with arteriovenous malformations.

Visual hallucinations can also be associated with lesions of the temporal and parietal areas of the brain. These hallucinations can be formed, in which case they represent specific objects or persons, or unformed, in which case they represent imaginary objects or things. It is felt that the complex hallucinations are related to irritation to the associational areas of the cortex and that the simple hallucinations result from abnormal stimulation of the neurons of the visual pathway. Hallucinations can occur either in the area of the field defect or in the area of the normal field, but more commonly are in the area of the field defect.

An important diagnostic clue in differentiating these patients with visual hallucinations from occipital lobe lesions from those with psychiatric or metabolic derangements is documentation that the portrayed images had actually been viewed recently and therefore represented a transposition in either time or space of an actual visual image.

MIGRAINE

The scintillating scotoma of migraine is a very common visual complaint. It typically lasts 20 to 30 minutes and starts in the central portion of the field and extends out to the periphery. Duration can be as short as a minute or as long as several hours, however. It can involve the entire visual field of a hemianopsic field. Patients sometimes describe the migraine as occurring in only one eye but often patients do not compare the vision of two eyes. The scintillating scotomas are usually still seen even when the eyelids are closed, look like irregular multicolored lightning streaks, and tend to form into a hemicircle. Often the jagged appearance is not seen but there is a haziness or waviness to the vision in the portion of the field that is having the scintillating scotoma.

A headache sometimes occurs after the scotoma is seen but it does not have to occur. Usually the headache is hemicranial and involves the side of the head opposite of the visual field loss. Although the headache tends to occur after the scotoma, neurologic symptoms, such as transitory aphasia, hemianesthesia, or paresthesia can occur along with the scotoma. Diplopia and partial hemiplegias have also been recorded.

OCCIPITAL LOBE EPILEPSY

Arteriovenous malformations cause occipital lobe epilepsy with focal seizures. Often there is a visual aura that sometimes last only seconds but occasionally they can last up to a few minutes. Commonly, a generalized seizure occurs afterward.

Toxic Amblyopias

From the standpoint of visual field testing, toxic amblyopias can present either with central scotomas or with peripheral visual field loss. Bilateral central scotomas can be caused by tobacco, nutritional deficiency, ethanol, methanol, lead, or some medications.

Tobacco amblyopia is more common in cigar and pipe smokers than in cigarette smokers. Visual field loss is in the centrocecal area with a horizontally oval central scotoma. The scotoma is usually bilateral and the size and the shape can vary, depending on the amount of tobacco consumption. The scotoma develops midway between the blind spot and fixation, and from there extends both nasally and temporally. Lateral extension of the scotoma greatly overshadows vertical extension. The borders of the scotoma tend to be rather vague. Color vision is usually affected early on, especially red perception.

Treatment is accomplished by noncyanide containing vitamin B_{12} and abstinence from tobacco. The scotoma will go away slowly with it receding in the opposite direction of its growth. Return of color vision is seen last.

Nutritional amblyopia is really not a toxic amblyopia, but a nutritional disease. Scotomas tend to be irregular in shape with steep margins and uniform density.

Ethanol amblyopia can occur acutely from drinking impure alcohol. More commonly it is associated with chronic alcoholism and presents with a picture more similar to nutritional amblyopias than to tobacco amblyopia. Vision is described as hazy and later on in the area of the scotoma as selectively missing. The characteristic visual field defect is a central scotoma, irregular in shape and varying in size from 2 to 5 degrees. Margins are steep and density is uniform. It can extend temporally and coalesce with the blind spot, giving a centrocecal defect. The area of greatest density in the scotoma, however, tends to be at fixation, rather than in the centrocecal portion, as is seen with tobacco amblyopia. Visual field loss is usually bilateral and the central scotomas are fairly symmetrical. Dietary deficiency is often found when histories are taken of these patients. Treatment consists of eliminating alcohol consumption and giving vitamin B_{12}.

Disulfiran, or antabuse, is used for the treatment of chronic alcoholism, but when alcohol is ingested in combination with its use, retrobulbar neuritis with central and centrocecal visual field defects can occur. This continuance of the drug usually leads to a return of a normal visual field.

Methyl alcohol poisoning can occur with doses as small as a third of an ounce. Systemic symptoms include nausea, vomiting, abdominal cramps, and headaches lasting up to a day or more. Visual symptoms range from slight haziness to a total loss of vision.

Only a small amount of methyl alcohol is needed for severe poisoning to result. Because methyl alcohol is metabolized very slowly, it remains in the body in significant concentration for many days. In the acute phase of poisoning, central and centrocecal scotomas develop. These can be transient, but more commonly are permanent.

The nervous system involvement in methyl alcohol poisoning consists of retinal edema, fixed and dilated pupils, blindness, and basal ganglion necrosis. The ocular damage is thought to be due to the slow oxidation of methanol to formaldehyde. Even with a small amount of methanol, the patient is usually so ill that visual field examination is impossible to perform. Visual field loss can proceed even while systemic recovery appears to be taking place. The central scotomas can become progressively larger and peripheral loss can increase.

Lead poisoning can affect all parts of the visual pathway, including the retina, the optic nerve, and the occipital cortex. Visual field loss manifests itself as depressed peripheral fields and bilateral central scotomas; one or both may be present. Lead poisoning is usually caused by a gradual accumulation of lead in the body and therefore is a chronic type of illness. It is frequently accompanied by increased intracranial pressure resulting in papilledema and optic atrophy. Occasionally, there is an acute onset of symptoms with a sudden loss of vision from which there can be recovery later on. When the loss of vision is acute, papilledema is usually also present.

Carbon monoxide causes cerebral anoxia. When the visual fields are affected, they are on a cerebral level resulting in homonymous hemianopsias. One or both sides of the vision can be affected. A small central island of vision can be spared in some patients.

Digitalis can cause a number of visual difficulties. Usually these occur within the first several weeks of therapy and usually they disappear within several weeks of the cessation of therapy. Visual symptoms include blurred vision, xanthopsia, photophobia, scintillating scotomas, and bilateral central scotomas.

Ethambutol causes a loss of central vision with bilateral central or bilateral temporal scotomas. There is also a marked impairment of color vision and peripheral visual field loss. Ethambutol toxicity is dose dependent.

Isoniazide, used for the treatment of tuberculosis, can produce optic neuritis and optic atrophy with bilateral central scotomas. Peripheral visual field loss can be caused by quinine, chloroquine, arsenic, salicylates, ethylhydrocupreine (Optochin), carbon monoxide, hyperbaric oxygen, and epinephrine.

Although quinine poisoning is rare, the onset of blindness is sudden and it can be either transient or permanent. It has a direct affect on the ganglion cells, nerve fiber cells, and rods and cones of the retina with a marked attenuation of the retinal vasculature. There is constriction of the peripheral field to within a few degrees of fixation. Field loss is usually permanent although partial recovery has been reported.

Chloroquine and hydroxychloroquine (Plaquenil), when used in large doses, can cause ocular problems. Corneal deposits with severe visual loss have been reported. A marked narrowing of the retinal arterioles and a pigmentary degeneration of the macula can lead to visual field loss. Field defects vary from a central scotoma to a ring scotoma to peripheral contraction, the most characteristic being the central scotoma associated with pigmentation. Symptoms are dose-related and are caused by the accumulation of the substances in the pigmented tissues of the body over time. It can be retained in the retinal pigment epithelium for long periods of time after discontinuance of the drug and, therefore, the retinopathy and field defects can proceed even after the drug has been stopped.

Evaluation of the Neurologic Patient with a Field Defect of Unknown Etiology

Computerized tomography should be performed on patients who show visual field defects that are suggestive of neurologic defects. Speiss[8] reported on 272 such patients. Seventy-eight patients showed a chiasmal lesion, 45 showed a lesion of the optic tract or lateral geniculate body, and 136 showed a lesion of the optic radiation or the occipital cortex. All of these patients were evaluated by computerized tomography and in 96 percent of them, topographical localization of the lesion corresponded to the known visual field defect.

It should be noted that in patients with demyelinating disease and previous bouts of optic neuritis, a small residual visual field defect can be present even if the visually evoked potential has returned to normal. Magnetic resonance imaging can be used to confirm the presence of a demyelinating plaque.

References

1. Patterson VH, Heron JR: Visual field abnormalities in multiple sclerosis. J Neurol Neurosurg Psychiatry 43:205–209, 1980.
2. Mienberg D, Flammer J, Ludin HP: Subclinical visual field defects in multiple sclerosis demonstration and quantification with automated perimetry, and comparison with visually evoked potentials. J Neurol 227:125–133, 1982.
3. Chamlin M, Davidoff LM: The 1/2000 field in chiasmal interference. Arch Ophthalmol 44:53–70, 1950.

4. Muller-Jensen A, Zschocke S, Dannheim F: VER analysis of the chiasmal syndrome. J Neurol 255:33–40, 1981.
   Bender MB, Battersby WS: Homonymous macular scotomata in cases of occipital be tumor. Arch Ophthalmol 60:928–938, 1958.
   ʼnes G, Lister WT: Disturbances of vision from cerebral lesions with special nce to the cortical representation of the macula. Brain 39:34, 1916.
   G: Dissociation of visual perception due to occipital injuries with especial ʼo appreciation of movement. Brain 40:15, 1917.
   mputerized tomography—results in affections of the chiasm and visual Monatsbl Augenheilkd 174:816–823, 1979.

pertensive male who suffered a right ulting in a total left homonymous hemianopsia med on an Octopus 201 using program 32. Each ss with essentially normal right-sided fields.

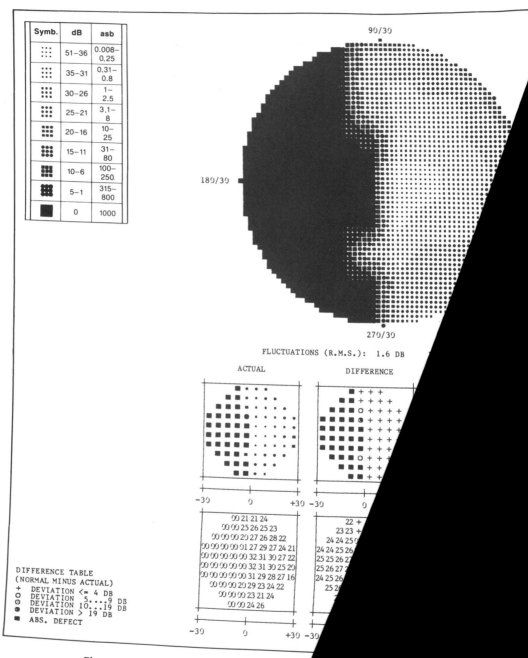

Symb.	dB	asb
⋮⋮⋮	51–36	0.008–0.25
⋮⋮⋮	35–31	0.31–0.8
▪▪▪	30–26	1–2.5
▪▪▪	25–21	3.1–8
▪▪▪	20–16	10–25
▪▪▪	15–11	31–80
▪▪▪	10–6	100–250
▪▪▪	5–1	315–800
▪	0	1000

90/30

180/30

270/30

FLUCTUATIONS (R.M.S.): 1.6 DB

ACTUAL

DIFFERENCE

-30   0   +30   -30   0

DIFFERENCE TABLE
(NORMAL MINUS ACTUAL)
+   DEVIATION <= 4 DB
◦   DEVIATION 5...9 DB
◉   DEVIATION 10...19 DB
●   DEVIATION > 19 DB
▪   ABS. DEFECT

```
            00 21 21 24
         00 00 25 26 25 23
      00 00 00 20 27 26 28 22
   00 00 00 00 01 27 29 27 24 21
   00 00 00 00 00 32 31 30 27 22
   00 00 00 00 00 32 31 30 25 29
   00 00 00 00 31 29 28 27 16
      00 00 00 20 29 23 24 22
         00 00 00 23 21 24
            00 00 24 26
```

```
         22 +
      23 23 +
   24 24 25
24 24 25 26
25 25 26 2
25 26 27 2
24 25 26
   25 2
```

-30   0   +30   -30

Figure 9–2A. Left field of a 59-year-old h
hemispheric cerebrovascular accident res
with macular splitting. Fields were perfo
eye demonstrated total left-sided field l
(continued)

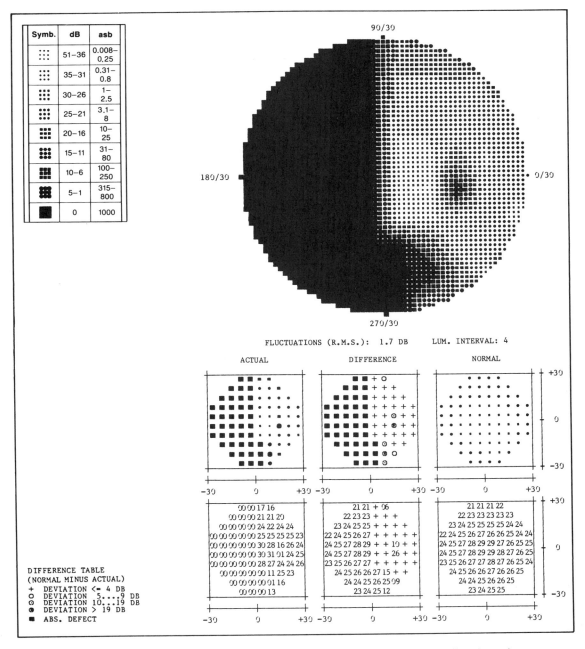

Figure 9–2B. Right field of a 59-year-old hypertensive male who suffered a right hemispheric cerebrovascular accident resulting in a total left homonymous hemianopsia with macular splitting. Fields were performed on an Octopus 201 using program 32. Each eye demonstrated total left-sided field loss with essentially normal right-sided fields.

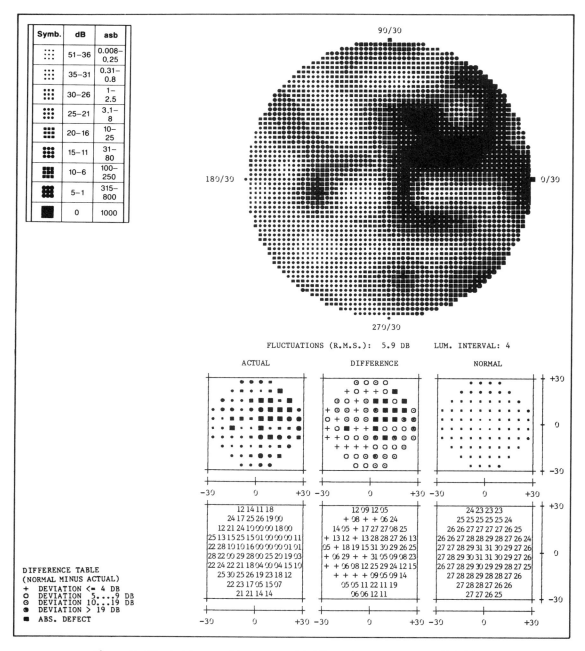

Figure 9–3A. A 44-year-old woman with bilateral optic neuritis. All fields were performed on an Octopus 201 using program 32. Field loss in the left eye is seen primarily in the left upper quadrant, however, generalized depression of the field exists. (continued)

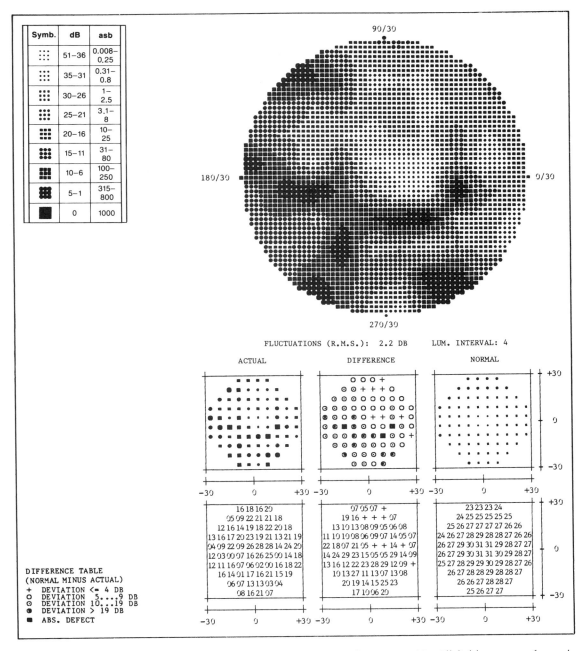

Figure 9–3B. *A 44-year-old woman with bilateral optic neuritis. All fields were performed on an Octopus 201 using program 32. There is generalized depression of the field in the right eye with the blind spot. (continued)*

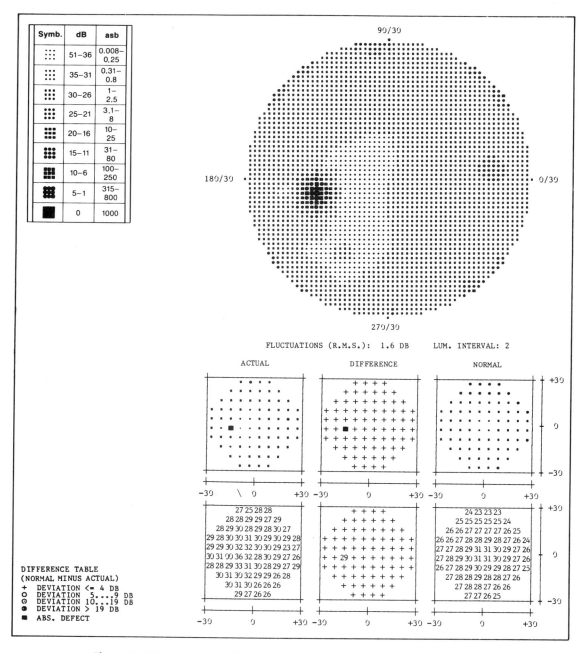

Figure 9–3C. A 44-year-old woman with bilateral optic neuritis. All fields were performed on an Octopus 201 using program 32. Fifth examination of the left eye shows total visual field recovery. (continued)

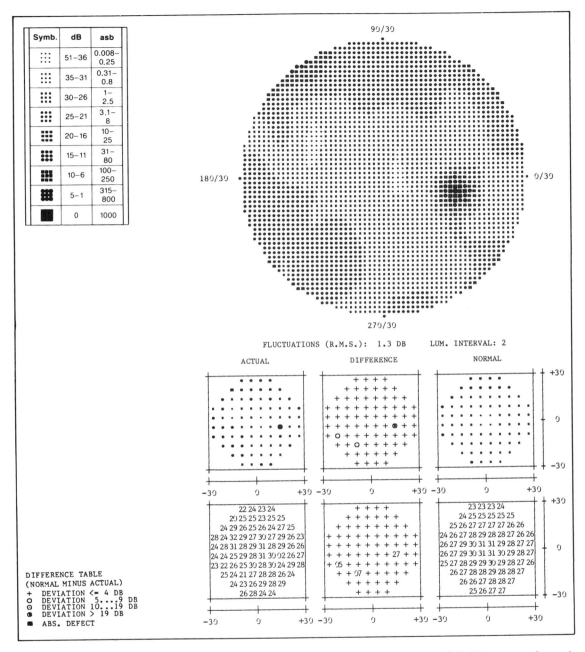

Figure 9–3D. *A 44-year-old woman with bilateral optic neuritis. All fields were performed on an Octopus 201 using program 32. Fifth examination of the right eye shows total visual field recovery. (continued)*

	EX1	EX2	EX3	EX4	EX5	SUMMARY
DATE OF EXAM : DAY	10.04	11.02	12.29	06.24	11.25	
YEAR	1982	1982	1982	1983	1983	
PROGRAM / EXAMINATION	32/01	32/02	32/03	32/04	32/05	
TOTAL LOSS (WHOLE FIELD)	873	129	79	5	12	219 ± 164
MEAN LOSS (PER TEST LOC)						
WHOLE FIELD	11.8	1.7	1.1	0.1	0.2	3.0 ± 2.2
QUADRANT UPPER NASAL	11.0	1.8	2.1	0.0	0.0	3.0 ± 2.1
LOWER NASAL	17.5	4.4	1.8	0.0	0.6	4.9 ± 3.2
UPPER TEMP.	5.1	0.0	0.3	0.3	0.0	1.1 ± 1.0
LOWER TEMP.	13.4	0.6	0.0	0.0	0.0	2.8 ± 2.6
ECCENTRICITY 0 - 10	11.7	0.4	0.9	0.0	0.0	2.6 ± 2.3
10 - 20	13.5	2.2	0.9	0.3	0.4	3.5 ± 2.5
20 - 30	11.1	1.9	1.2	0.0	0.1	2.9 ± 2.1
MEAN SENSITIVITY						
WHOLE FIELD (N: 27.1)	14.9	24.3	25.2	28.2	26.2	23.8 ± 2.3
QUAD.UPP.NAS.(N: 26.4)	15.3	23.2	23.1	27.8	26.3	23.1 ± 2.2
LOW.NAS.(N: 27.4)	9.9	21.8	24.6	29.1	25.3	22.1 ± 3.3
UPP.TMP.(N: 26.5)	20.4	25.4	25.9	26.7	26.0	24.9 ± 1.1
LOW.TMP.(N: 28.1)	14.4	26.9	27.3	29.2	27.4	25.1 ± 2.7
ECC. 0 - 10 (N: 29.9)	17.9	27.6	27.7	30.1	29.1	26.5 ± 2.2
10 - 20 (N: 27.9)	14.4	24.6	25.6	28.2	26.8	23.9 ± 2.4
20 - 30 (N: 26.0)	14.3	23.3	24.3	27.7	25.2	23.0 ± 2.3
NO. OF DISTURBED POINTS	66	14	13	1	2	19 ± 12
R.M.S. FLUCTUATION	2.2	3.3	2.1	1.0	1.3	2.0
TOTAL FLUCTUATION						6.0

Figure 9–3E. A 44-year-old woman with bilateral optic neuritis. All fields were performed on an Octopus 201 using program 32. Follow-up visual fields were performed on each eye at 1 month, 3 months, 6 months, and 15 months. These are summarized above by the series mode of the Delta program. Figures for total field loss and number of disturbed points show field recovery as the optic nerve inflammation improved in the left eye. By the second examination, only nasal loss persists. The nasal loss is reduced further and concentrated in the upper nasal quadrant by the third examination. Recovery is complete by the fourth examination. (continued)

	EX1	EX2	EX3	EX4	EX5	SUMMARY
DATE OF EXAM : DAY	10.04	11.02	12.29	06.24	11.25	
YEAR	1982	1982	1982	1983	1983	
PROGRAM / EXAMINATION	32/01	32/02	32/03	32/04	32/05	
TOTAL LOSS (WHOLE FIELD)	897	115	38	0	0	210 ± 173
MEAN LOSS (PER TEST LOC)						
WHOLE FIELD	12.1	1.6	0.5	0.0	0.0	2.8 ± 2.3
QUADRANT UPPER NASAL	20.9	3.4	1.3	0.0	0.0	5.1 ± 4.9
LOWER NASAL	15.4	2.6	0.4	0.0	0.0	3.7 ± 3.0
UPPER TEMP.	7.9	0.0	0.3	0.0	0.0	1.6 ± 1.6
LOWER TEMP.	3.6	0.0	0.0	0.0	0.0	0.7 ± 0.7
ECCENTRICITY 0 - 10	17.4	1.1	0.8	0.0	0.0	3.9 ± 3.4
10 - 20	14.3	2.7	0.4	0.0	0.0	3.5 ± 2.7
20 - 30	9.8	1.2	0.5	0.0	0.0	2.3 ± 1.9
MEAN SENSITIVITY						
WHOLE FIELD (N: 27.1)	14.7	25.2	27.6	28.7	28.8	25.0 ± 2.7
QUAD.UPP.NAS.(N: 26.4)	5.6	21.7	25.5	27.7	28.4	21.8 ± 4.2
LOW.NAS.(N: 27.4)	11.9	23.5	26.8	28.4	27.6	23.7 ± 3.0
UPP.TMP.(N: 26.5)	18.2	27.1	28.2	29.1	29.0	26.3 ± 2.1
LOW.TMP.(N: 28.1)	23.6	28.7	29.9	29.7	30.4	28.5 ± 1.3
ECC. 0 - 10 (N: 29.9)	12.2	27.7	28.7	30.0	31.0	25.9 ± 3.5
10 - 20 (N: 27.9)	13.0	25.0	28.7	29.1	29.5	25.1 ± 3.1
20 - 30 (N: 26.0)	16.0	24.6	26.8	28.2	28.0	24.7 ± 2.3
NO. OF DISTURBED POINTS	58	14	5	0	0	15 ± 11
R.M.S. FLUCTUATION	5.9	1.5	2.4	1.6	1.6	2.6
TOTAL FLUCTUATION						5.7

Figure 9–3F. *A 44-year-old woman with bilateral optic neuritis. All fields were performed on an Octopus 201 using program 32. Follow-up visual fields were performed on each eye at 1 month, 3 months, 6 months, and 15 months. These are summarized by the series mode of the Delta program. Figures for total field loss and number of disturbed points show field recovery as the optic nerve inflammation improved in the right eye. By the second examination, primarily nasal loss persists. This is improved further by the third examination and by the fourth examination the field is essentially normal.*

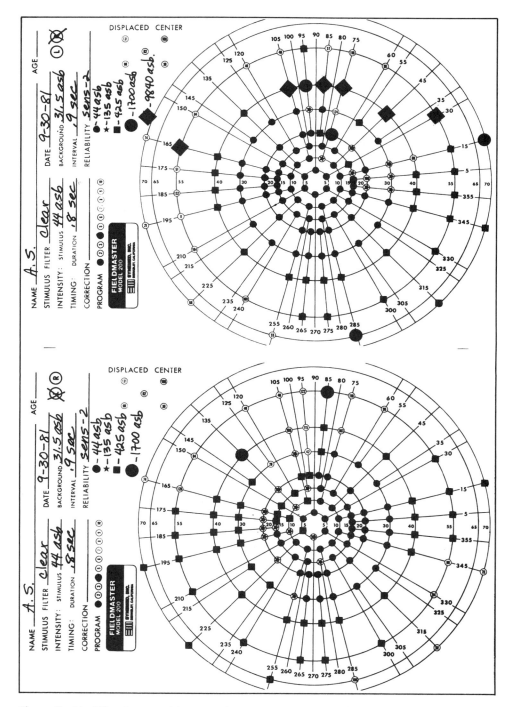

Figure 9–4A. Fifty-six-year-old man with pituitary adenoma. Visual fields were performed on a Fieldmaster 200 using a suprathreshold technique but repeating examination at several intensity levels. The data was then combined onto one report. Temporal field loss extending to, but not crossing, the verticle meridian is seen in both eyes. (continued)

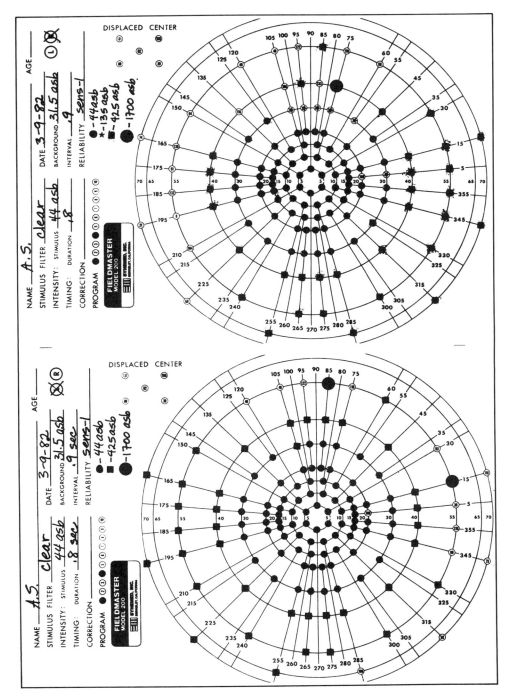

Figure 9–4B. *Postoperative field on patient in Figure 9–4A. The patient has recovered much of his field loss, especially in the periphery.*

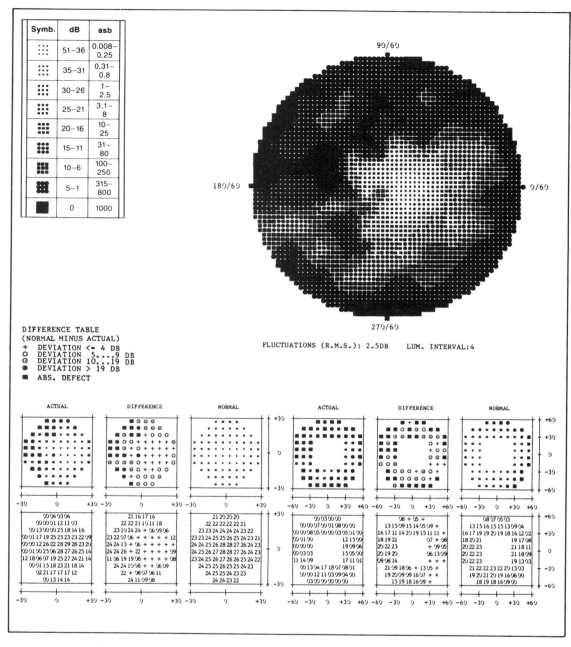

Figure 9–5A. Visual field of left eye of a 68-year-old man with a pituitary adenoma. Examination was performed on an Octopus 201 using programs 32 (central) and 42 (peripheral). Shown is a difference table for program 32 (bottom left), a difference table for program 42 (bottom right), and a grey scale combining the results of the two programs. Both peripheral constriction and temporal field loss can be seen. Temporal loss is greater superiorly than inferiorly. The temporal nature of the loss is not appreciated well in the peripheral field (program 42) but is clearly demonstrated in the central field (program 32). (continued)

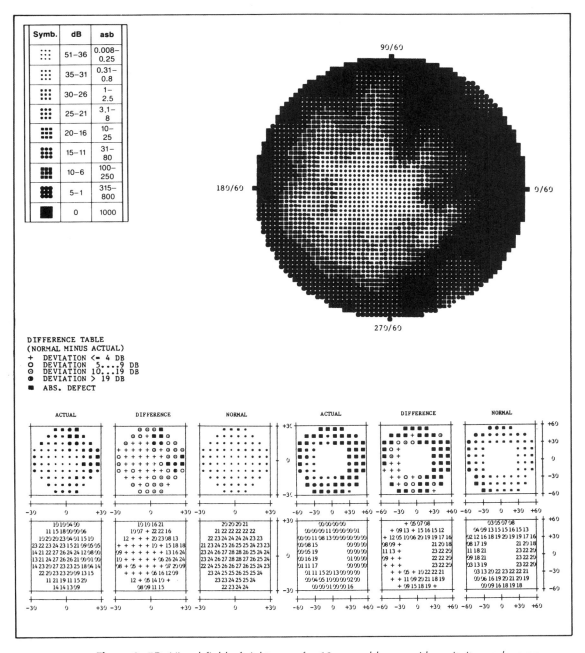

Figure 9–5B. *Visual field of right eye of a 68-year-old man with a pituitary adenoma. Examination was performed on an Octopus 201 using programs 32 (central) and 42 (peripheral). Shown is a difference table for program 32 (bottom left), a difference table for program 42 (bottom right), and a grey scale combining the results of the two programs. As in the left eye, there is both peripheral constriction and temporal field loss. The peripheral loss is worse in the temporal field so that a Chamlin step is clearly formed in both the peripheral and central fields.*

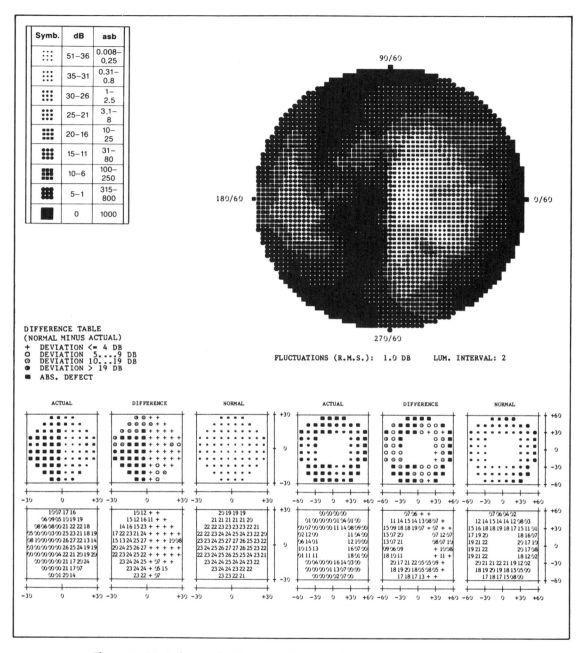

Figure 9–6A. Left eye of a 74-year-old man with a pituitary adenoma causing a classic bitemporal hemianopsia. Field was performed with an Octopus 201 using programs 32 and 42. Shown are difference tables for each program and a grey scale combining the results of the two programs. There is dense central temporal field loss and variable peripheral temporal loss with the extent of central loss exceeding the extent of peripheral loss. (continued)

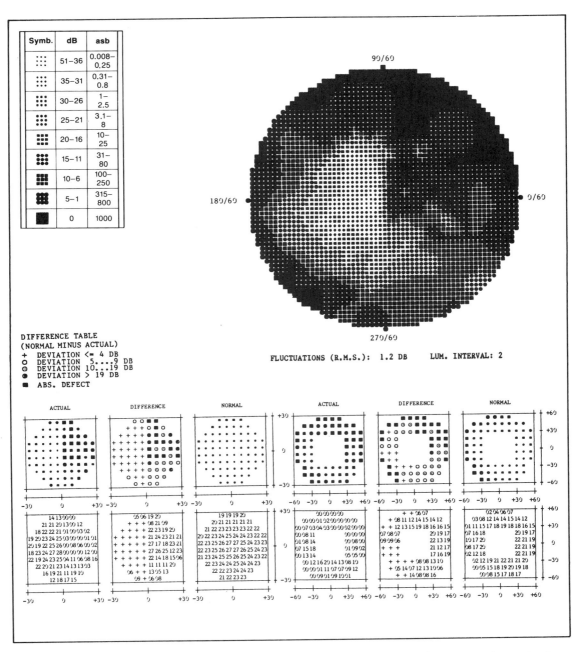

Symb.	dB	asb
⁞⁞⁞	51–36	0.008–0.25
⁞⁞⁞	35–31	0.31–0.8
⁞⁞⁞	30–26	1–2.5
⁞⁞⁞	25–21	3.1–8
⁞⁞⁞	20–16	10–25
⁞⁞⁞	15–11	31–80
⁞⁞⁞	10–6	100–250
⁞⁞⁞	5–1	315–800
■	0	1000

90/60

180/60

0/60

270/60

DIFFERENCE TABLE
(NORMAL MINUS ACTUAL)
+ DEVIATION <= 4 DB
o DEVIATION 5....9 DB
⊙ DEVIATION 10...19 DB
● DEVIATION > 19 DB
■ ABS. DEFECT

FLUCTUATIONS (R.M.S.): 1.2 DB   LUM. INTERVAL: 2

ACTUAL   DIFFERENCE   NORMAL   ACTUAL   DIFFERENCE   NORMAL

Figure 9–6B. Right eye of a 74-year-old man with a pituitary adenoma causing a classic bitemporal hemianopsia. Field was performed with an Octopus 201 using programs 32 and 42. Shown are difference tables for each program and a grey scale combining the results of the two programs. There is a superior Chamlin step, a dense superior temporal quadrantanopia, and a less dense inferior temporal quadrantanopia. There is generalized depression in the periphery, but the nasal half of the central field is intact. (continued)

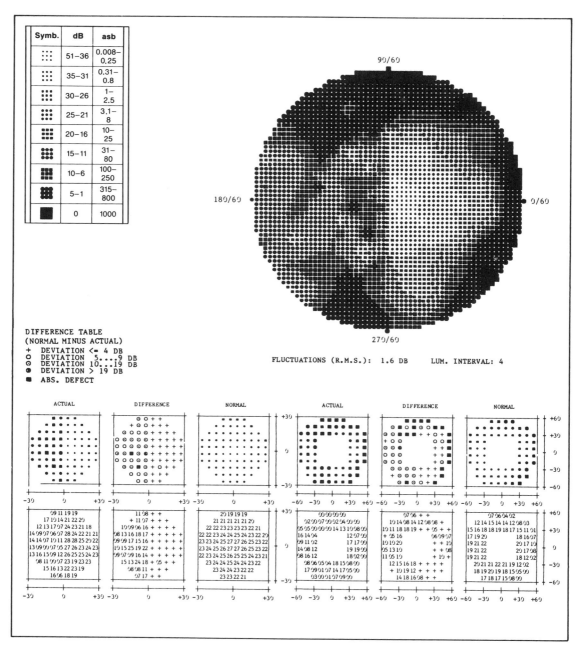

Figure 9–6C. Postoperative Octopus 201 visual field of patient in Figure 9–6A. Recovery of field loss in the temporal field can be seen. (continued)

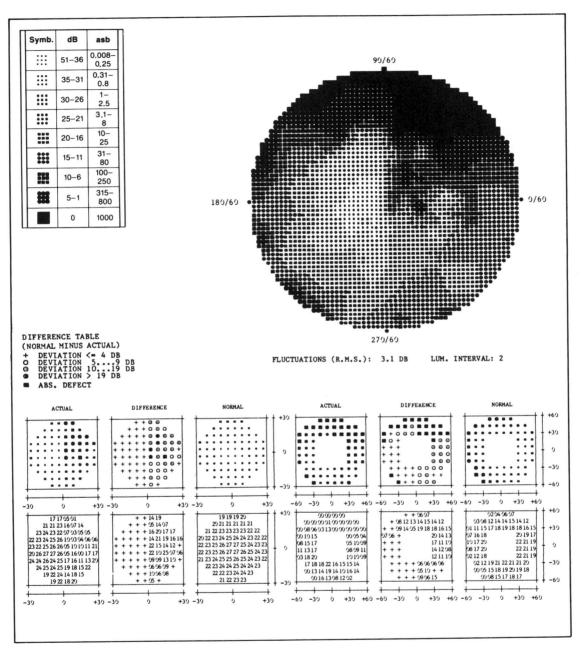

Figure 9–6D. *Postoperative Octopus 201 visual field of right eye of patient in Figure 9–6B. Generalized field loss recovery, especially in the periphery and superotemporally, can be seen. (continued)*

	EX1	EX2	SUMMARY
DATE OF EXAM : DAY	09.19	10.26	
YEAR	1984	1984	
PROGRAM / EXAMINATION	32/01	32/04	

| TOTAL LOSS (WHOLE FIELD) | 808 | 446 | 627 ± 181 |

MEAN LOSS (PER TEST LOC)

	EX1	EX2	SUMMARY
WHOLE FIELD	10.9	6.0	8.5 ± 2.4
QUADRANT UPPER NASAL	1.5	0.0	0.8 ± 0.8
LOWER NASAL	1.8	0.3	1.0 ± 0.8
UPPER TEMP.	17.8	11.1	14.4 ± 3.4
LOWER TEMP.	23.6	13.4	18.5 ± 5.1
ECCENTRICITY 0 – 10	12.6	8.6	10.6 ± 2.0
10 – 20	10.4	7.1	8.7 ± 1.6
20 – 30	10.7	4.9	7.8 ± 2.9

MEAN SENSITIVITY

	EX1	EX2	SUMMARY
WHOLE FIELD (N: 23.1)	11.4	16.9	14.2 ± 2.8
QUAD.UPP.NAS.(N: 22.4)	19.6	22.4	21.0 ± 1.4
LOW.NAS.(N: 23.4)	19.8	22.9	21.3 ± 1.6
UPP.TMP.(N: 22.5)	4.7	11.2	8.0 ± 3.3
LOW.TMP.(N: 24.1)	0.4	10.6	5.5 ± 5.1
ECC. 0 – 10 (N: 25.9)	12.9	17.9	15.4 ± 2.5
10 – 20 (N: 23.9)	12.4	16.7	14.6 ± 2.2
20 – 30 (N: 22.0)	10.5	16.8	13.6 ± 3.1

NO. OF DISTURBED POINTS	43	36	40 ± 4
R.M.S. FLUCTUATION	3.9	2.7	3.3
TOTAL FLUCTUATION			3.6

	EX1	EX2	SUMMARY
DATE OF EXAM : DAY	09.19	10.26	
YEAR	1984	1984	
PROGRAM / EXAMINATION	32/01	32/04	

| TOTAL LOSS (WHOLE FIELD) | 646 | 400 | 523 ± 123 |

MEAN LOSS (PER TEST LOC)

	EX1	EX2	SUMMARY
WHOLE FIELD	8.7	5.4	7.1 ± 1.7
QUADRANT UPPER NASAL	0.6	0.0	0.3 ± 0.3
LOWER NASAL	0.9	0.0	0.4 ± 0.4
UPPER TEMP.	19.9	14.7	17.3 ± 2.6
LOWER TEMP.	14.5	7.6	11.0 ± 3.5
ECCENTRICITY 0 – 10	11.7	7.7	9.7 ± 2.0
10 – 20	8.1	6.1	7.1 ± 1.0
20 – 30	8.2	4.5	6.3 ± 1.8

MEAN SENSITIVITY

	EX1	EX2	SUMMARY
WHOLE FIELD (N: 23.1)	13.8	17.8	15.8 ± 2.0
QUAD.UPP.NAS.(N: 22.4)	20.8	22.8	21.8 ± 1.0
LOW.NAS.(N: 23.4)	21.3	23.8	22.6 ± 1.3
UPP.TMP.(N: 22.5)	2.6	7.7	5.1 ± 2.6
LOW.TMP.(N: 24.1)	9.6	16.2	12.9 ± 3.3
ECC. 0 – 10 (N: 25.9)	14.3	18.3	16.3 ± 2.0
10 – 20 (N: 23.9)	15.1	18.1	16.6 ± 1.5
20 – 30 (N: 22.0)	13.1	17.5	15.3 ± 2.2

NO. OF DISTURBED POINTS	40	32	36 ± 4
R.M.S. FLUCTUATION	1.2	1.7	1.5
TOTAL FLUCTUATION			3.6

	EX1	EX2	SUMMARY
DATE OF EXAM : DAY	09.19	10.26	
YEAR	1984	1984	
PROGRAM / EXAMINATION	42/02	42/05	

| TOTAL LOSS (WHOLE FIELD) | 671 | 491 | 581 ± 90 |

MEAN LOSS (PER TEST LOC)

	EX1	EX2	SUMMARY
WHOLE FIELD	9.9	7.2	8.5 ± 1.3
QUADRANT UPPER NASAL	5.5	3.8	4.6 ± 0.8
LOWER NASAL	4.6	1.5	3.1 ± 1.6
UPPER TEMP.	13.5	11.5	12.5 ± 1.0
LOWER TEMP.	15.9	12.0	13.9 ± 1.9
ECCENTRICITY 30 – 40	10.8	8.3	9.6 ± 1.3
40 – 50	11.1	8.1	9.6 ± 1.5
50 – 60	8.6	6.1	7.4 ± 1.3

MEAN SENSITIVITY

	EX1	EX2	SUMMARY
WHOLE FIELD (N: 14.5)	4.4	6.8	5.6 ± 1.2
QUAD.UPP.NAS.(N: 11.4)	5.0	6.1	5.6 ± 0.6
LOW.NAS.(N: 10.9)	6.1	8.9	7.5 ± 1.4
UPP.TMP.(N: 16.0)	2.5	4.4	3.5 ± 0.9
LOW.TMP.(N: 19.8)	3.9	7.7	5.8 ± 1.9
ECC. 30 – 40 (N: 19.8)	8.6	10.3	9.4 ± 0.9
40 – 50 (N: 16.8)	5.8	8.5	7.1 ± 1.4
50 – 60 (N: 10.4)	1.4	3.9	2.7 ± 1.3

NO. OF DISTURBED POINTS	55	43	49 ± 6
R.M.S. FLUCTUATION	3.3	4.5	3.9
TOTAL FLUCTUATION			3.4

	EX1	EX2	SUMMARY
DATE OF EXAM : DAY	09.19	10.26	
YEAR	1984	1984	
PROGRAM / EXAMINATION	42/02	42/05	

| TOTAL LOSS (WHOLE FIELD) | 633 | 449 | 541 ± 92 |

MEAN LOSS (PER TEST LOC)

	EX1	EX2	SUMMARY
WHOLE FIELD	9.3	6.6	8.0 ± 1.4
QUADRANT UPPER NASAL	6.9	4.4	5.6 ± 1.3
LOWER NASAL	2.4	0.0	1.2 ± 1.2
UPPER TEMP.	15.4	14.1	14.7 ± 0.7
LOWER TEMP.	12.6	8.0	10.3 ± 2.3
ECCENTRICITY 30 – 40	10.9	8.2	9.5 ± 1.3
40 – 50.	10.8	7.8	9.3 ± 1.5
50 – 60	7.6	5.1	6.3 ± 1.3

MEAN SENSITIVITY

	EX1	EX2	SUMMARY
WHOLE FIELD (N: 14.5)	4.9	8.1	6.5 ± 1.6
QUAD.UPP.NAS.(N: 11.4)	3.6	5.6	4.6 ± 1.0
LOW.NAS.(N: 10.9)	8.1	13.6	10.9 ± 2.8
UPP.TMP.(N: 16.0)	0.6	1.9	1.3 ± 0.7
LOW.TMP.(N: 19.8)	7.2	11.4	9.3 ± 2.1
ECC. 30 – 40 (N: 19.8)	8.3	11.2	9.8 ± 1.4
40 – 50 (N: 16.8)	6.0	9.3	7.7 ± 1.7
50 – 60 (N: 10.4)	2.4	5.9	4.2 ± 1.7

NO. OF DISTURBED POINTS	50	40	45 ± 5
R.M.S. FLUCTUATION	2.2	2.1	2.1
TOTAL FLUCTUATION			3.9

Figure 9–6E. *Series Mode Delta examination of the preoperative and postoperative visual fields shown in Figures 9–6A through 9–6D. Program 32 is at the top and program 42 is at the bottom. Recovery can be seen in all quadrants of all examinations, especially in the temporal quadrants. (continued)*

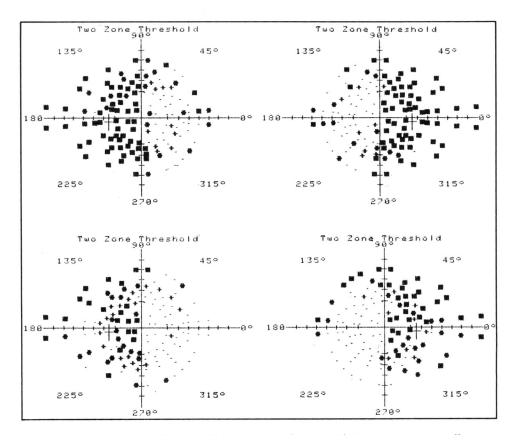

Figure 9–6F. *A 74-year-old man with a pituitary adenoma. The tumor was surgically resected. Preoperative (top) and postoperative fields (bottom) were performed on the Dicon AP 2000 using the two-zone program starting at the 100 asb level. A classic bitemporal hemianopsia is seen. Postoperative fields show some recovery of field loss. This is seen nasally in both eyes, superotemporally and inferotemporally in the left eye, and inferotemporally in the right eye. Recovery is seen primarily in the peripheral fields and not the central fields.*

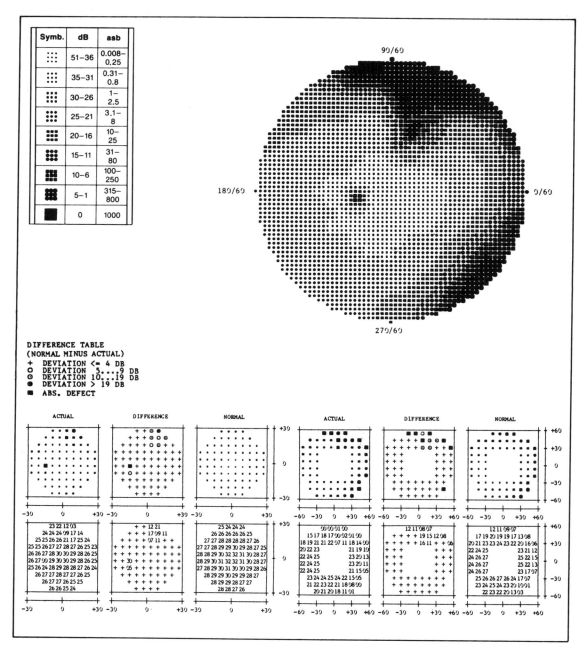

Figure 9–7A. *Thirty-two-year-old man with presumed optic tract lesion. Visual field examination was performed on an Octopus 201 using programs 32 and 42. Shown is a combined grey scale and comparison tables for both program. A small right superior sector defect, which does not cross the midline, is demonstrated in the left eye. (continued)*

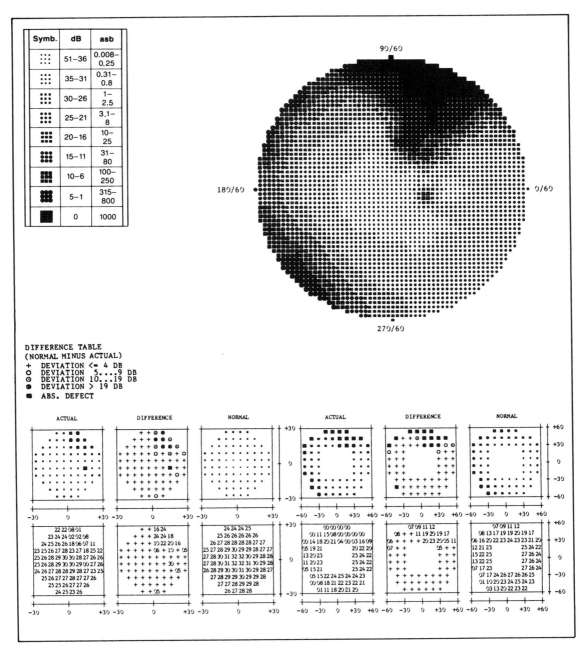

Figure 9–7B. *Examination of the right eye of the patient in Figure 9–7A shows a somewhat congruous but slightly larger right upper quadrant sectoral defect.*

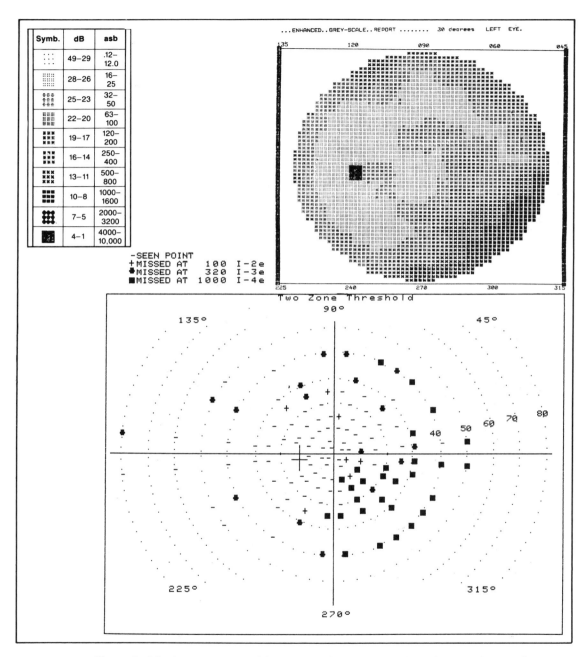

Figure 9–8A. *A seventy-year-old woman with a left parietal cerebrovascular accident. Visual field examination was performed on a Dicon AP 2000 using program 32. Examination of the left eye shows a dense inferior quadrantinopia. (continued)*

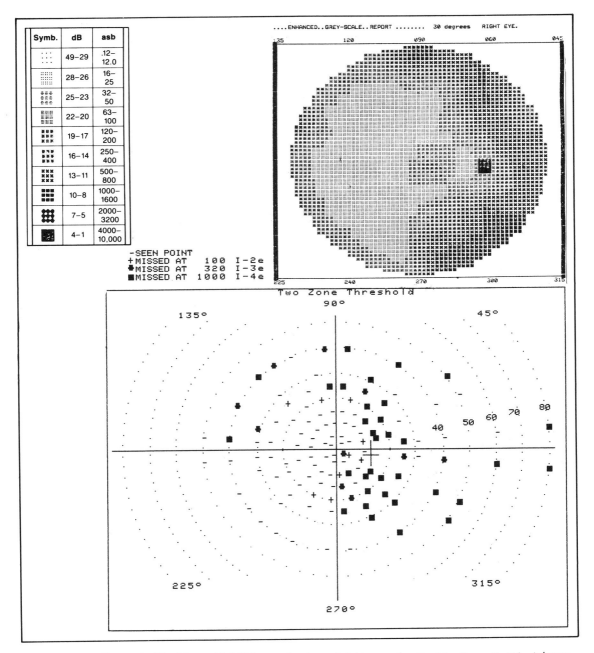

Figure 9–8B. Dicon AP 2000 examination of right eye of patient in Figure 9–8A. A larger area of right-sided field involvement is seen, although the greatest amount of loss is seen inferiorly.

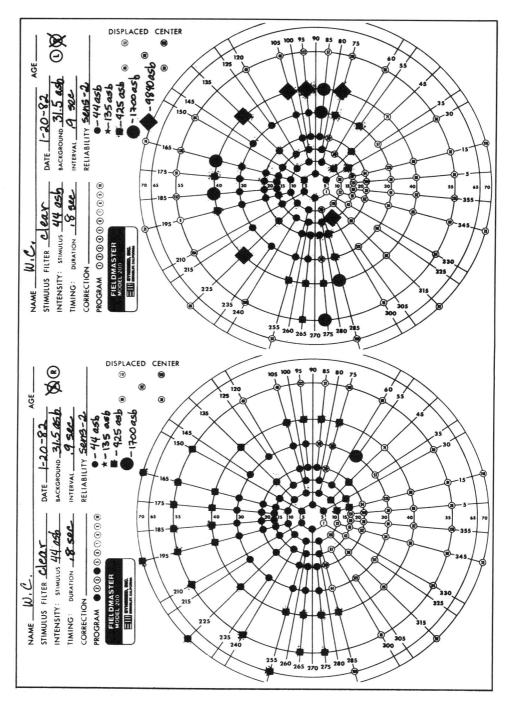

Figure 9–9. Fieldmaster 200 examination of a sixty-four-year-old man who suffered a left parietal cerebrovascular accident with temporal lobe involvement. A dense right homonymous hemianopsia can be seen.

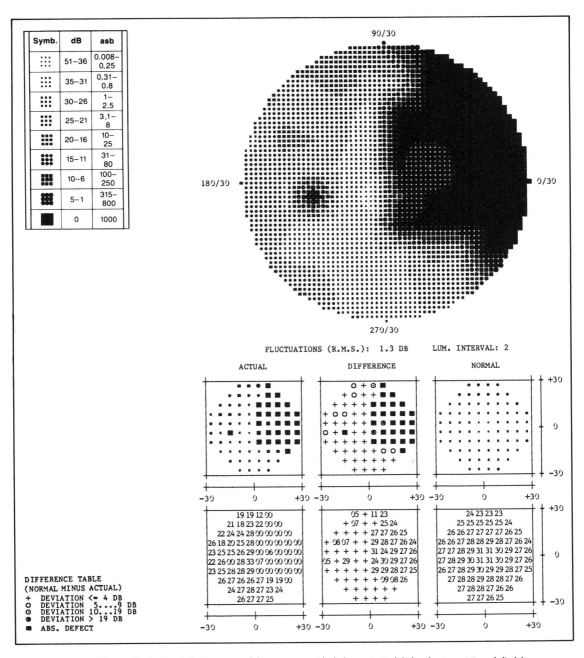

Symb.	dB	asb
⋮⋮⋮	51–36	0.008–0.25
⋮⋮⋮	35–31	0.31–0.8
∷∷	30–26	1–2.5
∷∷	25–21	3.1–8
▪▪▪	20–16	10–25
▪▪▪	15–11	31–80
▪▪▪	10–6	100–250
▓	5–1	315–800
■	0	1000

FLUCTUATIONS (R.M.S.): 1.3 DB   LUM. INTERVAL: 2

ACTUAL

DIFFERENCE

NORMAL

DIFFERENCE TABLE
(NORMAL MINUS ACTUAL)
+ DEVIATION <= 4 DB
○ DEVIATION 5...9 DB
◎ DEVIATION 10..19 DB
● DEVIATION > 19 DB
■ ABS. DEFECT

```
        19 19 12 00            05 + 11 23          24 23 23 23
      21 18 23 22 00 00        + 07 + + 25 24     25 25 25 25 24
    22 24 24 28 00 00 00 00    + + + + 27 27 26 25   26 26 27 27 27 27 26 25
  26 18 20 25 28 00 00 00 00 00  + 08 07 + + 29 28 27 26 24  26 26 27 28 28 29 28 27 26 24
  23 25 25 26 29 00 06 00 00 00  + + + + + 31 24 29 27 26  27 27 28 29 31 31 30 29 27 26
  22 26 00 28 33 07 00 00 00 00  05 + 29 + + 24 30 29 27 26  27 28 29 30 31 31 30 29 27 26
  23 25 28 28 29 00 00 00 00 00  + + + + + 29 29 28 27 25  26 27 28 29 30 29 29 28 27 25
    26 27 26 26 27 19 19 00    + + + + + 09 08 26   27 28 28 29 28 28 27 26
      24 27 28 27 23 24        + + + + + +       27 28 28 27 26
        26 27 27 25            + + + +            27 27 26 25
```

Figure 9–10A. *A forty-year-old woman with left occipital lobe lesion. Visual field examination was performed on an Octopus 201 using program 32. A dense right hemianopsia is demonstrated in the left eye, greater superiorly than inferiorly. The midline was not crossed. (continued)*

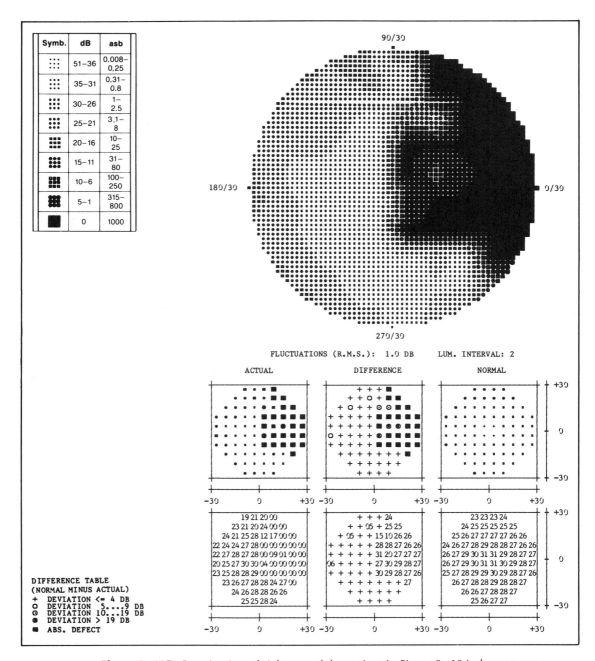

Figure 9–10B. Examination of right eye of the patient in Figure 9–10A shows a very congruous right hemianopsia.

10

The Visual Field in Other Diseases

Diseases of the Retina

Diseases of the retina that interfere with its vascular supply or cause inflammation within the retina can produce visual field defects. In addition, trauma to the retina or the underlying choroid, the accumulation of toxic substances within the retina, tumors of the retina or the choroid, detachments of the retina, and retinoschisis can all produce visual field defects.

Any disease that causes localized damage to the retina yields a localized defect in the area of the damage. Therefore, in such patients, the visual field is supportive of the information gained in a good retinal examination.

A loss of the arteriolar circulation to the retina produces an absolute defect in the area nourished by the involved branches. A central retinal artery occlusion yields a complete loss of vision. If only a branch of the artery is affected, only the area of the retina fed by that branch will be affected and the resulting field defect will point toward and usually be contiguous with the blindspot (Fig. 10–1). Those patients having a cilioretinal artery will have the area supplied by the cilioretinal artery spared when either a branch or complete central retinal artery occlusion occurs (Fig. 10–2).

Retinal vein occlusions, in their early stage of development, cause a depression of the visual field. When they reach a more advanced stage, with frank hemorrhage and exudate, severe visual field loss occurs (Fig. 10–3). Vein occlusions often can be accompanied by arterial occlusions with corresponding field defects. They also can be confined to a branch of the vein with a corresponding sector field loss (Fig. 10–4).

Arteriosclerotic, hypertensive, and diabetic retinopathies yield visual field defects that are usually secondary to the pathology in the retina itself. Areas of hemorrhage, exudate, or scarring yield localized visual field loss.

Macular edema causes metamorphopsia or distortion of the central 5 to 10 degrees of field and depression of the field corresponding to the area of the edema. Some investigators have maintained that blue colored test objects are the best for bringing out this type of field defect, but it has been our experience that the most effective method is the use of an Amsler grid (Chap. 2). When macular edema persists for a long period of time, regardless of the cause, damage to the retinal receptor cells within the macula can cause a patchwork pattern of visual field loss with areas of absolute and relative scotomas that are very tiny in size. These also can be outlined best by an Amsler grid examination.

Macular holes yield absolute scotomas. These can be the result of trauma, long-standing macular disease, vitreous disease, or the end stages of solar retinopathy (Fig. 10–5). Macular degeneration yields a range of field defects from mild central depression to a large absolute defect (Fig. 10–6).

Trauma to the retina can produce commotio retinae, choroidal ruptures, or retinal tears. Commotio retinae causes a depression of the visual field in the corresponding area of the field that usually resolves as the retinal edema resolves. Choroidal ruptures and tears in the retina yield absolute permanent scotomas.

Retinitis pigmentosa involves the retinal rods and is first noticed by the patient as night blindness. Visual field loss usually starts as a ring scotoma in the area between 20 and 25 degrees from fixation. This loss then progresses both into the periphery and toward the center yielding a visual field of only a few degrees (Fig. 10–7).

Many retinitis pigmentosa patients also develop macular degeneration. In these patients the central visual field can also be lost. Visual fields can be useful in retinitis pigmentosa patients in following their progression, however, for diagnosis and classification, electrophysiologic studies are essential.

Papilledema produces an increase in the size of the blind spot. Long-standing papilledema causes an overall depression in the visual field especially in the peripheral field inferonasally. Paracentral and arcuate can also be seen.

Absolute scotomas can be seen due to retinal tumors including angiomas and retinoblastomas. The visual field loss is localized to the area of the tumor. Likewise, colobomata yield an area of absolute visual field loss localized to the area of the coloboma.

Retinal detachments cause a relative visual field loss in the area of the detachment, which is seen as a depression of the visual field in that area. This is contrasted to retinoschisis, where the anatomic defect is within the layers of the retina with a resultant destruction of the receptor cell connections. The visual field defect in retinoschisis, therefore, is an absolute scotoma extending to the edge of the retinoschisis (Fig. 10–8). The visual field examination, therefore, can be extremely useful when the differentiation between retinoschisis and retinal detachment is unclear on ophthalmoscopic examination.

Diseases of the Choroid

Visual field loss can be caused by choroidal inflammation and tumors. Visual field defects are seen corresponding to the exact sites of the choroidal inflammation and/or scarring. The visual field examination in diseases of the choroid is useful in seeing the progression of the lesions by following the size of the field defect.

Very often a normal visual field can be seen in areas where there is a great deal of choroidal inflammation. In such cases, as the inflammation spreads into the retina, visual field defects can appear. In juxtapapillary choroiditis, the inflammation adjacent to the blind spot causes an enlargement of the blind spot and a baring of the blind spot.

Choroidal tumors, such as melanomas, tend to cause a deep, if not absolute, defect with steep margins. This is contrasted to a nevus that usually shows no visual field defect, but can, in some cases, cause absolute defects. It is useful to follow the visual fields in patients with possible melanomas, but a visual field test can only be supportive of the other clinical information gained from studies such as fluorescein angiography and ultrasonography.

Opacities of the Media

Opacities can occur in the cornea, the lens, the anterior chamber, or the vitreous, which will cause visual field defects by direct interruption of the light rays entering the eye. Dense corneal scarring, cataracts, vitreous hemorrhages, and hyphemas all cause a generalized depression of the visual field.

Partial opacities of the media, such as a developing cataract or a resolving hemorrhage, cause a variety of visual field defects related to the partial obstruction of light rays. The transient variability of the pathology is reflected in variable field defects.

Any obstruction to the rays of light entering the eye reduces the ability of those rays of light to be seen in the retina. Opacities in the media must be taken into consideration when evaluating a visual field. A patient who is being evaluated for glaucoma or neurologic disease, for example, can also have cataracts causing defects in the visual fields. Because therapeutic decisions are often made on the basis of field defects in glaucoma and in neurologic disease, it is important to reevaluate the patient clinically.

A miotic or small pupil can cause a generalized visual field depression and can accentuate the effect of opacities in the media. An abnormal appearing visual field related mainly to pupil size can be so produced. Therefore, it is always important to note the pupil size when the visual field examination is performed. If visual field defects are present with a small pupil, the visual field examination should be repeated with the pupil dilated.

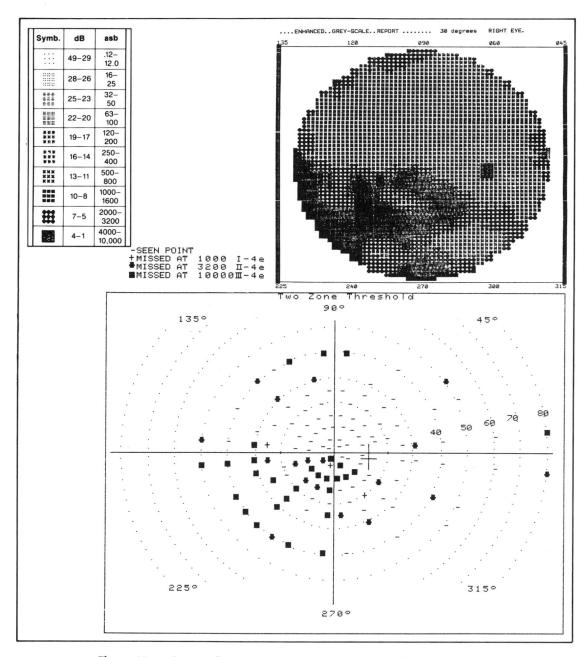

Figure 10–1. *Seventy-five-year-old woman with long-standing right superotemporal branch vein occlusion. Visual field examination was performed on a Dicon AP 2000 using the two-zone testing strategy. Starting intensity was 1000 asb. A dense inferonasal quadrant loss, which extends to the blind spot, is seen. There is also some superior constriction that was related to the patient's eyelid.*

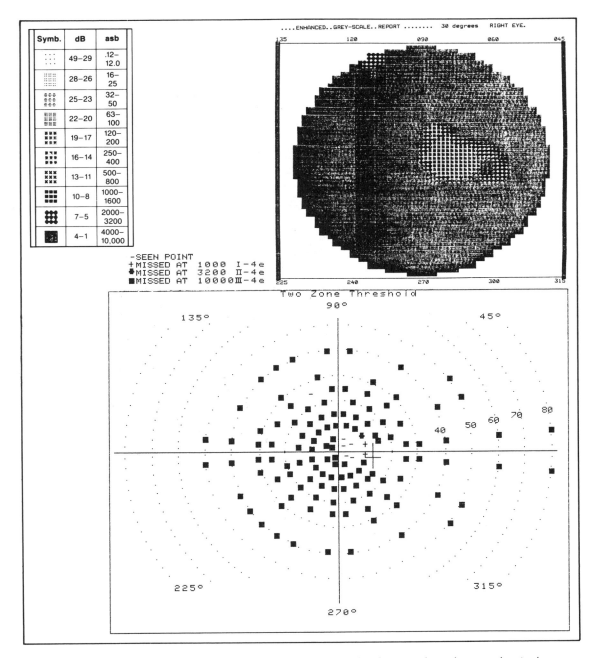

Figure 10–2. *Seventy-seven-year-old aphake with a history of a right central retinal artery occlusion. The patient had a patent cilioretinal artery. Visual field examination was performed on a Dicon AP 2000 using the two-zone testing strategy. Starting intensity was 1000 asb. The old area of remaining field corresponds to the distribution of the cilioretinal artery and extends from the edge of the disk to the macula.*

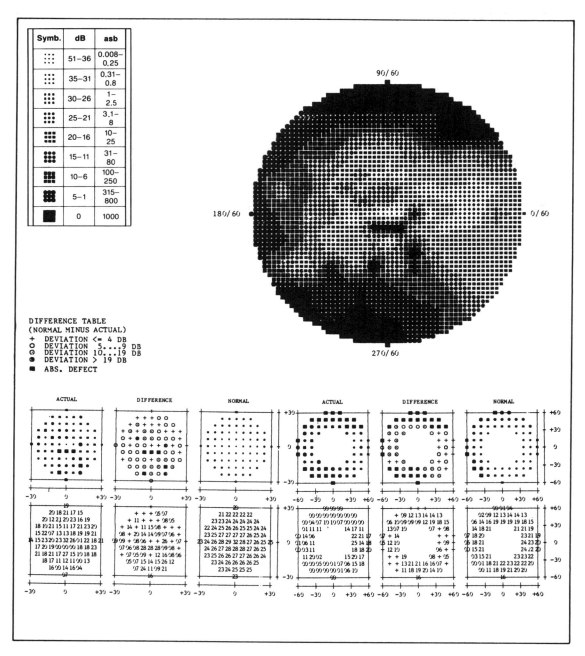

Figure 10–3. Fifty-six-year-old man with right central retinal vein thrombosis. Visual field examination was performed on an Octopus 201 using programs 32 and 42. The field shows diffuse, patchy loss with a dense central scotoma. This corresponds to the scattered hemorrhages and exudate in the patient's retina.

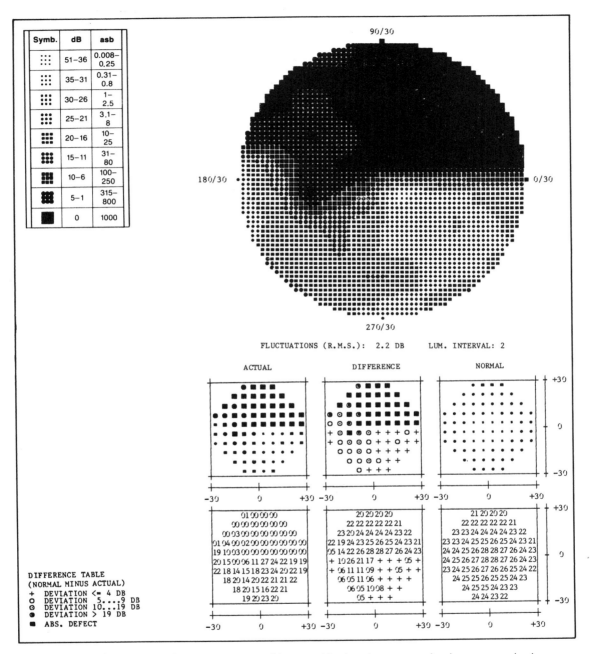

Symb.	dB	asb
⠿	51–36	0.008–0.25
⠿	35–31	0.31–0.8
⠿	30–26	1–2.5
⠿	25–21	3.1–8
⠿	20–16	10–25
⠿	15–11	31–80
⠿	10–6	100–250
⠿	5–1	315–800
■	0	1000

90/30

180/30

0/30

270/30

FLUCTUATIONS (R.M.S.): 2.2 DB   LUM. INTERVAL: 2

ACTUAL   DIFFERENCE   NORMAL

DIFFERENCE TABLE
(NORMAL MINUS ACTUAL)
+   DEVIATION <= 4 DB
○   DEVIATION   5...:9 DB
⊙   DEVIATION 10...:19 DB
◉   DEVIATION > 19 DB
■   ABS. DEFECT

```
        01 00 00 00
     00 00 00 00 00 00
  00 03 00 00 00 00 00 00
01 04 00 02 00 00 00 00 00 00
19 10 03 00 00 00 00 00 00 00
20 15 00 06 11 27 24 22 19 19
22 18 14 15 18 23 24 29 22 19
   18 20 14 20 22 21 21 22
   18 20 15 16 22 21
      19 20 23 20
```

```
        20 20 20 20
     22 22 22 22 22 21
  23 20 24 24 24 24 23 22
22 19 24 23 25 26 25 24 23 21
05 14 22 28 28 28 27 26 24 23
 + 19 26 21 17 + + + 05 +
 + 06 11 11 09 + + + 05 + +
   06 05 11 06 + + + +
      06 05 10 08 + +
         05 + + +
```

```
        21 20 20 20
     22 22 22 22 22 21
  23 23 24 24 24 24 23 22
23 23 24 25 25 26 25 24 23 21
24 24 25 26 28 27 26 24 23
24 25 26 27 28 28 27 26 24 23
23 24 25 26 27 26 26 25 24 22
   24 25 25 25 25 24 23
   24 25 25 24 23 23
      24 24 23 22
```

Figure 10–4. *Seventy-two-year-old man with chronic open-angle glaucoma and a long-standing inferior branch vein occlusion. Visual field examination was performed on an Octopus 201 using program 32. There is total loss of the superior field corresponding to the branch vein occlusion. There is also some inferior temporal arcuate area depression.*

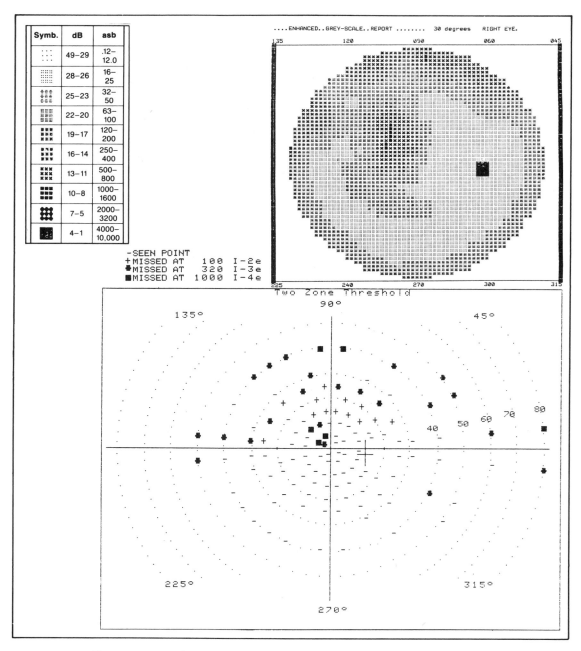

Symb.	dB	asb
	49–29	.12–12.0
	28–26	16–25
	25–23	32–50
	22–20	63–100
	19–17	120–200
	16–14	250–400
	13–11	500–800
	10–8	1000–1600
	7–5	2000–3200
	4–1	4000–10,000

....ENHANCED..GREY-SCALE..REPORT .... 30 degrees   RIGHT EYE.

-SEEN POINT
+MISSED AT   100 I-2e
✱MISSED AT   320 I-3e
■MISSED AT   1000 I-4e

Two Zone Threshold

Figure 10–5. Eighty-two-year-old woman with a full thickness retinal hole at the inferior temporal aspect of the right macula. Visual field examination was performed on a Dicon AP 2000 using the two-zone testing strategy. A dense paracentral scotoma is seen in the corresponding superonasal central field. In addition there is some superior constriction.

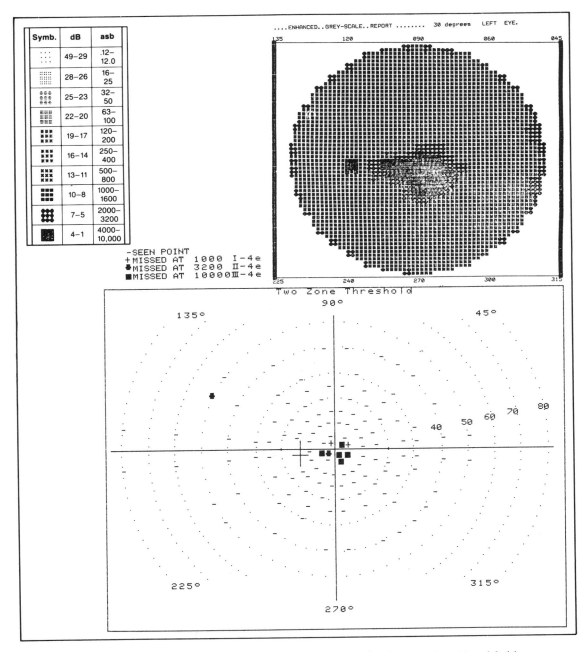

Figure 10–6. *Fifty-four-year-old woman with macular degeneration. Visual field examination was performed on a Dicon AP 2000 using the two-zone testing strategy. A dense central scotoma is present corresponding to the area of macular destruction.*

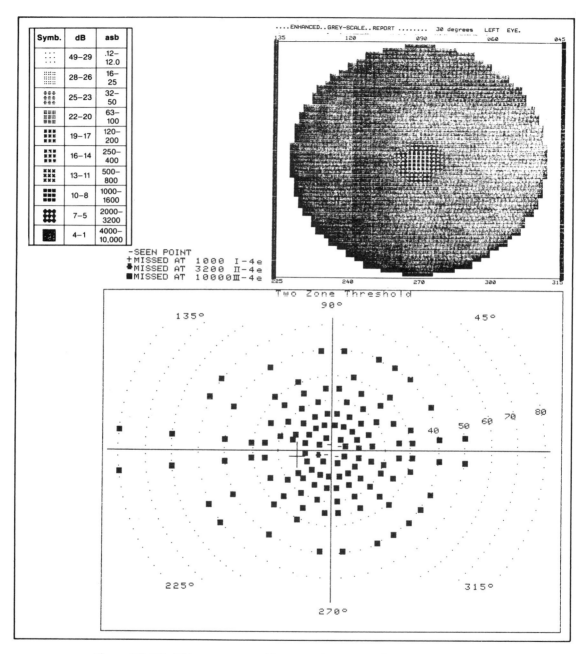

Figure 10–7A. *Thirty-two-year-old-man with autosomal recessive retinitis pigmentosa. Visual acuity was 20/30, o.u. Visual field examination was performed on a Dicon AP 2000 using the two-zone testing strategy. Left shows severe constriction with a 2.5-degree central field remaining. (continued)*

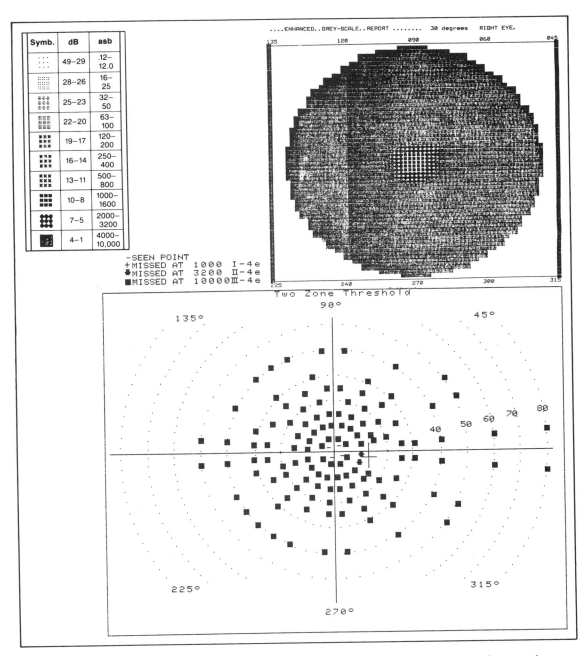

Figure 10–7B. *Right eye of retinitis pigmentosa patient in Fig. 10–7A. Only a 2.5-degree central field remains in this eye also.*

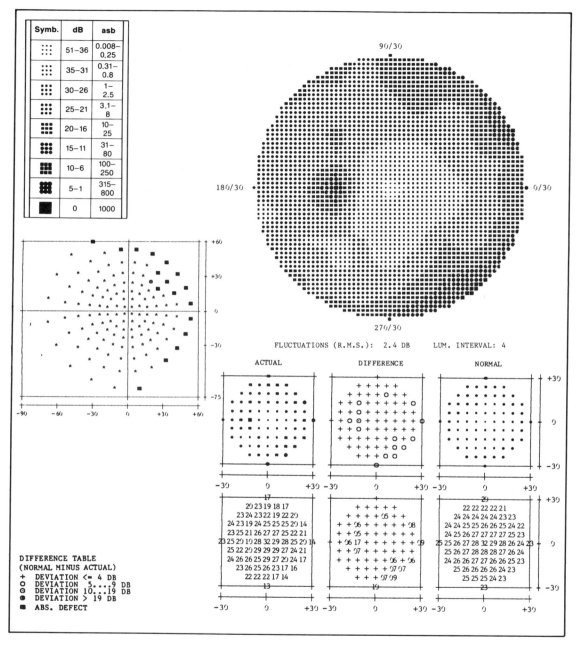

Figure 10–8A. Fifty-seven-year-old man with temporal retinoschisis, o.u. Visual field examination was performed on an Octopus 201 using programs 31 and 7. Dense peripheral nasal scotomas are seen corresponding to the area of retinoschisis. The field is normal until the edge of the schisis is encountered at which point the defect appears and is absolute. The defect is seen primarily in the program 7 field, which extends out to 60 degrees. (continued)

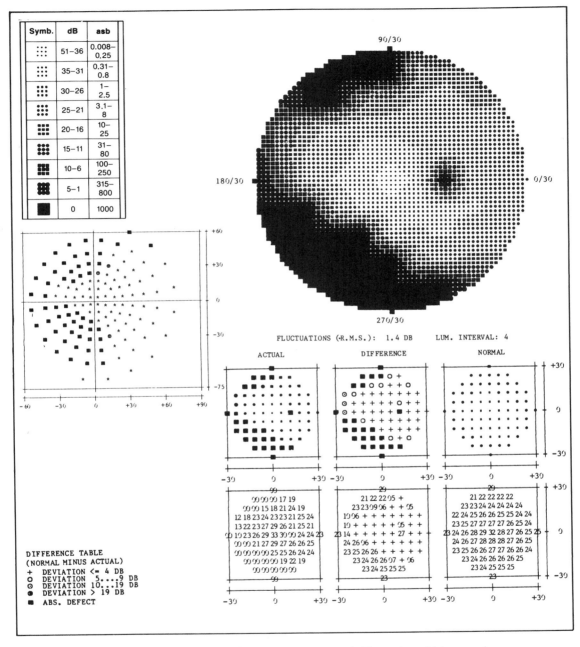

Figure 10–8B. *Right eye of patient in Fig. 10–8A. The retinoschisis extends more posteriorly in the right eye than in the left eye and can be seen clearly in the central field study of program 31 as well as in program 7. The appearance of the defect in the field corresponds exactly to the area of retinal involvement.*

11
Future Directions

Quantitative measurement of visual fields provides a significant advance in the measurement and the evaluation of visual fields. Not only are the advantages of more rigorous measurements significant for clinical purposes, new opportunities for eye research also emerge. Some automated visual field machines have the ability to store individual examinations for several patients on a single floppy diskette. Most currently available automated visual field machines, however, provide very limited access to information (usually only a few files [examinations] at a time). This severely limits the usefulness of many currently available automated perimeters for large sample research purposes, or for time series analyses on a single patient. This limitation is overcome, however, by transmission of individual examinations to a host computer equipped with a large data storage device, operating system, and a computer language. Transmission software is now available for some machines that will transmit files to a microcomputer such as the IBM PC or to any other host computer with software to receive the files. These technical advances in automated perimetry make possible a new era in clinical research involving large and carefully identified groups of patients and fields, as well as new opportunities in clinical practice to access and analyse any desired field or set of fields.

New directions in research may modify some of the current views of field loss. For example, although isolated reports documenting cases where field loss in glaucoma was reversed have previously been reported, abnormalities in the visual field of glaucoma patients are generally considered irreversible. Recent studies, however, suggest that field dynamics (both progression and regression) may constitute a new facet of field analysis. For example, it has been suggested that early defects may be best identified by threshold variation rather than by an absolute reduction in visual sensitivity. J. Flammer[1] has recently proposed that some defects may not necessarily be localized scotomas, but rather be described as a distributed defect without a clear border. Such a defect would be identified as "diffuse" damage rather than a specific area of loss.

Current directions for development include new techniques to extract more clinically relevant information from a field. New field indices such as mean defect, loss variance, and corrected loss variance have been proposed by J. Flammer and Hans Bebie[2] to probe local and diffuse field changes. Specifically, mean defect (MD) and loss variance (LV) provide first and second moment descriptions of the field loss. These indices require that a set of expected normal values be known and all observed thresholds are compared against these values. For example, the mean defect index is described by the following notation:

$$MD = \frac{\sum\limits_{i=1}^{n} (N_i - X_i)}{n}$$

where N_i and X_i refer to the expected normal and observed values respectively at a location i, and n refers to the number of locations in the field examination. This index provides a summary of the over-all average defect and a useful measure of diffuse loss.

The loss variance (LV) index is the variance associated with the mean defect, and is described by the following notation:

$$LV = \frac{\sum\limits_{i=1}^{n} (Z_i - MD)^2}{n - 1}$$

where Z_i refers to the quantity $(N_i - X_i)$ at location i, and all other symbols are as described above. Although this index is useful as an index of location fluctuations, it is problematic in that fluctuations due to true physiologic variation are not separated from variation due to measurement error (short-term fluctuation). However, this limitation is overcome by an index called the corrected loss variance (CLV) and is described by the following notation:

$$CLV = LV - (RMS)^2$$

where RMS refers to the root mean square determined for an individual field examination as an index of measurement reliability. The advantage of the CLV is that at least some component of fluctuation due to the short-term (measurement) conditions is extracted from the total variance. The remaining variance, CLV, provides a better estimate of the extent to which local fluctuations in threshold (relative to a normal standard) occur in the visual field. Flammer and Bebie have found that the corrected loss variance statistic provides a field evaluation that is independent of loss statistics, and may document field disturbances in some cases prior to the observation of a sensitivity deficit.

The new set of indices: mean defect, loss variance, and corrected loss variance potentially offer new dimensions in field evaluations. Several other new approaches to field interpolation have also recently been suggested. For example, J. Hirsch[3] has recently proposed a factorial type analysis to compare multiple fields over time. This analysis yields global information about both field variations with time and field variations over area. R. Shields[4] has presented a potentially very useful technique to compare local (point by point) threshold changes over time. W. Herman and colleagues[5] have developed a three-dimensional retinal map to assess macular function by both static thresholds and cone ERGs. Quantitative visual fields coupled with powerful computing facilities will undoubtedly serve to link sensory changes with underlying physiology. The goal of these additional analyses is to extract more information from the visual field that reflects field dynamics associated with disease processes.

In addition to providing more information about the visual field and physiologic processes associated with eye disease, future directions in automated visual field testing may also include information resources along the lines of expert systems to assist with interpretation and application of complex field information. Sorting out combined influences, such as pupil size, measurement error, response biases, and deviations from expected values, are complex issues that can potentially be managed by a supporting computer. The expert systems approach could also integrate field information with other relevant clinical information including history, medications, acuity, eye pressure, and appearance of the disc. S. Feldon[6] has recently proposed a coding system to standardize the coding of additional clinical information along with the field report. Improved quantification of normal population values and interindividual variations constitutes a very significant future objective. Currently a large interinstitutional study (directed by R. LaBlanc) is in progress to assess normal fields for different age groups. Results of this study will provide an invaluable baseline to compare and interpret patient fields.

Management of diverse clinical information as well as the identification and extraction of new field information is technically achievable. Future directions, however, depend upon creative and systematic efforts by clinicians and medical investigators to effectively use the new tools.

References

1. Flammer J: First experiences with the Octopus Glaucoma Program G1. Presented at the Octopus Users' Society Meeting, San Diego, Ca., 1985.
2. Bebie H: Computerized techniques of visual field comparisons, in Automated Perimetry: A Practical Guide. New York, Grune & Stratton, 1984.
3. Hirsch J: Comparison of multiple visual fields obtained over extended periods of time. Presented at the Octopus Users' Society Meeting, San Diego, Ca., 1985.
4. Shields RL: Status Report—IBM PC/XT Software. Presented at the Octopus Users' Society Meeting, San Diego, Ca., 1985.
5. Herman WK, Birch DGS, Defaller JM, Disbrow DT: 3-D foveal static threshold mapping and cone ERGs in the assessment of macular function. Presented at the Octopus Users' Society Meeting, San Diego, Ca., 1985.
6. Feldon S: Diagnostic Filing System for Octopus records on the IBM PC. Presented at the Octopus Users' Society Meeting, San Diego, Ca., 1985.

Bibliography

Accornero N, Beradelli A, Cruccu G, Manfredi M: Computerized video screen perimetry. Arch Ophthalmol 102:40–41, 1984.

Akiyama K, Sugai M, Akiyama H: The determination of normal visual fields of children in primary and junior high school. Acta Soc Ophthalmol Jpn 77:516–519, 1973. (In Japanese with English abstract.)

Albert ML, Reches A, Silverberg R: Hemianopic colour blindness. J Neurology Neurosurg Psychiatry 43:546–549, 1975.

Alexander GL: Diagnostic value of colour fields in neurosurgery. Trans Ophthalmol Soc UK 76:235–244, 1956.

American Academy of Ophthalmology: Selective Perimetry—A Strategy for Detection of Glaucomatous Visual Field Defects. Ophthalmology Basic and Clinical Science Course. Section 8: Glaucoma, lens, and anterior segment trauma. San Francisco, American Academy of Ophthalmology, 60–61, 1981.

Amsler M. Earliest symptoms of diseases of the macula: Br J Ophthalmol 57:521–537, 1953.

Anderson DR: Testing the Field of Vision. St. Louis, Toronto, London, C.V. Mosby, 1982.

Anderson DR: Programmed visual field testing. Trans Am Ophthalmol Soc 80:326–348, 1982.

Aoyama T: Visual field change examined by pupillography in glaucoma. Doc Ophthalmol Proc Ser 19:265–271, 1979.

Armaly MF: Ocular pressure and visual fields. Arch Ophthalmol 81:25–40, 1969.

Armaly MF: Reversibility of glaucomatous defects of the visual field. Doc Ophthalmol Proc Ser 19:177–185, 1979.

Armaly MF: Selective perimetry for glaucomatous defects in ocular hypertension. Arch Ophthalmol 87:518–524, 1972.

Armaly MF: The size and location of the normal blind spot. Arch Ophthalmol 81:192–201, 1969.

Armon H, Weinman J, et al: Automatic testing of the visual field using electro-oculographic potentials. Doc Ophthalmol 43:51–63, 1977.

Aulhorn E: Comparative visual field study in patients with primary open angle glaucoma and anterior ischemic optic neuropathy. Doc Ophthalmol Proc Ser 22:3–13, 1980.

Aulhorn A: Visual field defects in vitamin B12–avitaminosis. Doc Ophthalmol Proc Ser 14:259–265, 1977.

Aulhorn E, Durst W: Comparative investigation of automatic and manual perimetry in different visual field defects. Doc Ophthalmol Proc Ser 14:17–22, 1977.

Aulhorn E, Durst W, Gauger E: A new quick-test for visual field examination in glaucoma. Doc Ophthalmol Proc Ser 22:57–64, 1980.

Aulhorn E, Harms H: Visual perimetry, in Jameson D, Hurvich LM (eds): Handbook of Sensory Physiology, Vol VII/4: Visual Psychophysics. 1972, pp 102–145.

Aulhorn E, Harms H, Karmeyer H: The influence of spontaneous eye-rotation on the perimetric determination of small scotomas. Doc Ophthalmol Proc Ser 19:363–367, 1979.

Aulhorn E, Karmeyer H: Frequency distribution in early glaucomatous visual field defects. Doc Ophthalmol Proc Ser 14:75–83, 1977.

Aulhorn E, Tanzil M: Comparison of visual field defects in glaucoma and in acute anterior ischemic optic neuropathy. Doc Ophthalmol Proc Ser 19:73–79, 1979.

Bagolini B, Campos EC: Binocular campimetry in small angle concomitant esotropia. Doc Ophthalmol Proc Ser 14:399–409, 1977.

Bajandas FJ, McBeath, Smith JL: Clinical features of congenital homonymous hemianopia: A study of eight cases. Doc Ophthalmol Proc Ser 14:349–353, 1977.

Barlow HB, Levick WR, Westheimer G: Computer-plotted receptive fields. Science 154:920, 1966.

Bartl G, Hofmann H, Wocheslaender E, Faschinger C: Electroophthalmological, fluorescence angiographical and computer perimetrical examinations in cases of contusio bulbi. Klin Monatsbl Augenheilk 177:858–863, 1980. (In German with English abstract.)

Bartoli F, Liuzzi L: Laser light in static perimetry (a preliminary report). Doc Ophthalmol Proc Ser 14:445–448, 1977.

Batko KA, Anctil JL, Anderson DR: Detecting glaucomatous damage with the Friedmann analyzer compared with the Goldmann perimeter and evaluation of stereoscopic photographs of the optic disk. Am J Ophthalmol 95:435–447, 1983.

Bebie H, Fankhasuer F: A statistical program for determining fields of vision. Klin Monatsbl Augenheilk 177:417–422, 1980. (In German with English abstract.)

Bebie H, Fankhauser F: Statistical program for the analysis of perimetric data. Doc Ophthalmol Proc Ser 26:9–10, 1981.

Bebie H, Fankhauser F, Jenni A, Haeberlin H: The New Software Package. Schlieren, Switzerland, Interzeag, 1979, pp 155–178.

Bebie H, Fankhauser F, Spahr J: Static perimetry: Accuracy and fluctuations. Acta Ophthalmol 54:339–348, 1976.

Bebie H, Fankhauser F, Spahr J: Static perimetry: Strategies. Acta Ophthalmol 54:325–338, 1976.

Bec P, Greite JH, et al: Importance of automatic computerized perimetry in the examination of ocular function. Bull Mem Soc Fr Ophthalmol 93:314–319, 1981. (In French with English abstract.)

Bec P, Wetterwald N, et al: Perimetrie automatique computerisée (OCTOPUS)—premiers resultats. Bull Soc Ophthalmol Fr 81:941–943, 1981. (In French with English abstract.)

Bechetoille A, Dauzat M, Brun Y: Presentation of an automated system of analysis of the central visual field. Bull Soc Ophthalmol Fr 82:491–493, 1982. (In French with English abstract.)

Bedwell C: The design of instrumentation for the efficient investigation of the visual field. Am J Optom Physiol Opt 44:609–633, 1967.

Bedwell CH, Davies SA: The effect of pupil size on multiple static quantitative visual field threshold. Doc Ophthalmol Proc Ser 14:363–366, 1977.

Bender MB, Battersby WS: Homonymous macular scotomata in cases of occipital lobe tumor. Arch Ophthalmol 60:928–938, 1958.

Bender MB, Furlow LT: Phenomenon of visual extinction in homonymous fields and psychologic principles involved. AMA Arch Neurol Psychiatry 53:29–32, 1945.

Bender MB, Strauss I: Defects in visual field of one eye only in patients with a lesion of one optic radiation. Arch Ophthalmol 17:765–787, 1937.

Bengtsson G, Holmin C, Krakau CET: Disc haemorrhagae and glaucoma. Acta Ophthalmol 59:1–14, 1981.

Bengtsson G, Krakau CET: Automatic perimetry in a population survey. Acta Ophthalmol 57:929–937, 1979.

Berry V, Drance SM, et al: An evaluation of differences between two observers plotting and measuring visual fields. Can J Ophthalmol 1:297–300, 1966.

Bjerrum JP: An addition to the general examination of the field of vision. Eye, Ear, Nose & Throat Month 13:221, 1934, in Lebensohn JE (ed): An Anthology of Ophthalmic Classics. Baltimore, Williams & Wilkins, 1969.

Blackwell HR: Studies of psychophysical methods for measuring visual thresholds. J Opt Soc Am 42:606–616, 1952.

Blair LH: Some fundamental physiologic principles in study of the visual field. Arch Ophthalmol 24:10–20, 1940.

Block MA, Goree JA, Jimenez JP: Craniopharyngioma with optic canal enlargement simulating glioma of the optic chaism. J Neurosurg 39:523–527, 1973.

Blondeau P, Phelps CD: Acuity perimetry: Standardization of test parameters. Invest Ophthalmol Vis Sci Suppl ARVO 20:22, 1981.

Blum FG, Gates LK, Janes BR: How important are peripheral fields? Arch Ophthalmol 61:1–8, 1959.

Bobrow JC, Drews RC: Clinical experience with the Fieldmaster perimeter. Am J Ophthalmol 93:238–241, 1982.

Brais P, Drance SM: The temporal field in chronic simple glaucoma. Arch Ophthalmol 99:518–522, 1972.

Bresky RH, Charles S: Pupil motor perimetry. Am J Ophthalmol 68:108–112, 1969.

Buchanan W, Gloster W: An automatic device for rapid assessment of the central visual field. Br J Ophthalmol 49:57–70, 1965.

Bynke H: Krakau's computerized perimeter in neuroophthalmology. Neuro-Ophthalmol 1:45–52, 1980.

Bynke H: Statistical analysis of normal visual fields and hemianopsias recorded by a computerized perimeter. Doc Ophthalmol Proc Ser 35:287–288, 1983.

Bynke H, Heijl A: Automatic computerized perimetry in the detection of neurological visual field defects. Pilot study. Albrecht von Graefes Arch klin exp Ophthalmol 206:11–15, 1978.

Bynke H, Heijl A: A portable hemianopsia tester. Doc Ophthalmol Proc Ser 14:353–354, 1977.

Bynke H, Heijl A, Holmin C: Automatic computerized perimetry in neuro-ophthalmology. Doc Ophthalmol Proc Ser 19:319–325, 1979.

Bynke H, Holmin C, Krakau CET: Computerized perimetry in follow-up studies. Acta Ophthalmol 59:798–799, 1981.

Bynke H, Krakau CET: A modified computerized perimeter and its use in neuro-ophthalmological patients. Neuro-Ophthalmol 2:105–116, 1981.

Bynke H, Vestergren-Brenner L: Visual field defects in congenital hydrocephalus. Doc Ophthalmol Proc Ser 19:87–94, 1979.

Calabria G, Gandolfo E, Ciurlo G, Rossi P: Flicker fusion in pericoecal area. Doc Ophthalmol Proc Ser 26:107–110, 1981.

Campos EC, Jacobson SG: Receptive field-like properties tested with critical flicker fusion frequency. Premetric analysis. Doc Ophthalmol Proc Ser 26:103–106, 1981.

Caprioli J, Spaeth GL: Comparisons of visual field defects in the low-tension glaucomas with those in the high-tension glaucomas. Am J Ophthalmol 97:730–737, 1984.

Caprioli J, Spaeth GL: Static threshold examination of the peripheral nasal visual field in glaucoma. Arch Ophthalmol 103:1150–1154, 1985.

Carella G, Vallavanti C, et al: Computerized perimetry in the detection of glaucoma. Bull Mem Soc Fr Ophthalmol 93:309–313, 1981.

Carenini BB, Luizzi L, Cembrano S, Musso D: Friedmann visual field analyzer: Efficacy of the screening of glaucomatous visual field defects. Glaucoma 5:488–498, 1980.

Carlow TJ, Flynn JT, Shipley T: Color perimetry parameters. Doc Ophthalmol Proc Ser 14:427–429, 1977.

Cassidy V, Havener WH: Evaluation of a screening procedure in the detection of eye disease. Arch Ophthalmol 61:589–598, 1959.

Chamlin M: Minimal defects in visual field studies. Arch Ophthalmol 42:126–139, 1949.

Chamlin M, Davidoff LM: Choice of test objects in visual field studies. Am J Ophthalmol 35:381–393, 1952.

Chamlin M, Davidoff LM: The 1/2000 field in chiasmal interference. Arch Ophthalmol 44:53–70, 1950.

Chamlin M, Davidoff LM, Feiring EH: Ophthalmologic changes produced by pituitary tumors. Am J Ophthalmol 40:353–368, 1955.

Chaplin GBB, Edwards JH, et al: Automated system for testing visual fields. Proc IEEE 120:1321–1327, 1977.

Charlier JR: A new instrument for automatic subjective and objective perimetry. Med Progr Technol 7:125–129, 1980.

Charlier JR, Moussu L, Hache JC: Optimization of computer-assisted perimetry. Doc Ophthalmol Proc Ser 35:359–364, 1983.

Cornsweet TN: Luminance discrimination of brief flashes under various conditions of adaptation. J Physiol 176:294–310, 1965.

Coughlan M, Friedmann AI: The frequency distribution of early visual field defects in glaucoma. Doc Ophthalmol Proc Ser 26:345–349, 1981.

Crick JCP, Crick RP: The sine-bell stimulus in perimetry. Doc Ophthalmol Proc Ser 26:239–246, 1981.

Crick JCP, Ripley LJ, Crick RP: The principles involved in the design of a visual field computer and automatic transcriber. Ann Ther Clin Ophthalmol 25:355–363, 1974.

Crick RP, Crick JCP: The sine-bell screener. Doc Ophthalmol Proc Ser 26:233–237, 1981.

Crick RP, Crick JCP, Ripley L: The representation of the visual field. Doc Ophthalmol Proc Ser 35:193–203, 1983.

Crick RP, Crick JCP, Ripley L: Some aspects of perimetry in glaucoma. Glaucoma 7:27–34, 1985.

Crick RP, Daubs JG: Epidemiological aids to clinical decision making in primary open angle glaucoma. Int Ophthalmol Clin 3:37–41, 1980.

Crick RP, et al: The relationship between intraocular pressure and visual field progress in chronic simple glaucoma and ocular hypertension. Glaucoma 7:208–221, 1985.

Czechowicz-Janicka K, Majewska K, et al: Visual field changes in glaucoma examined by means of electronic computer techniques. Klin Oczna 45:897–901, 1975.

Dannheim F: Clinical experiences with a new automated perimeter "Peritest." Doc Ophthalmol Proc Ser 35:309–312, 1983.

Dannheim F: Clinical experiences with a new automated perimeter "Peritest." Presented at the V. International Visual Field Symposium, Sacramento, California, October 20–23, 1982.

Dannheim F: Clinical experiences with a semi-automated perimeter (Fieldmaster). Int Ophthalmol 2:11–18, 1980.

Dannheim F: Color perimetry in chiasmal lesions. Doc Ophthalmol Proc Ser 14:449–455, 1977.

Dannheim F: Kinetic perimetry with supra-threshold stimuli. Doc Ophthalmol Proc Ser 14:385–388, 1977.

Dannheim F: Liminal and supraliminal stimuli in the perimetry of chronic simple glaucoma. Doc Ophthalmol Proc Ser 19:151–157, 1979.

Dannheim F: Non-linear projection in visual field charting. Doc Ophthalmol Proc Ser 35:217–220, 1983.

Dannheim F: Non-linear projection in visual field charting. Presented at the V. International Visual Field Symposium, Sacramento, California, October 20–23, 1982.

Dannheim F: Patterns of visual field alterations for liminal and supraliminal stimuli in chronic simple glaucoma. Doc Ophthalmol Proc Ser 26:97–102, 1981.

Dannheim F: Perimetry in glaucoma I: Methods. Doc Ophthalmol Proc Ser 22:29–38, 1980.

Dannheim F: Perimetry in glaucoma II: Peristat, Fieldmaster, Octopus. Doc Ophthalmol Proc Ser 22:39–56, 1980

Dannheim F: Zur Anwender-Software fuer die neuen Rodenstock-Perimeter. Der Augenspiegel 28:15–27, 1981. (In German.)

Dannheim F, Luedecke D, Kuehne D: Visual fields before and after transnasal removal of a pituitary tumor. Doc Ophthalmol Proc Ser 19:43–51, 1979.

Dannheim F, Mueller-Jensen A, Zschocke S: Perimetry and pattern—VECP in chiasmal lesions. Doc Ophthalmol Proc Ser 26:71–77, 1981.

De Boer RW, Van Den Berg TJTP: The Competer automatic campimeter. I. Technical description and evaluation. Doc Ophthalmol 53:295–302, 1982.

De Boer RW, Van Den Berg TJTP, Beintema MR, Greve EL, Hoeppner J, Verduin WM: The Friedmann Visual Field Analyser Mark II—technical evaluation and clinical results. Doc Ophthalmol 53:331–342, 1982.

De Boer RW, Van Den Berg TJTP, Greve EL, Bos HJ: The Fieldmaster 101PR automatic visual field screener—technical evaluation and clinical results. Doc Ophthalmol 53:311–320, 1982.

De Boer RW, Van Den Berg TJTP, et al: The Ocuplot semi-automatic visual field screener—Technical evaluation and clinical results. Doc Ophthalmol 53:321–330, 1982.

De Boer RW, Van Den Berg TJTP, et al: Concepts for automatic perimetry as applied to the Scoperimeter, an experimental automatic perimeter. Int Ophthalmol 5:192–200, 1982.

Demailly PH, Papoz L: Long-term study of visual capability in relation to intra-ocular pressure in chronic open angle glaucoma. Doc Ophthalmol Proc Ser 14:141–145, 1977.

Dennehy J: Concepts for Examination—and Research—Programs. Schlieren, Switzerland, Interzeag, 1979, pp 149–153.

Doden W, Schnaudigel O-E: Visual field defects in glaucoma, a long follow-up study, in ACTA: XXIV International Congress of Ophthalmology, Volume I. Philadelphia, Lippincott, 1983, pp 176–179.

Doroszewski J, Majewska K, Czechowicz-Janicka K: Selected applications of the digital image transformer in ophthalmology (editorial). Mater Med Pol 10:150–151, 1978.

Douglas GR: Automatic perimetry (editorial). Can J Ophthalmol 15:107–108, 1980.

Dowling JE: Foveal receptors of monkey retina: Fine structure. Science 147:57–59, 1965.

Drance SM: Automatic perimetry: The current state of the art, in ACTA: XXIV International Congress of Ophthalmology, Volume I. Philadelphia, Lippincott, 1983, pp 160–161.

Drance SM: Discussion of presentations by Drs. Johnson, et al, McCrary, et al, and Li, et al. Ophthalmol 86:1313–1316, 1979.

Drance SM: The glaucomatous visual field. Invest Ophthalmol 11:85–97, 1972.

Drance SM: Richard Cross Lecture. Early disturbances of colour vision in chronic open angle glaucoma. Doc Ophthalmol Proc Ser 26:155–159, 1981.

Drance SM: Visual field defects, in Duane TD (ed): Clinical Ophthalmology. Philadelphia, Harper & Row, 1981, pp 1–21.

Drance SM, Anderson D (eds): Automated Perimetry in Glaucoma: A Practical Guide. Orlando, Fl, Gruen and Stratton, 1985.

Drance SM, Bryett J, Schulzer M: The effects of surgical pressure reduction on the glaucomatous field. Doc Ophthalmol Proc Ser 19:153–157, 1977.

Drance SM, Fairclough M, et al: The early visual field defects in glaucoma and the significance of nasal steps. Doc Ophthalmol Proc Ser 19:119–126, 1979.

Drance SM, Keltner JL, Johnson CA: Module 11: Automated Perimetry. Focal points: Clinical Modules for Ophthalmologists. San Francisco, Am Academy Ophthalmology, 1984.

Drasdo N, Peaston WC: Sampling systems for visual field assessment and computerised perimetry. Br J Ophthalmol 64:705–712, 1980.

Drews RC: Concepts in practical office perimetry: Manual and computer-assisted techniques. Glaucoma 7:110–115, 1985.

Dubois-Poulsen A: Retinal photocoagulation as a physiological experiment. Doc Ophthalmol Proc Ser 14:275–279, 1977.

Dubois-Poulsen A: The enlargement of the blind spot in binocular vision. Doc Ophthalmol Proc Ser 19:423–426, 1979.

Duke-Elder S (ed): The Visual Field. System of Ophthalmology. Vol. VII: The Foundations of Ophthalmology. Heredity, Pathology, Diagnosis and Therapeutics. London, Henry Kimpton, 1962, pp 393–425.

Dugan C, et al: Automated differential threshold perimetry for detecting glaucomatous visual field loss. Am J Ophthal 100:420–423, 1985.

Dunn PM, Lakowski R: Fully-photopic and -scotopic spatial summation in chromatic perimetry. Doc Ophthalmol Proc Ser 26:199–206, 1981.

Dunn PM, Massof RW: Temporal resolution in the peripheral visual field. Doc Ophthalmol Proc Ser 35:433–438, 1983.

Dyster-Aas K, Heijl A, Lundgvist L: Computerized visual field screening in the management of patients with ocular hypertension. Acta Ophthalmol 58:918–928, 1980.

Ellenberger C: Modern perimetry in neuro-ophthalmic diagnosis. Arch Neurology 30:193–201, 1974.

Ellenberger C, Ziegler SB: Visual-evoked potentials and quantitative perimetry in multiple sclerosis. Ann Neurology 1:561–564, 1977.

Ellenberger C Jr: Perimetry: Principles, Technique, and Interpretation. New York, Raven Press, 1980.

Ellenberger C Jr, Ziegler SB: Quantitative perimetry and visual evoked potentials in multiple sclerosis. Doc Ophthalmol Proc Ser 14:203–207, 1977.

Endo N: The relation between depression in the Bjerrum area and nasal step in early glaucoma (DBA & NS). Doc Ophthalmol Proc Ser 19:167–176, 1979.

Enoch JM: Automation of perimetry and modern methods of subjective eye examination, in ACTA: XXIV International Congress of Ophthalmology, vol. I. Philadelphia, Lippincott, 1983, pp 136–146.

Enoch JM, Campos EC: Analysis of patients with open-angle glaucoma using perimetric techniques reflecting receptive field-like properties. Doc Ophthalmol Proc Ser 19:137–149, 1979.

Enoch JM, Fitzgerald CR, Campos EC: The relationship between fundus lesions and areas of functional change. Doc Ophthalmol Proc Ser 19:381–401, 1979.

Enoch JM, Johnson CA, Fitzgerald CR: Human psychophysical analysis of receptive field-like properties. VII: Initial clinical trials of the psychophysical transient-like function. Doc Ophthalmol Proc Ser 14:373–379, 1977.

Enoch JM, Johnson CA, Fitzgerald CR: The effect of pupil size on multiple static quantitative visual field-like properties. VII: Initial clinical trials of the psychophysical transient-like function. Doc Ophthalmol Proc Ser 14:373–338, 1977.

Enoch JM, Moses RA, Nygaard RW, Allen D: Perimetric techniques used to assess retinal strain during accommodation. Doc Ophthalmol Proc Ser 35:413–420, 1983.

Enoksson P: A study of the visual fields with white and coloured objects in cases of pituitary tumors with especial reference to early diagnosis. Acta Ophthalmol 31:505–515, 1953.

Ernest JT: Recovery of visual function during elevation of the intraocular pressure. Doc Ophthalmol Proc Ser 19:205–210, 1979.

Ernst W, Faulkner DJ, et al: An automated static perimeter/adaptometer using light emitting diodes. Br J Ophthalmol 67:431–442, 1983.

Esterman B: Functional scoring of the binocular visual field. Doc Ophthalmol Proc Ser 35:187–192, 1983.

Esterman B: Functional scoring of the binocular field. Ophthalmol 89:1226–1234, 1982.

Esterman B: Grids for functional scoring of visual fields. Doc Ophthalmol Proc Ser 26:373–380, 1981.

Evans JN: An Introduction to Clinical Scotometry. New Haven, Yale University Press, 1938.

Evans JN: Transient fluctuations in the scotoma of glaucoma. Am J Ophthalmol 18:333–347, 1935.

Falconer MA, Wilson JL: Visual field changes following anterior temporal lobectomy. Their significance in relation to "Meyer's loop" of the optic radiation. Brain 81:1–14, 1958.

Fankhauser F: Adaptive High Resolution Programs. Schlieren, Switzerland, Interzeag, 1979, p 154.

Fankhauser F: Automated perimetry, in Heilman K, Richardson KT (eds): Glaucoma, Conceptions of a Disease. Philadelphia, W.B. Saunders, 1978, pp 204–211.

Fankhauser F: Detection of Scotomata by Computer Logic and Human Search Strategies. Schlieren, Switzerland, Interzeag, 1979, pp 130–148.

Fankhauser F: Developmental milestones of automatic perimetry, in ACTA: XXIV International Congress of Ophthalmology, vol. I. Philadelphia, Lippincott, 1983, pp 147–150.

Fankhauser F: (Letter to the Editor) re: editorial, "Automated perimetry minimizes bias in visual field testing" [Halberg GP. Ophthalmol Times 1982; p 59]. Ophthalmol Times 15:3–4, 1982.

Fankhauser F: Problems related to the design of automatic perimeters. Doc Ophthalmol 46:89–138, 1979.

Fankhauser F: The automatic perimeter Octopus in clinical and research. Buch Augen-arzt 90:1–12, 1982. (In German with English abstract.)

Fankhauser F, Bebie H: Threshold fluctuations, interpolations and spatial resolution in perimetry. Doc Ophthalmol Proc Ser 19:295–309, 1979.

Fankhauser F, Enoch JM: The effects of blur upon perimetric thresholds. Arch Ophthalmol 68:240–251, 1962.

Fankhauser F, Haeberlin H: Dynamic range and stray light. An estimate of the falsifying effects of stray light in perimetry. Doc Ophthalmol 50:143–167, 1980.

Fankhauser F, Haeberlin H, Jenni A: Octopus programs SAPRO and F. Two new principles for the analysis of the visual field. Albrecht von Graefes Arch klin exp Ophthalmol 216:155–165, 1981.

Fankhauser F, Jenni A: Programs SARGON and DELTA: Two new principles for the automated analysis of the visual field. Albrecht von Graefes Arch klin exp Ophthalmol 216:41–48, 1981.

Fankhauser F, Koch P, Roulier A: On automation of perimetry. Albrecht von Graefes Arch klin exp Ophthalmol 184:126–150, 1972.

Fankhauser F, Roehler F: The physical stimulus, the quality of the retinal image and foveal brightness discrimination in one amblyopic and two normal eyes. Doc Ophthal-mol 23:149–188, 1967.

Fankhauser F, Spahr J, Bebie H: Some aspects of the automation of perimetry. Surv Ophthalmol 22:131–141, 1977.

Fankhauser F, Spahr J, Bebie H: Three years of experience with the Octopus automatic perimeter. Doc Ophthalmol Proc Ser 14:7–15, 1977.

Faschinger C, Brunner H: Visual field examinations using the Octopus computerized perimeter following laser therapy of central serous chorioretinitis (Wessing Type I). Klin Monatsbl Augenheilk 181:376–378, 1982. (In German with English abstract.)

Faschinger C, Hofmann H, Bartl G, Gruber H: Initial experience with the computerized Octopus perimeter. Klin Monatsbl Augenheilk 177:753–758, 1980. (In German with English abstract.)

Faschinger C, Wutz W, Schumann G, Brunner H: Qualitative rapid screening of glaucoma outpatients with the Octopus computer perimeter. Klin Monatsbl Augenheilk 179:521–523, 1981. (In German with English abstract.)

Feldman M, Todman L, Bender MB: "Flight of colours" in lesions of the visual system. J Neurol Neurosurg Psychiatry 37:1265–1272, 1974.

Ferree CE, Rand G: Interpretation of refractive conditions in the peripheral field of vision. Arch Ophthalmol 9:925–938, 1933.

Ferree CE, Rand G: Methods for increasing the diagnostic sensitivity of perimetry and scotometry with the form field stimulus. Am J Ophthalmol 13:118–120, 1930.

Finkelstein D, Gouras P, Hoff M: Human electroretinogram near the absolute threshold of vision. Invest Ophthalmol 7:214–218, 1968.

Fischer FW: Manual projection perimetry combined with a pattern. Klin Monatsbl Augenheilk 178:392–396, 1981.

Fitzgerald CR, Enoch JM, Temme LA: Kinetic perimetry (in the plateau region of the field) as a sensitive indication of visual fatigue or saturation-like defects in retrobulbar anomalies. Doc Ophthalmol Proc Ser 26:293–303, 1981.

Flammer J, Drance SM: Correlation between color vision scores and quantitative perimetry in suspected glaucoma. Arch Ophthalmol 102:38–39, 1984.

Flammer J, Drance SM, et al: Differential light threshold in automated static perimetry. Arch Ophthalmol 102:876–879, 1984.

Flammer J, Drance SM, Schulzer M: The estimation and testing of the components of long-term fluctuations of the differential light threshold. Doc Ophthalmol Proc Ser 35:383–389, 1983.

Flammer J, Eppler E, Niesel P: Quantitative perimetry in the glaucoma patient without local visual field defects. Albrecht von Graefes Arch klin exp Ophthalmol 219:92–94, 1982.

Flammer J, Nagel G, et al: Detection and definition of scotomata of the central visual field by computer methods. Doc Ophthalmol Proc Ser 26:33–41, 1981.

Flocks M, Rosenthal AR, Hopkins JL: Mass visual screening via television. Ophthalmol 85:1141–1149, 1978.

Foerster MH: The recording of the scotopic and photopic DC-ERG by means of local stimulation with white light and coloured background. Doc Ophthalmol Proc Ser 14:189–195, 1977.

Fonda S, Campos EC: Patterned evoked potentials in objective perimetry. Doc Ophthalmol Proc Ser 14:197–201, 1977.

Foulds WS: Optic nerve function in the toxic amblypoias and related conditions. Doc Ophthalmol Proc Ser 26:269–277, 1981.

French LA: Studies on the optic radiations. The significance of small field defects in the region of the vertical meridian. J Neurosurg 19:522–528, 1962.

Friedman AI: A modern strategy for visual field examination. Jpn J Clin Ophthalmol 34:395–397, 1980.

Friedman AI: Experiences with a prototype 100-hole front plate for the visual field analyser in glaucoma. Doc Ophthalmol Proc Ser 14:87–92, 1977.

Friedman AI: Experiences with a prototype 100-hole front plate for the visual field analyser in neuro-ophthalmology. Doc Ophthalmol Proc Ser 14:343–347, 1977.

Friedman AI: Outline of visual field analyzer Mark II. Doc Ophthalmol Proc Ser 22:65–67, 1980.

Friedman AI: Serial analysis of changes in visual field defects employing a new instrument to determine the activity of diseases involving the visual pathways. Ophthalmologica 152:1–12, 1966.

Friedman AI: The relationship between visual field changes and intra-ocular pressure. Doc Ophthalmol Proc Ser 19:263–264, 1979.

Frisen L: A versatile color confrontation test for the central visual field. Arch Ophthalmol 89:3–9, 1973.

Frisen L: Funduscopic correlates of visual field defects due to lesions of the anterior visual pathway. Doc Ophthalmol Proc Ser 19:5–16, 1979.

Frisen L: Visual field defects due to hypoplasia of the optic nerve. Doc Ophthalmol Proc Ser 19:81–87, 1979.

Frisen L, Frisen M: Objective recognition of abnormal isopters. Acta Ophthalmol 53:378–392, 1975.

Frisen L, Holm M: Visual field defects associated with chorioretinal folds. Doc Ophthalmol Proc Ser 14:327–330, 1977.

Frisen L, Schoeldstroem G: Relationship between perimetric eccentricity and retinal locus in a human eye. Doc Ophthalmol Proc Ser 19:409–410, 1979.

Frisen M: Evaluation of perimetric procedures: A statistical approach. Doc Ophthalmol Proc Ser 19:427–431, 1979.

Fulmek R: Perimetric detection of chiasmal injury after contusion of the skull and brain. Doc Ophthalmol Proc Ser 14:337–343, 1977.

Fulmek R, Friedrich F: Visual field defect characteristics in cases of hyperprolactinaemia. Doc Ophthalmol Proc Ser 26:329–335, 1981.

Funkhouser A, Wetterwald N, Fankhauser F: The accuracy of screening programs. A preliminary report on an on-going longitudinal investigation to ascertain the quantitativeness of qualitative 2-niveau-test procedures. Doc Ophthalmol Proc Ser 35:345–350, 1983.

Furuno F: Some aetiological aspects of the homonymous hemianoptic scotoma. Doc Ophthalmol Proc Ser 14:303–313, 1983.

Furuno F, Matsuo H: Early stage progression in glaucomatous visual field changes. Doc Ophthalmol Proc Ser 19:247–253, 1979.

Futenma M: A screening of the visual field on 13,357 school children. Acta Soc Ophthalmol Jpn 77:19–30, 1973.

Gandolfo E, Calabria G, Zingirian M: The perioecal area in optic sub-atrophy. Doc Ophthalmol Proc Ser 26:287–292, 1981.

Gandolfo E, Zingirian M, Capris P: The role of perimetry in retinal detachment. Doc Ophthalmol Proc Ser 35:465–471, 1983.

Gans JA: Considerations in the design of an automatic visual field tester. Med Res Eng 10:7–11, 1971.

Gauger E: Computer simulation of examination procedures for the automatic 'Tuebinger perimeter.' Doc Ophthalmol Proc Ser 14:31–36, 1977.

Genio C, Friedmann AI: A comparison between white light and blue light on about 70 eyes of patients with early glaucoma using the Mark II Visual Field Analyser. Doc Ophthalmol Proc Ser 26:207–214, 1981.

Gerber DS, Brothers DM, et al: Automated visual field plotters vs. tangent screen kinetic perimetry (letter to the editor). Arch Ophthalmol 98:930–931, 1980.

Gloor B, Faessler A, Luedin B: Glaucomatous visual fields: Observation of development with the Octopus automatic perimeter. Klin Monatsbl Augenheilk 177:748–752, 1980. (In German with English abstract.)

Gloor B, Schmied U: Findings in glaucomatous visual fields under observation using the "Octopus" automatic perimeter. Klin Monatsbl Augenheilk 176:545–546, 1980.

Gloor BP, Schmied U, Faessler A: Changes of glaucomatous field defects. Analysis of OCTOPUS fields with Programme Delta. Doc Ophthalmol Proc Ser 26:11–15, 1981.

Gloor B, Schmied U, Faessler A: Changes of glaucomatous field defects. Degree of accuracy of measurements with the automatic perimeter Octopus. Int Ophthalmol 3:5–10, 1980.

Gloor B, Schmied U, Faessler A: Glaucomatous visual fields—Analysis of Octopus observations with statistical material. Klin Monatsbl Augenheilk 177:423–436, 1980. (In German with English abstract.)

Gloster J: Automatic visual field tests. Proc R Soc Med 60:65–68, 1967.

Gloster J: Flash perimetry. Br J Ophthalmol 54:649–658, 1970.

Goldmann H: Interaction Between Science and Technology. Schlieren, Switzerland, Interzeag, 1979, pp 60–65.

Goolkasian P: Retinal location and its effect on the processing of target and distractor information. J Exp Psychol (Human Percept) 7:1247–1257, 1981.

Graham CH: Area and the intensity-time relation in the peripheral retina. Am J Physiol 113:299–305, 1935.

Gramer E, Gerlach R, Krieglstein GK: Zur Sensitivitaet des Computerperimeters Competer bei fruehen glaukomatoesen Gesichtsfeldausfaellen. Eine kontrollierte Studie. Klin Monatsbl Augenheilk 180:203–209, 1982. (In German.)

Gramer E, Gerlach R, Krieglstein GK, Leydhecker W: Topography of early glaucomatous visual field defects in computerized perimetry. Klin Monatsbl Augenheilk 180:515–523, 1982.

Gramer E, Jeschke R, Krieglstein GK: Computerized perimetry in infants treated with ethambutol. Klin Padiatr 194:52–55, 1982. (In German with English abstract.)

Gramer E, Kontic D, Krieglstein GK: Die computerperimetrische Darstellung glaukomatoeser Gesichts felddefekte in Abhaegigkeit von der Stimulusgroesse. Ophthalmologica 183:162–167, 1981. (In German with English abstract.)

Gramer E, Krieglstein GK: Follow-up of retrobulbar neuritis with the Octopus computer perimeter. Klin Monatsbl Augenheilk 179:418–423, 1981. (In German with English abstract.)

Gramer E, Krieglstein GK: Specificity of suprathreshold computer perimetry. Klin Monatsbl Augenheilk 181:373–375, 1982. (In German with English abstract.)

Gramer E, Proell M, Krieglstein GK: Reproducibility of central visual field testing using kinetic or computerized static perimetry. Klin Monatsbl Augenheilk 176:374–384, 1980. (In German with English abstract.)

Gramer E, Proell M, Krieglstein GK: The perimetry of the blind spot. A comparison of kinetic and static, computerized strategies. Ophthalmologica 179:201–208, 1979. (In German with English abstract.)

Gramer E, Steinhauser, Krieglstein GK: The specificity of the automated suprathreshold perimeter Fieldmaster 200. Graefes Arch klin exp Ophthalmol 218:253–255, 1982.

Graniewski-Wijands H, Greve EL, Bakker D, Moed JL: The Competer automatic campimeter. II: Clinical experience. Doc Ophthalmol 53:303–310, 1982.

Greenblat SH: Posttraumatic transient cerebral blindness association with migraine and seizure diatheses. JAMA 225:1073–1076, 1973.

Grehn F, Knorr-Held S, Kommerell G: Glaucomatouslike visual field defects in chronic papilledema. Albrecht von Graefes Arch klin exp Ophthalmol 217:99–109, 1981.

Grehn F, Stange D: The influence of short-term IOP elevation and hypoxia on the impulse conduction in the nerve fibre layer of the cat retina. Doc Ophthalmol Proc Ser 14:147–150, 1977.

Greite JH: Octopus Perimetry in Diabetic Retinopathy. Schlieren, Switzerland, Interzeag, 1979, pp 107–116.

Greite JH, Zumbansen HP, Adamczyk R: Automated perimetry in diabetic retinopathy. Buch Augenarzt 90:34–38, 1982. (In German with English abstract.)

Greite JH, Zumbansen HP, Adamczyk R: Visual field in diabetic retinopathy (DR). Doc Ophthalmol Proc Ser 26:25–32, 1981.

Greve EL: Automated perimetry and its clinical value, in Heilman K, Richardson KT (eds): Glaucoma, Conceptions of a Disease. Philadelphia, Saunders, 1978, pp 196–204.

Greve EL: Automatic and Non-Automatic Perimetry. Schlieren, Switzerland, Interzeag, 1979, pp 81–88.

Greve EL: Automatic and non-automatic perimetry. Int Ophthalmol 2:19–22, 1980.

Greve EL: Automation of perimetry. Doc Ophthalmol 40:234–254, 1976.

Greve EL: Clinical evaluation of the Scoperimeter, an experimental automatic perimeter. Int Ophthalmol 5:193–200, 1982.

Greve EL: Comparative examinations of visual function and fluorescein angiography in early stages of senile disciform macular degeneration. Doc Ophthalmol Proc Ser 19:371–380, 1979.

Greve EL: Differential perimetric profiles in disciform macular degeneration: Stages of development. Doc Ophthalmol Proc Ser 9:327–339, 1976.

Greve EL: Myopia and glaucoma. Albrecht von Graefes Arch klin exp Ophthalmol 213:33–41, 1980.

Greve EL: Performance of computer assisted perimeters. Doc Ophthalmol 53:343–380, 1982.

Greve EL: Peritest. Doc Ophthalmol Proc Ser 22:71–74, 1980.

Greve EL: Single and multiple stimulus static perimetry in glaucoma: The two phases of perimetry. Doc Ophthalmol 36:1–355, 1973.

Greve EL: Single stimulus and multiple stimulus thresholds. Vision Res 12:1533–1543, 1972.

Greve EL: Some aspects of visual field examination related to strategies for detection and assessment phase. Doc Ophthalmol Proc Ser 22:15–29, 1980.

Greve EL: The Peritest. Doc Ophthalmol Proc Ser 26:17–18, 1981.

Greve EL: The Peritest, a new automatic and semi-automatic perimeter. Int Ophthalmol 5:201–214, 1982.

Greve EL: Visual field analyzer and threshold. Br J Ophthalmol 55:704–708, 1971.

Greve EL: Visual fields, glaucoma and cataract. Doc Ophthalmol Proc Ser 22:79–89, 1980.

Greve EL, Bakker D: Some possibilities of the Peritest automatic and semi-automatic perimeter. Doc Ophthalmol Proc Ser 35:313–321, 1983.

Greve EL, Bos PKM, Bakker D: Photopic and mesopic central static perimetry in maculopathies and central neuropathies. Doc Ophthalmol Proc Ser 14:243–257, 1977.

Greve EL, Dannheim F, Bakker D: The Peritest, a new automatic and semi-automatic perimeter. Int Ophthalmol 5:201–214, 1982.

Greve EL, De Boer RW, Pijnappel-Groothuyse HTHJN: Perimetron. Doc Ophthalmol Proc Ser 22:69–70, 1980.

Greve EL, Furuno F, Verduin WM: A critical phase in the development of glaucomatous visual field defects. Doc Ophthalmol Proc Ser 19:127–135, 1979.

Greve EL, Furuno F, Verduin WM: The clinical significance of reversibility of glaucomatous visual field defects. Doc Ophthalmol Proc Ser 19:197–203, 1979.

Greve EL, Geijssen HC: The relation between excavation and visual field in glaucoma patients with high and with low intraocular pressures. Doc Ophthalmol Proc Ser 35:34–42, 1983.

Greve EL, Groothuyse MTHJN, Bakker P: Simulated automatic perimetry. Doc Ophthalmol Proc Ser 14:23–29, 1977.

Greve EL, Raakman MAC: On atypical chiasmal visual field defects. Doc Ophthalmol Proc Ser 14:315–325, 1977.

Greve EL, Van Veenendaal WG, Van Den Berg TJTP: Hardware considerations in automatic perimetry, in ACTA: XXIV International Congress of Ophthalmology, vol. I. Philadelphia, Lippincott, 1983, pp 156–159.

Greve EL, Verduin WM: Detection of early glaucomatous damage. Part I: Visual field examination. Doc Ophthalmol Proc Ser 103–114, 1977.

Greve EL, Verduin WM: Detection of early glaucomatous damage. Part II: Cupping and visual field. Doc Ophthalmol Proc Ser 14:115–120, 1977.

Greve EL, Verduin WM: Mass visual field investigation in 1,834 persons with supposedly normal eyes. Albrecht von Graefes Arch klin exp Ophthalmol 183:286–293, 1972.

Grignolo A, Tagliasco V, Zingirian M: Preliminary results about a new remotely controlled projection campimeter. Ophthalmologica 171:432–438, 1975.

Grignolo A, Zingirian M, et al: The visual field examination and its automation. Doc Ophthalmol 43:45–50, 1977.

Grignolo A, Zingirian M, et al: Proceedings: Simulation of the visual field examination on a computer. Exp Eye Res 20:183, 1975.

Gruber H: Multifocal ischemic lesions of the visual pathways. Klin Monatsbl Augenheilk 179:36–37, 1981. (In German with English abstract.)

Gruber P: Experiences with Automated Perimetry in Neurological Disease. Schlieren, Switzerland, Interzeag, 1979, pp 117–129.

Guilino G: Zur Anwender-Software fuer die neuen Rodenstock-Perimeter. A) Konzept des (Glaukom-) Untersuchungsprogramms. Der Augenspiegel 28:3–13, 1981. (In German.)

Gunderson CH, Hoyt WF: Geniculate hemianopia: Incongruous homonymous field defects in two patients with partial lesions of the lateral geniculate nucleus. J Neurol Neurosurg Psychiatry 34:1–6, 1971.

Haeberlin H, Fankhauser F: Adaptive programs for analysis of the visual field by automatic perimetry—Basic problems and solutions. Efforts oriented towards the realization of the generalized spatially adaptive Octopus program. Doc Ophthalmol 50:123–141, 1980.

Haeberlin H, Fankhauser F: Analysis of paracentral scotomata with spatially adaptive computer methods. Klin Monatsbl Augenheilk 176:533–535, 1980. (In German with English abstract.)

Haeberlin H, Funkhouser A, Fankhauser F: Angioscotoma: Preliminary results using the new spatially adaptive program SAPRO. Doc Ophthalmol Proc Ser 35:337–344, 1983.

Haeberlin H, Jenni A, Fankhauser F: Researches on adaptive high resolution programming for automatic perimeter. Principles and preliminary results. Int Ophthalmol 2:1–9, 1980.

Haefliger E: First Results of a Comparative Study with Octopus and Tuebingen Perimetry. Schlieren, Switzerland, Interzeag, 1979, pp 89–106.

Halberg GP: Automated Perimetry: The Safe Limits. Translated from French, as delivered at the Congress of the French Society of Ophthalmology, Paris, May 11, 1980.

Halberg GP: Automatic perimetry: The limits of dependability. Bull Men Soc Fr Ophthalmol 92:139–142, 1980. (In French).

Hallet BE: Spatial summation. Vision Res 3:9–24, 1963.

Hamazaki S, Matsuo H: Quantitative perimetry and local ERG in the diseases of macular area and Bjerrum area. Doc Ophthalmol Proc Ser 14:173–187, 1977.

Hamazaki S, Yokota T, et al: Semi-automatic campimeter with graphic display. Doc Ophthalmol Proc Ser 19:311–317, 1979.

Hansen E: Hereditary dominant optic atrophy. Doc Ophthalmol Proc Ser 26:315–322, 1981.

Hansen E: Investigation of retinitis pigmentosa by use of specific quantitative perimetry. Doc Ophthalmol Proc Ser 14:461–472, 1977.

Hansen E, Seim T: Loss of inhibitory mechanisms as a measure of cone impairment: A method applied in static colour perimetry. Doc Ophthalmol Proc Ser 35:405–411, 1983.

Hara T: Visual field changes in mesopic and scotopic conditions using Friedmann visual field analyser. Doc Ophthalmol Proc Ser 19:403–416, 1979.

Harms H: Advantages and limitations of automatic perimetry. Ber Zusammenkunft Dtsch Ophthalmol Ges 75:555–556, 1978. (In German.)

Harms H: Visual field defects in diseases of the fasciculus opticus. Doc Ophthalmol Proc Ser 14:289–298, 1977.

Harms H: Visual field defects in diseases of the fasciculus opticus. Doc Ophthalmol Proc Ser 14:289–297, 1977.

Harrington DO: The Bjerrum scotoma. Am J Ophthalmol 59:646–656, 1965.

Harrington DO: The Visual Fields. A Textbook and Atlas of Clinical Perimetry, ed 3. Saint Louis, Mosby, 1971.

Harrington DO: Visual field character in temporal and occipital lobe lesions. Arch Ophthalmol 66:779–792, 1961.

Harrington DO, Flocks M: The multiple-pattern method of visual field examination. Arch Ophthalmol 61:755–765, 1959.

Harrington DO, Flocks M: Visual field examination by a new tachystoscopic multiple-pattern method. Am J Ophthalmol 37:719–723, 1954.

Hart MH Jr: Computer processing of visual data. II: Automated pattern analysis of glaucomatous visual fields. Arch Ophthalmol 99:133–136, 1981.

Hart MH Jr: Three-dimensional topography of the central visual field. Sparing of foveal sensitivity in macular disease, in ACTA: XXIV International Congress of Ophthalmology, vol. I. Philadelphia, Lippincott, 1983, pp 184–189.

Hart MH Jr, Becker B: Visual field changes in ocular hypertension. A computer-based analysis. Arch Ophthalmol 95:1176–1179, 1977.

Hart MH Jr, Burde RM: Three-dimensional topography of the central visual field. Sparing of foveal sensitivity in macular disease. Ophthalmol 90:1028–1038, 1983.

Hart MH Jr, Gordon MO: Calibration of the Dicon Auto Perimeter 2000 compared with that of the Goldmann perimeter. Am J Ophthalmol 96:744–750, 1983.

Hart MH Jr, Gordon MO: Color perimetry of glaucomatous visual field defects. Ophthalmol 91:338–346, 1984.

Hart MH Jr, Hartz, RK: Computer-generated display for three-dimensional static perimetry. Arch Ophthalmol 100:312–318, 1982.

Hart MH Jr, Hartz RK: Computer processing of visual field data. I. Recording, storage, and retrieval. Arch Ophthalmol 99:128–132, 1981.

Hart MH Jr, Hartz RK, Hagen RW, Clark K: Color contrast perimetry. Invest Ophthalmol Vis Sci 25:400–413, 1984.

Hart WM: Computer generated display for three-dimensional static perimetry. Invest Ophthalmol Vis Sci suppl ARVO 20:22, 1981.

Hart WM Jr, Kolker AE: Computer-generated display for three-dimensional static perimetry: Correlation of optic disc changes with glaucomatous defects. Doc Ophthalmol Proc Ser 35:43–49, 1983.

Harth E, Tzanakou E: Alopex: A stochastic method for determining visual receptive fields. Vision Res 14:1475–1482, 1974.

Hayreh SS, Podhajsky P: Visual field defects in anterior ischemic optic neuropathy. Doc Ophthalmol Proc Ser 19:53–71, 1979.

Hayreh SS, Woolson RF, Kohler JA: A procedure for the computer coding of visual fields. Doc Ophthalmol Proc Ser 26:381–388, 1981.

Hecht S, Shlaer S, Pirenne MH: Energy, quanta, and vision. J Gen Physiol 25:819–840, 1942.

Hedin A, Verriest G: Is clinical colour perimetry useful? Doc Ophthalmol Proc Ser 26:161–184, 1981.

Heijl A: Automatic perimetry in glaucoma visual field screening: A clinical study. Albrecht von Graefes Arch klin exp Ophthalmol 200:21–37, 1976.

Heijl A: Computer test logics for automatic perimetry. Acta Ophthalmol 55:837–853, 1977.

Heijl A: Computerized glaucoma visual field screening. Doc Ophthalmol Proc Ser 14:47–51, 1977.

Heijl A: Evaluation of automatic perimetry in glaucoma screening, in ACTA: XXIV International Congress of Ophthalmology, vol. I. Philadelphia, Lippincott, 1983, pp 162–165.

Heijl A: Studies on computerized perimetry. Acta Ophthalmol (Suppl) 132:1–42, 1977.

Heijl A: Time changes of contrast thresholds during automatic perimetry. Acta Ophthalmol 55:696–708, 1977.

Heijl A, Airaksinen PJ: Correlation between computerized perimetry and retinal nerve fibre layer photography after optic disc haemorrhage. Doc Ophthalmol Proc Ser 35:19–25, 1983.

Heijl A, Drance SM: A clinical comparison of three computerized automatic perimeters in the detection of glaucoma defects. Arch Ophthalmol 60:832–836, 1981.

Heijl A, Drance SM: A clinical comparison of three computerized automatic perimeters in the detection of glaucoma defects. Doc Ophthalmol Proc Ser 26:43–48, 1981.

Heijl A, Drance SM: Computerized profile perimetry in glaucoma. Arch Ophthalmol 98:2199–2201, 1980.

Heijl A, Drance SM: Deterioration of threshold in glaucoma patients during perimetry. Doc Ophthalmol Proc Ser 35:129–136, 1983.

Heijl A, Drance SM, Douglas GR: Automatic perimetry (COMPETER). Ability to detect early glaucomatous field defects. Arch Ophthalmol 98:1560–1563, 1980.

Heijl A, Drance SM, Douglas GR: The value of an automatic perimeter (Competer) in detecting early glaucomatous field defects. Arch Ophthalmol 95:1560–1563, 1980.

Heijl A, Krakau CET: A note on fixation during perimetry. Acta Ophthalmol 55:854–861, 1977.

Heijl A, Krakau CET: An automatic perimeter. Acta Ophthalmol (Suppl) 125:23–24, 1975.

Heijl A, Krakau CET: An automatic perimeter for glaucoma visual field screening and control. Construction and clinical cases. Albrecht von Graefes Arch klin exp Ophthalmol 97:13–23, 1975.

Heijl A, Krakau CET: An automatic static perimeter, design and pilot study. Acta Ophthalmol 53:293–310, 1975.

Heijl A, Krakau CET: Preliminary experiences with an automatic static perimeter. Ann Ther Clin Ophthalmol 25:364–370, 1974.

Heijl A, Lundqvist L: The location of earliest glaucomatous visual field defects documented by automatic perimetry. Doc Ophthalmol Proc Ser 35:153–158, 1983.

Hellner KA, Jensen W, Mueller-Jensen A: Video-processing pupillography as a method for objective perimetry in pupillary hemiakenisia. Doc Ophthalmol Proc Ser 14:221–226, 1977.

Henkind P: Technology: Its role in our conception of glaucoma. Ophthalmol 90:753–757, 1983.

Herbert H: Subconjunctival fistula operation in the treatment of primary chronic glaucoma. Trans Ophthalmol Soc UK 23:324–347, 1903.

Herzau V: Perimetry of suppression scotomas with phase difference haploscopy. Doc Ophthalmol Proc Ser 14:399–403, 1977.

Herzau V: The Aulhorn-extinction phenomenon. Suppression scotomas in normal and strabismic subjects. Doc Ophthalmol Proc Ser 26:131–138, 1981.

Hicks BC, Anderson DR: Quantitation of glaucomatous visual field defects with the Mark II Friedmann analyzer. Am J Ophthalmol 95:692–700, 1983.

Hills JF, Wirtschafter, Maeder P: Boundary curves for dividing visual fields into sectors corresponding to a retinoptic projection onto the optic disc. Doc Ophthalmol Proc Ser 35:459–464, 1983.

Hilton GF: The multiple-pattern visual field screener—An evaluation. Am J Ophthalmol 35:314–320, 1958.

Hitchings RA, Anderton SA: A comparative study of visual field defects seen in patients with low-tension glaucoma and chronic simple glaucoma. Br J Ophthalmol 67:818–821, 1983.

Hitchings RA, Powell DJ, Arden GB, Carter RM: Contrast sensitivity gratings in glaucoma family screening. Br J Ophthalmol 65:515–517, 1981.

Hoff JT, Patterson RH: Craniopharygiomas in children and adults. J Neurosurg 36:299–302, 1972.

Holmin C: Optic disc evaluation versus the visual field in chronic glaucoma. Acta Ophthalmol 60:275–283, 1982.

Holmin C, Krakau CET: Automatic perimetry in the control of glaucoma. Glaucoma 3:154–159, 1981.

Holmin C, Krakau CET: Computerized medidian perimetry. A preliminary report. Acta Ophthalmol 58:33–39, 1980.

Holmin C, Krakau CET: Regression analysis of the central visual field in chronic glaucoma cases. A follow-up study using automatic perimetry. Acta Ophthalmol 60:267–274, 1982.

Holmin C, Krakau CET: Short-term effects of timolol in chronic glaucoma. A double blind study using computerized perimetry. Acta Ophthalmol 60:337–346, 1982.

Holmin C, Krakau CET: Variability of glaucomatous visual field defects in computerized perimetry. Albrecht von Graefes Arch klin exp Ophthalmol 210:235–250, 1979.

Holmin C, Krakau CET: Visual field decay in normal subjects and in cases of chronic glaucoma. Albrecht von Graefes Arch klin exp Ophthalmol 213:291–298, 1980.

Honda Y, Negi A, Miki M: Eye movements during peripheral field tests monitored by electro-oculogram. Doc Ophthalmol Proc Ser 19:433–437, 1979.

Hong C, Kitazawa Y, Shirato S: Use of Fieldmaster automated perimeter for the detection of early visual field changes in glaucoma. Int Ophthalmol 4:151–156, 1982.

Horrax G: Visual hallucinations as a cerebral localizing phenomenon with special reference to their occurrence in tumors of the temporal lobes. Arch Neurology Psychiatry 10:532–547, 1923.

Hoyt WF: Cortical blindness with partial recovery following acute cerebral anoxia from cardiac arrest. Arch Ophthalmol 60:1061–1069, 1958.

Hoyt WF, Schlicke B, Eckelhoff RJ: Fundoscopic appearance of a nerve-fibre bundle defect. Br J Ophthalmol 56:577–583, 1972.

Huber C: Pattern evoked cortical potentials and automated perimetry in chronic glaucoma. Doc Ophthalmol Proc Ser 27:87–101, 1981.

Hughes EBC: Some observations of the visual fields in hydrocephalus. J Neurol Neurosurg Psychiatry 9:30–39, 1946.

Iinuma I: An attempt of flicker perimetry using coloured light in simple glaucoma. Doc Ophthalmol Proc Ser 22:215–218, 1980.

Iinuma I: Reversibility of visual field defects in simple glaucoma. Doc Ophthalmol Proc Ser 19:229–232, 1979.

Inatomi A: A simple fundus perimetry with fundus camera. Doc Ophthalmol Proc Ser 19:359–362, 1979.

Isayama Y: Visual field defects due to tumors of the sellar region. Doc Ophthalmol Proc Ser 19:27–42, 1979.

Isayama Y, Tagami Y: Quantitative maculometry using a new instrument in cases of optic neuropathies. Doc Ophthalmol Proc Ser 14:237–242, 1977.

Israel A, Verriest G: Normal results of kinetic colour perimetry by means of the Goldmann apparatus. Doc Ophthalmol Proc Ser 14:435–439, 1977.

Iwata K: Reversible cupping and reversible field defect in glaucoma. Doc Ophthalmol Proc Ser 19:233–239, 1979.

Jenni A, Fankhauser F, Bebie H: New programs for the Octopus automatic perimeter. Klin Monatsbl Augenheilk 176:536–544, 1980. (In German with English abstract.)

Jenni A, Flammer J, Funkhouser A, Fankhauser F: Special Octopus software for clinical investigation. Doc Ophthalmol Proc Ser 35:351–356, 1983.

Jernigan, ME: Visual field plotting using eye movement response. IEEE Trans Biomed Eng 26:601–606, 1979.

Johnson CA: Automated suprathreshold static perimetry. Am J Ophthalmol 89:731–741, 1980.

Johnson CA: The test logic of automated perimetry, in ACTA: XXIV International Congress of Ophthalmology, vol. I. Philadelphia, Lippincott, 1983, pp 151–155.

Johnson CA, Enoch JM: Human psychophysical analysis of receptive field-like properties. VI: Current summary and analysis of factors affecting the psychophysical transient-like function. Doc Ophthalmol Proc Ser 14:367–372, 1977.

Johnson CA, Keltner JL: Comparative evaluation of the Autofield-I, CFA-120, and Fieldmaster Model 101-PR automated perimeters. Ophthalmol 87:777–783, 1980.

Johnson CA, Keltner JL: Comparison of manual and automated perimetry in 1000 eyes. Computers in Ophthalmol 178–181, April 1979.

Johnson CA, Keltner JL: Computer analysis of visual field loss and optimization of automated perimetric test strategies. Ophthalmol 88:1058–1065, 1981.

Johnson CA, Keltner JL: Properties of scotomata in glaucoma and optic nerve disease: Computer analysis. Doc Ophthalmol Proc Ser 35:281–286, 1983.

Johnson CA, Keltner JL: Static and acuity profile perimetry in optic neuritis. Doc Ophthalmol Proc Ser 22:305–312, 1980.

Johnson CA, Keltner JL: The incidence of visual field loss in 20,000 eyes and its relationship to driving performance. Arch Ophthalmol 107:371–375, 1983.

Johnson CA, Keltner JL, Balestrery FG: Suprathreshold static perimetry in glaucoma and other optic nerve disease. Ophthalmol 86:1278–1286, 1979.

Kampik A, Lund OE, Greite JH: Automatic perimeter "Octopuse" (according to Fankhauser). A clinical comparison with the visual field device of Goldmann. Klin Monatsbl Augenheilk 175:72–81, 1979. (In German with English abstract.)

Kani K, Eno N, Abe K, Ono T: Perimetry under television ophthalmoscopy. Doc Ophthalmol Proc Ser 14:231–236, 1977.

Kani K, Ogita Y: Fundus controlled perimetry. The relation between the position of a lesion in the fundus and in the visual field. Doc Ophthalmol Proc Ser 19:341–350, 1979.

Kathol RG, Cox TA, Corbett JJ, Thompson S: Functional visual loss: Follow-up of 42 cases. Arch Ophthalmol 101:729–735, 1983.

Kaul SN, Du Goulay GH, et al: Relationship between visual field defect and arterial occlusion in the posterior cerebral circulation. J Neurosurg Psychiatry 37:1022–1030, 1974.

Kazutaka K, Inui T, Haruta R, Mimura O: Lateral inhibition in the fovea and parafoveal regions. Doc Ophthalmol Proc Ser 35:391–396, 1983.

Kearns TP, Rucker CW: Arcuate defects in the visual fields due to chromophobe adenoma of the pituitary gland. Am J Ophthalmol 45:505–507, 1958.

Keeny AH: Discussion of mass visual field screening in a driving population. Paper by J L Keltner and C A Johnson. Ophthalmol 87:791–792, 1980.

Keltner JL: Comments on automated perimetry papers. Ophthalmol 86:1317–1319, 1979.

Keltner JL, Johnson CA: Automated perimetry. I: A consumer's guide (Glaucoma editorial, edited by Thom J Zimmerman, New Orleans). Ann Ophthalmol 13:275–279, 1981.

Keltner JL, Johnson CA: Automated perimetry. West J Med 130:543, 1979.

Keltner JL, Johnson CA: Automated perimetry. II: Devices manufactured in the United States and abroad (Thom J Zimmerman (ed): Glaucoma editorial, New Orleans). Ann Ophthalmol 13:395–397, 1981.

Keltner JL, Johnson CA: Capabilities and limitations of automated suprathreshold static perimetry. Doc Ophthalmol Proc Ser 22:49–55, 1980.

Keltner JL, Johnson CA: Comparative material on automated and semi-automated perimeters. Ophthalmol 10S:67–69, 1981.

Keltner JL, Johnson CA: Comparative material on automated and semi-automated perimeters—1982. Ophthalmol (Instrument and Book Suppl) 65–76, 1982.

Keltner JL, Johnson CA: Comparative material on automated and semi-automated perimeters—1983. Ophthalmol (Suppl) 1–35, 1983.

Keltner JL, Johnson CA: Comparative material on automated and semi-automated perimeters—1984. Ophthalmol (Instrument and Book Suppl) 27–57, 1984.

Keltner JL, Johnson CA: Comparative material on automated and semi-automated perimeters—1985. Ophthalmol (Suppl) 34–57, 1985.

Keltner JL, Johnson CA: Effectiveness of automated perimetry in following glaucomatous visual field progression. Ophthalmol 89:247–254, 1982.

Keltner JL, Johnson CA: Mass visual field screening in a driving population. Ophthalmol 87:785–790, 1980.

Keltner JL, Johnson CA: Preliminary examination of the Squid automated perimeter. Doc Ophthalmol Proc Ser 35:371–377, 1983.

Keltner JL, Johnson CA: Screening for visual field abnormalities with automated perimetry. Surv Ophthalmol 28:175–183, 1983.

Keltner JL, Johnson CA: Automated and manual perimetry—A six-year overview. Special emphasis on neuro-ophthalmic problems. Ophthalmol 91:68–85, 1983.

Keltner JL, Johnson CA, Balestrery FG: Suprathreshold static perimetry. Initial clinical trials with the Fieldmaster automated perimeter. Arch Ophthalmol 97:260–272, 1979.

Kitahara H, Kitahara K, et al: Extrafoveal stiles' pi5-mechanism. Doc Ophthalmol Proc Ser 22:185–191, 1980.

Kitahara H, Kitahara K, Matsuzaki H: Trial of a color perimeter. Doc Ophthalmol Proc Ser 19:439–445, 1979.

Kitahara K, Tamaki R, et al: Extrafoveal Stiles' pi mechanisms. Doc Ophthalmol Proc Ser 35:397–403, 1983.

Kitahara Y, Takahashi O, Ohiwa Y: The mode of development and progression of field defects in early glaucoma—A follow-up study. Doc Ophthalmol Proc Ser 19:211–221, 1979.

Koch P, Roulier A, Fankhauser F: Perimetry—The information theoretical basis for its automation. Vision Res 12:1619–1630, 1972.

Koerner F, Fankhauser F, Bebie H, Spahr J: Threshold noise and variability of field defects in determination by manual and automatic perimetry. Doc Ophthalmol Proc Ser 14:53–59, 1977.

Kosaki H: A new screening method for the detection of glaucomatous field changes. The flicker triple circle method. Doc Ophthalmol Proc Ser 22:253–258, 1980.

Kosaki H: The earliest visual field defects (IIa Stage) in glaucoma by kinetic perimetry. Doc Ophthalmol Proc Ser 19:255–259, 1979.

Kosaki H, Nakatani H: Computer analysis of kinetic field data determined with a Goldmann perimeter. Doc Ophthalmol Proc Ser 35:473–477, 1983.

Kosaki H, Nakatani H, Tsukamato H, Nakauchi M: Topographical studies of field defects in various stages of primary chronic glaucoma. Doc Ophthalmol Proc Ser 14:121–129, 1977.

Koch P, Roulier A, Fankhauser F: Perimetry—The information theoretical basis for its automation. Vision Res 12:1619–1630, 1972.

Krakau CET: A feasible development of computerized perimetry. Acta Ophthalmol 59:485–494, 1981.

Krakau CET: Aspects on the design of an automated perimeter. Acta Ophthalmol 56:389–405, 1978.

Krakau CET: On automatic testing of the visual field. Acta Ophthalmol 51:745, 1972.

Krieglstein GK, Glaab E, Gramer E: The Fieldmaster-200 computer perimeter: A comparative, controlled clinical study of its sensitivity and specificity in glaucomatous field defects. Klin Monatsbl Augenheilk 179:340–345, 1981. (In German with English abstract.)

Krieglstein GK, Glaab E, Gramer E: The Perimetry of the Glaucoma Visual Field with the Kinetic and Automatic, Suprathreshold Examination Method. 1978 meeting of the DOG in Kiel, 21–24 Sept.

Krieglstein GK, Schrems W, Gramer E, Leydhecker W: Detectability of early glaucomatous field defects. A controlled comparison of Goldmann versus Octopus perimetry. Doc Ophthalmol Proc Ser 22:19–24, 1980.

Kronfeld PC: Perimetry, in Clinical Ophthalmology, vol. 3. Philadelphia, Harper & Row, 1981, pp 1–21.

Kubota S: Videopupillographic perimetry perimetric findings with rabbit eyes. Doc Ophthalmol Proc Ser 19:447–452, 1979.

Kuhn HS: Glaucoma detection in industry, multiple field pattern test. Indust Med Surg 26:327–330, 1957.

Lakowski R, Drance SM: Acquired dyschromatopsias, the earliest functional losses in glaucoma. Doc Ophthalmol Proc Ser 19:159–165, 1979.

Lakowski R, Dunn P: A new interpretation of the relative central scotoma for blue stimuli under photopic conditions. Doc Ophthalmol Proc Ser 19:411–416, 1979.

Lakowski R, Dunn PM: An instrument for the establishment of chromatic perimetry norms. Doc Ophthalmol Proc Ser 26:193–197, 1981.

Lakowski R, Wright WD, Oliver K: High luminance chromatic Goldmann perimeter. Doc Ophthalmol Proc Ser 14:441–443, 1977.

Leblanc RP: Peripheral nasal field defects. Doc Ophthalmol Proc Ser 14:131–133, 1977.

Leibowitz H, Johnson CA, Guez JR: Differences in the processing of peripheral stimuli. Doc Ophthalmol Proc Ser 14:299–302, 1977.

Leydhecker W: Perimetry update. Ann Ophthalmol 15:511–543, 1983.

Li SG, Spaeth GL, Scimeca HA, Schatz NJ: Clinical experiences with the use of an automated perimeter (Octopus) in the diagnosis of patients with glaucoma and neurologic diseases. Ophthalmol 86:1302–1312, 1979.

Lichter PR, Standardi CL: Early glaucomatous visual field defects and their significance to clinical ophthalmology. Doc Ophthalmol Proc Ser 19:111–118, 1979.

Logan N, Anderson DR: Detecting early glaucomatous visual field changes with a blue stimulus. Am J Ophthalmol 95:432–434, 1983.

Lueddeke H, Aulhorn E: On the luminance and size of test-points in 'multiple-stimulus' perimetry. Doc Ophthalmol Proc Ser 14:379–384, 1977.

Lund OE, Greite JH, Kampik A: Clinical Experiences With the Automated Perimeter Octopus. Schlieren, Switzerland, Interzeag, 1979, pp 72–80.

Maeda S: Screening of visual field defect among healthy adults. A preliminary trial of population survey of ocular disease. Doc Ophthalmol Proc Ser 26:365–371, 1981.

Maeda S, Usuba S, Nagata K, Matsuyama S: Visual field investigation in cerebrovascular accident. Doc Ophthalmol Proc Ser 26:351–357, 1981.

Majewska K: Proposal of computer processing of data concerning the visual fields. Klin Oczna 48:137–139, 1978. (In Polish with English abstract.)

Mariotte PE: A new discovery touching vision. Philosophical Trans 3:668–671, 1668, in JE Lebensohn (ed): An Anthology of Ophthalmic Classics. Baltimore, Williams & Wilkins, 1969.

Marmion VJ: A report on colour normals on the Friedmann Mark II Analyser. Doc Ophthalmol Proc Ser 26:227–231, 1981.

Marmion VJ: An evaluation of the Baylor semi-automated device. Doc Ophthalmol Proc Ser 35:379–381, 1983.

Marmion VJ: An evaluation of the Friedmann analyser Mark II. Doc Ophthalmol Proc Ser 26:265–267, 1981.

Marmion VJ: The results of a comparison of the hundred hue test and static colour perimetry. Doc Ophthalmol Proc Ser 14:473–474, 1977.

Maruo T: Electroencephalographic perimetry clinical applications of vertex potentials elicited by focal retinal stimulation. Doc Ophthalmol Proc Ser 19:461–468, 1979.

Massof RW, Finkelstein D: Subclassifications of retinitis pigmentosa from two-colour scotopic static perimetry. Doc Ophthalmol Proc Ser 26:219–225, 1981.

Matsudaira K, Suzuki R: Visual field changes after photocoagulation in retinal branch vein occlusion. Doc Ophthalmol Proc Ser 19:395–401, 1979.

Matsuo H, Kikuchi G, et al: Automatic perimeter with graphic display. Doc Ophthalmol Proc Ser 26:1–7, 1981.

Matsuno K, Haruta R, Mimura O, Kani K: Photocoagulation and retinal sensitivity, in ACTA: XXIV International Congress of Ophthalmology, vol. I. Philadelphia, Lippincott, 1983, pp 190–194.

McCrary MA, Feigon J: Computerized perimetry in neuro-ophthalmology. Ophthalmol 86:1287–1301, 1979.

Michel EM, Troost BT: Palinopia: Cerebral localization with computed tomography. Neurology 30:887–889, 1980.

Mienberg D, Flammer J, Ludin H-P: Subclinical visual field defects in multiple sclerosis demonstration and quantification with automated perimetry, and comparison with visually evoked potentials. J Neurol 227:125–133, 1982.

Miles PW: Flicker fusion fields: Technique and interpretation. Am J Ophthalmol 33:1060–1077, 1950.

Mills DW: Visual field defects in pregnancy. Can J Ophthalmol 5:16–21, 1970.

Mills RP: A comparison of Goldmann, Fieldmaster 200, and Dicon AP 2000 perimeters used in a screening mode. Ophthalmol 91:347–354, 1984.

Mimura O, Kani K, Inui T: Spatial summation in the foveal and parafoveal region. Doc Ophthalmol Proc Ser 26:139–146, 1981.

Mindel JS, Safir A, Schare PW: Visual field testing with red targets. Arch Ophthalmol 101:927–929, 1983.

Mizokami K, Tagami Y, Isayama Y: The reversibility of visual field defects in the juvenile glaucoma cases. Doc Ophthalmol Proc Ser 19:241–246, 1979.

Moreland JD, Maione M, et al: The clinical assessment of the chromatic mechanisms of the retinal periphery. Doc Ophthalmol Proc Ser 14:413–421, 1977.

Motolko M, Drance SM, Douglas GR: The early psychophysical disturbances in chronic open-angle glaucoma. A study of visual functions with asymmetric disc cupping. Arch Ophthalmol 100:1632–1634, 1982.

Mueller-Jensen A, Zschocke S, Dannheim F: VER analysis of the chiasmal syndrome. J Neurol 255:33–40, 1981.

Nakatani H, Shimizu Y, Kikkawa A, Suzuki N: Moire topographic method for measuring the depth of papillary excavation. Doc Ophthalmol Proc Ser 14:135–140, 1977.

Nakatani H, Suzuki N: Correlation between the stereographic shape of the disc excavation and the visual field of glaucomatous eyes. Doc Ophthalmol Proc Ser 26:337–344, 1981.

Nakatani H, Suzuki N: Correlation between the stereographic shape of the ocular fundus and the visual field in glaucomatous eyes. Doc Ophthalmol Proc Ser 35:51–58, 1983.

Nakatani H, Suzuki N, Sato H: Correlation between the stereographic shape of the disc excavation and the visual field, in ACTA: XXIV International Congress of Ophthalmology, vol. I. Philadelphia, Lippincott, 1983, pp 180–183.

Natsikos VE, Dean Hart JC, Raistrick ER: Residual field changes in patients with idiopathic central serous retinopathy. Doc Ophthalmol Proc Ser 26:323–328, 1981.

Neuhann T, Greite JH: Reliability of visual field examination in clinical routine. Doc Ophthalmol Proc Ser 26:57–61, 1981.

Nielsen NV: A diurnal study of the ocular hypotensive effect of metoprolol mounted on ophthalmic rods compared to timolol eye drops in glaucoma patients. Acta Ophthalmol 59:495–502, 1981.

Niesel P: Planimetric evaluation of kinetic perimetry with the Goldman perimeter. Klin Monatsbl Augenheilk 180:17–19, 1982. (In German with English abstract.)

Norren DV: Automation of perimetry: The scoperimeter. Ophthalmologica 173:227–229, 1976.

Octopus system: Visual Field Atlas, ed 2. Schlieren, Switzerland, Interzeag, 1979.

Ogata H, Miyamoto F, et al: Instrument for mass examination of visual field and ocular movement. Preliminary report. Acta Soc Ophthalmol Jpn 77:1266–1269, 1973. (In Japanese with English abstract.)

Ogawa T, Furuno F, Seki A, Miyamoto T, Ohta Y: Kinetic quantitative perimetry of retinal nerve fiber layer defects in glaucoma by fundus photo-perimeter. Doc Ophthalmol Proc Ser 35:27–34, 1983.

Ogawa T, Suzuki R: Relationship between central and peripheral visual field changes with kinetic perimetry. Doc Ophthalmol Proc Ser 19:469–474, 1979.

Ogita Y, Sotani T, Kani K, Imachi J: Fundus controlled perimetry in optic neuropathy. Doc Ophthalmol Proc Ser 26:279–285, 1981.

Ogle KN: Foveal contrast thresholds with blurring of the retinal image and increasing size of the test stimulus. J Opt Soc Am 51:862–869, 1961.

Ogle KN: Peripheral contrast thresholds and blurring of the retinal image for a point light source. J Opt Soc Am 51:1265–1268, 1961.

Ohnuma T, Tagami Y, Isayama Y: Visual fields versus visual evoked potentials in optic nerve disorders. Doc Ophthalmol Proc Ser 35:239–244, 1983.

Ohta Y, Miyamoto T, Harasawa K: Experimental fundus photo perimeter and its application. Doc Ophthalmol Proc Ser 19:351–358, 1979.

Ohta Y, Tomonaga M, Miyamoto T, Harasawa K: Visual field studies with fundus photo-perimeter in postchiasmatic lesions. Doc Ophthalmol Proc Ser 26:119–126, 1981.

Ostertag CB, Unsoeld R: Correlation of infarctions of the visual cortex with homonymous visual field defects. A computer tomographic study. Arch Psychiatr Nervenkr 230:265–274, 1981. (In German with English abstract.)

Otori T, Hohki T, Ikeda M: Central field screener. A new tool for screening and quantitative campimetry. Doc Ophthalmol Proc Ser 26:247–252, 1981.

Otori T, Hohki T, Nakao Y: Central critical fusion frequency in neuro-ophthalmological practice. Doc Ophthalmol Proc Ser 19:95–100, 1979.

Ourgaud M: Static circular perimetry in open-angle glaucoma. J Fr Ophthalmol 5:387–391, 1982.

Owen WG: Spatiotemporal integration on the human peripheral retina. Vision Res 12:1011–1026, 1972.

Pashley JC: BIPAS—Binocular instantly programmable automatic screener. Doc Ophthalmol Proc Ser 14:37–45, 1977.

Patterson VH, Heron JR: Visual field abnormalities in multiple sclerosis. J Neurol Neurosurg Psychiatry 43:205–209, 1980.

Peter J, Zajicek G, Barzel I: Computerized evaluation of visual fields. Br J Ophthalmol 67:50–53, 1983.

Peter LC. A simplified conception of visual field changes in chronic glaucoma. Arch Ophthalmol 56:337–343, 1927.

Phelps CD: Visual field defects in open-angle glaucoma: progression and regression. Doc Ophthalmol Proc Ser 19:187–196, 1979.

Phelps CD, Remijan PW, Blondeau P: Acuity perimetry. Doc Ophthalmol Proc Ser 26:111–117, 1981.

Piccolino FC, Parodi GC, Beltrame F: Optic disc analysis by computerized image subtraction and perimetry. Doc Ophthalmol Proc Ser 35:87–91, 1983.

Pirenne MH: Vision and the Eye, ed 2. London, Chapman and Hall Ltd, 1967.

Portney GL, Krohn MA: Automated perimetry: Background, instruments and methods. Surv Ophthalmol 22:271–278, 1978.

Portney GL, Krohn MA: The limitations of kinetic perimetry in early scotoma detection. Ophthalmology 85:287–293, 1978.

Rabin S, Kolesar P: Mathematical optimization of glaucoma visual field screening protocols. Doc Ophthalmol 45:361–380, 1978.

Rabin S, Kolesar P, Podos SM, Wilensky JT: A visual field screening protocol for glaucoma. Am J Ophthalmol 92:530–535, 1981.

Radius RL: Perimetry in cataractous patients. Arch Ophthalmol 96:1574–1579, 1978.

Ratliff F, Hartline HK: The responses of limulus optic nerve fibers to patterns of illumination of the receptor mosaic. J Gen Physiol 42:1241–1255, 1963.

Ratliff F, Hartline HK, Miller WM: Spatial and temporal aspects of retinal inhibitory interaction. J Opt Soc Am 53:110–120, 1963.

Ratliff F, Riggs LA: Involuntary motions of the eye during monocular fixation. J Exp Psychol 40:687–701, 1950.

Reed H: The Essentials of Perimetry. Oxford, Oxford University Press, 1960.

Regan D, Beverley KI: Visual fields described by contrast sensitivity by acuity, and by relative sensitivity to different orientations. Invest Ophthalmol 24:754–759, 1983.

Richardson KT: Octopus Perimetry: A Preliminary Report. Schlieren, Switzerland, Interzeag, 1979, pp 66–71.

Richardson KT, Kurtzman C: New Dimensions in Interpretation of Visual Function in Glaucoma. Symposium on Glaucoma. Transactions of the New Orleans Academy of Ophthalmology. St. Louis, Mosby, 1981, pp 54–61.

Riddoch G: Dissociation of visual perception due to occipital injuries with especial reference to appreciation of movement. Brain 40:15–57, 1917.

Rinaldi I, Botton JE, Troland CE: Cortical visual disturbances following ventriuclography and/or ventricular decompression. J Neurosurg 19:569–576, 1962.

Rock WJ, Drance SM, Morgan RW: Visual field screening in glaucoma. Arch Ophthalmol 89:287–290, 1973.

Ronchi L, Galassi F: Absolute thresholds for monochromatic stimuli of various sizes and durations across the visual field. Doc Ophthalmol Proc Ser 14:423–426, 1977.

Ronchi LR, Barca L: Refraction scotomata and absolute peripheral sensitivity. Doc Ophthalmol Proc Ser 26:359–364, 1981.

Rossi P, Ciurlo G, Burtolo C, Calabria G: Temporal resolution and stimulus intensity in the central visual field. Doc Ophthalmol Proc Ser 35:439–441, 1983.

Salmon JH: Transient postictal hemianopsia. Arch Ophthalmol 79:523–524, 1968.

Schindler S, McCrary JA: Automated perimetry in a neuro-ophthalmologic practice. Ann Ophthalmol 13:691–697, 1981.

Schmied U: Automatic (Octopus) and Manual (Goldmann) Perimetry in Glaucoma: First Experience. Schlieren, Switzerland, Interzeag, 1979, pp 53–59.

Schmied U: Automatic (Octopus) and manual (Goldmann) perimetry in glaucoma. Albrecht von Graefes Arch klin exp Ophthalmol 213:239–244, 1980.

Schmied U: Introduction into Technique and Clinical Application of Octopus Perimetry. Schlieren, Switzerland, Interzeag, 1979, pp 16–23.

Scott GI: Traquair's Clinical Perimetry. St. Louis, Mosby, 1957.

Schwartz B, Sonty S: Differences in the visual evoked potentials between normals and open-angle glaucomas. Doc Ophthalmol Proc Ser 26:91–96, 1981.

Scobey RP: Psychophysical and electrophysiological determinants of motion detection. Doc Ophthalmol Proc Ser 26:63–69, 1981.

Serra A, Mascia C: Quantitative perimetry in optic subatrophy from previous optical neuritis in multiple sclerosis. Doc Ophthalmol Proc Ser 26:85–90, 1981.

Shevelev IA, Sharaev GA, et al: Dynamics of the receptive fields of visual cortex and lateral geniculate body neurons in the cat. Neirofiziologiia 14:622–630, 1982.

Shinoda Y, Ohnishi Y, et al: Empty sella syndrome with visual field disturbance. Jpn J Ophthalmol 27:248–254, 1983.

Shinzato E, Matsuo H: Clinical experiences with a new multiple dot plate. Doc Ophthalmol Proc Ser 19:453–460, 1979.

Shinzato E, Suzuki R, Furuno F: The central visual field changes in glaucoma using Goldmann perimeter and Friedmann visual field analyser. Doc Ophthalmol Proc Ser 14:93–101, 1977.

Sinclair AHH: A collapsible apparatus for testing the field of vision. Ophthalmol Rev 26:217, 1907.

Sinclair AHH: Bjerrum's method of testing the field of vision, the advantages of the method in clinical work, and its special value in the diagnosis of glaucoma. Trans Ophthalmol Soc UK 25:384–412, 1905.

Sloan LL: Area and luminance of test object as variable in examination of the visual field by projection perimetry. Vision Res 1:121–138, 1961.

Smith J: Diurnal variation in intraocular pressure: Correlation to automated perimetry. Ophthalmology 92:858–861, 1985.

Spaeth GL, Li SG, Scimeca HA: Clinical experiences with the use of Octopus automated perimeter in the detection of visual field loss in early glaucoma. Schlieren, Switzerland, Interzeag, 1979, pp 40–52.

Spahr J: Automation of the perimeter. I: Application of a computer-regulated perimeter. Albrecht von Graefes Arch klin exp Ophthalmol 188:328–338, 1972. (In German with English abstract.)

Spahr J: Optimization of the presentation pattern in automatic static perimetry. Vision Res 15:1275–1281, 1975.

Spahr J, Fankhauser F: Automation of perimetry. Ophthalmologica 170:106–107, 1975. (In German with English abstract.)

Spahr J, Fankhauser F, Bebie H: Advances in the automation of perimetry. Klin Monatsbl Augenheilk 168:84–86, 1976.

Spahr J, Fankhauser F, Jenni A, Bebie H: Practical experiences with the Octopus perimeter. Klin Monatsbl Augenheilk 172:470–477, 1978. (In German with English abstract.)

Spalding JMK: Wounds of the visual pathway. Part II: The striate cortex. J Neurol Neurosurg Psychiatry 15:169–183, 1952.

Spector RH, Glaser JS, David NJ, Vining Q: Occipital lobe infarctions: Perimetry and computed tomography. Neurol 31:1098–1106, 1981.

Spector RH, Glaser JS, Schatz NJ: Demyelinative chiasmal lesions. Arch Neurol 37:757–762, 1980.

Speiss H: Computerized tomography—Results in affections of the chiasm and visual pathway. Klin Monatsbl Augenheilk 174:816–823, 1979. (In German with English abstract.)

Spinelli DN: Computer-plotted receptive fields. Science 154:920–921, 1966.

Springer DA, Alexander LJ: Automated perimetry. Am J Optom Physiol Opt 55:725–727, 1878.

Stensaas SS, Eddington DK, Dobelle WH: The topography and variability of the primary visual cortex in man. J Neurosurg 40:747–755, 1974.

Sumie K, Nakatani H, Maeda H: Clinical trials with the Fieldmaster-101 perimeter. Folia Ophthalmologica Jpn 31:483–490, 1980. (In Japanese with English abstract.)

Suzuki R, Tomonaga M: Analysis of angioscotoma testing with Friedmann visual field analyser and Tuebinger perimeter. Doc Ophthalmol Proc Ser 19:369, 1979.

Suzumura A: Prototype campimeter AS-2 and its applicability with both eyes open. Doc Ophthalmol Proc Ser 26:259–264, 1981.

Symonds C, MacKenzie I: Bilateral loss of vision from cerebral infarction. Brain 80:415–455, 1957.

Tagami Y: Correlations between atrophy of maculopapillar bundles and visual functions in cases of optic neuropathies. Doc Ophthalmol Proc Ser 19:17–26, 1979.

Tagami Y, Onuma T, Mizokami K, Isayama Y: Comparison of spatial contrast sensitivity with visual field in optic neuropathy and glaucoma. Doc Ophthalmol Proc Ser 26:147–154, 1981.

Tate GW, Lynn JR: Principles of Quantitative Perimetry: Testing and Interpreting the Visual Field. New York, San Francisco, Grune & Stratton, 1977.

Teuber HL, Battersby WS, Bender MB: Visual Field Defects After Penetrating Missle Wounds of the Brain. Cambridge, Harvard University Press, 1960.

Ticho U, Zauberman H, et al: Oculographic automatic perimetry in glaucoma visual field screening: a clinical study—Preliminary results in glaucoma patients. Doc Ophthalmol 47:5–17, 1979.

Traquair HM: Perimetry in the study of glaucoma. Trans Ophthalmol Soc UK 51:585–599, 1903.

Traquair HM: The quantitative method in perimetry, with notes on perimetric apparatus. Ophthalmol Rev 33:65–83, 1914.

Trobe JA, Lorber ML, Schlezinger NS: Isolated homonymous hemianopia. Arch Ophthalmol 89:377–381, 1973.

Trobe JD: Chromophobe adenoma presenting with a hemianopic temporal arcuate scotoma. Am J Ophthalmol 77:388–392, 1974.

Trobe JD: How effective is perimetry in current practice? Ophthalmol 90:1380–1383, 1983.

Trobe JD: Neuro-Ophthalmology: Automated Perimetry, in Hughes WF (ed): The Year Book of Ophthalmology 1980. Chicago, London, Year Book Medical, 1980, pp 267–276.

Trobe JD, Acosta PC, Shuster JJ, Krischer JP: An evaluation of the accuracy of community-based perimetry. Am J Ophthalmol 90:645–660, 1980.

Trobe JD, Glaser JS: The Visual Fields Manual. A Practical Guide to Testing and Interpretation. Gainesville, Fla, Triad, 1983.

Trost DC, Woolson RF, Hayreh SS: Quantification of visual fields for statistical analysis. Arch Ophthalmol 97:2175–2180, 1979.

Van Buran J, Baldwin M: The architecture of the optic radiation in the temporal lobe of man. Brain 81:15–40, 1958.

Van Dalen JTW: Automated perimetry in aviation medicine. Visual field examination in 2500 flying personnel. Doc Ophthalmol Proc Ser 35:331–335, 1983.

Van Dalen JTW: Automated visual field screening in the flying dutch population. Aviat Space Environ Med 53:1006–1010, 1982.

Van Dalen JTW, Spekreyse H, Greve EL: Visual field (VF) versus visual evoked cortical potential (VECP) in multiple sclerosis patients. Doc Ophthalmol Proc Ser 26:79–83, 1981.

Van De Kraats J, Smit EP, Slooter JH: Objective perimetric measurements by the pupil balance method. Doc Ophthalmol Proc Ser 14:213–219, 1977.

Van Dijk HJL: Pituitary lesions and visual field defects: Selected cases. Doc Ophthalmol Proc Ser 14:331–335, 1977.

Van Lith GHM: Perimetry and electrophysiology. Doc Ophthalmol Proc Ser 14:169–172, 1977.

Van Veenendaal WG, Langerhorst CT, et al: New programs of the scoperimeter. Doc Ophthalmol Proc Ser 35:323–329, 1983.

Verduin WM, Bakker D: Modification of the Friedmann Visual Field Analyzer (model I) to cover 104 points of measurement. Doc Ophthalmol 52:429–433, 1982.

Verriest G: Modern trends in perimetry. Br J Physiol Opt 33:19–31, 1979.

Verriest G: Report on colour perimetry. Doc Ophthalmol Proc Ser 19:483–484, 1979.

Verriest G (ed): Barca L, Dubois-Poulsen A, Houtmans MJM, Inditsky B, Johnson C, Overington I, Ronchi L, Villani S. The occupational visual field. I: Theoretical aspects: the normal functional visual field. Doc Ophthalmol Proc Ser 35:165–186, 1983.

Verriest G, Uvijls A: A note on the spectral increment thresholds on a white background in different age groups of normal subjects. Doc Ophthalmol Proc Ser 14:431–432, 1977.

Verriest G, Uvijls A: An outline of the clinical interest of the spectral increment thresholds on a white background in acquired ocular diseases. Doc Ophthalmol Proc Ser 14:457–460, 1977.

Vodovozov AM, Andidalova GB, et al: Perimetric and visumetric methods for measuring individually tolerated intraocular pressure in glaucoma. Klin Monatsbl Augenheilk 180:548–550, 1982. (In German with English abstract.)

Vola JL, Jayle GE, et al: Differential kinetic thresholds according to test-luminance on the inferior temporal meridian at three background luminances (photopic, mesopic and scotopic). Doc Ophthalmol Proc Ser 14:389–394, 1977.

Von Graefe A: Examination of the visual field in amblyopic disease. Eye, Ear, Nose & Throat Monthly 14:117–196, 1935, in Lebensohn JE (ed): An Anthology of Ophthalmic Classics. Baltimore, Williams & Wilkins, 1969.

Wall M, Hart WM Jr, Burde RM: Visual field defects in idiopathic intracranial hypertension (pseudotumor cerebri). Am J Ophthalmol 96:654–669, 1983.

Walker CB: Color interlacing and perimetry. Trans Am Ophthalmol Soc 14:684–718, 1916.

Walker CB: Quantitative perimetry: Practical devices and errors. Arch Ophthalmol 46:537–561, 1917.

Walsh TJ: Field Defects, in Neuro-ophthalmology: Clinical Signs and Symptoms. Philadelphia, Lea & Febiger, 1978, pp 275–285.

Walsh TJ: Paracentral scotoma testing. Ophthalmol Surg 4:72–74, 1973.

Weale RA: A note on stray light in the Tuebingen perimeter. Doc Ophthalmol Proc Ser 14:361–362, 1977.

Weber B, Spahr J: Automation of perimetry. Demonstration methods of results of perimetric examinations. Acta Ophthalmol 54:349–362, 1976. (In French with English abstract.)

Welsh RC: Finger counting in four quadrants as a method of visual field gross screening. Arch Ophthalmol 66:94–95, 1961.

Werner EB: Peripheral nasal field defects in glaucoma. Doc Ophthalmol Proc Ser 19:223–228, 1979.

Werner EB, Drance SM: The effect of trabeculectomy on the progression of glaucomatous visual field defects. Doc Ophthalmol Proc Ser 14:67–73, 1977.

Whalen WR, Spaeth, GL (eds.): Computerized Visual Fields: What They Are and How to Use Them. Thorofare, N.J., Slack, 1985.

Wilensky JT, Joondeph BC: Variation in visual field measurements with an automated perimeter. Am J Ophthalmol 97:328–331, 1984.

Wilson JR, Sherman SM: Receptive-field characteristics of neurons in cat striate cortex: Changes with visual field eccentricity. J Neurophysiol 39:512–533, 1976.

Wilson P, Falconer MA: Patterns of visual failure with pituitary tumors. Clinical and radiological correlations. Br J Ophthalmol 52:94–110, 1968.

Wilson R, Walker AM, Dueker DK, Crick RP: Risk factors for rate of progression of glaucomatous visual field loss. Arch Ophthalmol 100:737–741, 1982.

Wirtschafter JD, Prater BN: A simplified stimulus value notation using preferred stimulus combinations for Goldmann quantitative perimetry. Surv Ophthalmol 23:177–182, 1978.

Wirtschafter JD, Becker WL, Howe JB, Younge BR: Glaucoma visual field analysis by computed profile of nerve fiber function in optic disc sectors. Ophthalmol 89:255–267, 1982.

Young SE, Walsh FB, Knox DL: The tilted disk syndrome. Am J Ophthalmol 82:16–23, 1976.

Young T: The Bakerian lecture. On the mechanism of the eye. Philos Trans R Soc Lond 91:23–88, 1801.

Younge BR: Computer-assisted perimetry results in neuro-ophthalmology problem cases. Doc Ophthalmol Proc Ser 35:271–279, 1983.

Younge BR: Midline tilting between seeing and nonseeing areas in hemianopia. Mayo Clinic Proc 51:562–567, 1976.

Younge BR: Quantitative analysis in glaucoma with computer-assisted perimetry (Octopus), in ACTA: XXIV International Congress of Ophthalmology, vol. I. Philadelphia, Lippincott, 1983, pp 166–175.

Younge BR, Trautmann JC: Computer-assisted perimetry in neuro-ophthalmic disease. Mayo Clinic Proc 55:207–222, 1980.

Zappia RJ, Enoch JM, et al: The Riddoch phenomenon revealed in non-occipital lobe lesions. Br J Ophthalmol 55:416–420, 1971.

Zingirian M, Calabria G, Gandolfo E: The nasal step: An early glaucomatous defect? Doc Ophthalmol Proc Ser 19:273–278, 1979.

Zingirian M, Calabria G, Gandolfo E, Sandini G: The normal pericoecal area. A static method for investigation. Doc Ophthalmol Proc Ser 26:393–403, 1981.

Zingirian M, Ciurlo G, Rossi P, Burtolo C: Flicker fusion and spatial summation. Doc Ophthalmol Proc Ser 26:127–130, 1981.

Zingirian M, Gandolfo E, Orciuolo M: Automation of the Goldmann perimeter. Doc Ophthalmol Proc Ser 35:365–369, 1983.

Zingirian M, Pisano E, Gandolfo E: Visual field damage after photocoagulative treatment for diabetic retinopathy. Doc Ophthalmol Proc Ser 14:265–274, 1977.

Zingirian M, Rolando M, Cardillo Piccolino F: Relationship between fundus densitometric analysis and perimetry. Doc Ophthalmol Proc Ser 26:389–392, 1981.

Zingirian M, Tagliasco V: Problems of automated perimetry. Klin Monatsbl Augenheilk 170:542–546, 1977. (In German with English abstract.)

Zingirian M, Tagliasco V, Gandolfo E: Automated perimetry: Minicomputers or microprocessors? Doc Ophthalmol Proc Ser 19:327–331, 1979.

Zuhlke GG: New kinetic automation. Ophthalmology Times, February 1982.

Index